CANCER SOURCEBOOK for Women

Health Reference Series

Volume Ten

CANCER SOURCEBOOK for Women

Basic Information about Specific Forms of Cancer that Affect Women, Featuring Facts about Breast Cancer, Cervical Cancer, Ovarian Cancer, Cancer of the Uterus and Uterine Sarcoma, Cancer of the Vagina, and Cancer of the Vulva; Statistical and Demographic Data; Treatments, Self-Help Management Suggestions, and Current Research Initiatives

Edited by
Alan R. Cook and Peter D. Dresser

Omnigraphics, Inc.
Penobscot Building / Detroit, MI 48226

BIBLIOGRAPHIC NOTE

This volume contains individual publications issued by the National Institutes of Health (NIH), its sister agencies, and sub-agencies. Numbered publications in this category are: NIH 94-1556, 93-1562, 92-2401, 91-2675, 91-2151, 91-659, 91-658, 87-2877, 87-657. Also included are numbered information sheets from the National Cancer Institute's NCI Cancerfax service: 208/ 0000103, 0000950, 0001038, 0001055, 0001163, 0003125, 0003371, 0004728, 0005145, 0400020, 0400077, 0400079, 0600036, 0600056, 0600075, 0600156, 0600313, 0600332, 0600342, 0600513, 0600514, 6000062; other numbered NCI publications: K60, K67, and PF4730(1094)•D14502; and one unnumbered NCI document dated November 1991 (Questions to Ask Your Doctor About Breast Cancer). The volume also includes FDA Consumer Reprints from DHHS numbered FDA: 94-8284, 93-1206, 91-1176, 90-1159; and a June 1994 FDA Update with revisions. It also includes extracts from two NIH Consensus statements (June 18-21, 1990 and August 15, 1994) and from the 1992 DHHS/CDC Progress Report to Congress, along with selected articles from National Center for Research Resources *Reporter*, the CDC's *Morbidity and Mortality Weekly Report,* and the FDA's *Consumer*. In addition, the volume includes one copyrighted article from Y-ME Publications and one from the American Cancer Institute. These documents are used by permission.

Edited by Allan R. Cook
Karen Bellenir, Series Editor, *Health Reference Series*
Peter D. Dresser, Managing Editor, *Health Reference Series*

Omnigraphics, Inc.

Matthew P. Barbour, *Production Coordinator*
Laurie Lanzen Harris, *Vice President, Editorial*
Peter E. Ruffner, *Vice President, Administration*
James A. Sellgren, *Vice President, Operations and Finance*
Jane J. Steele, *Vice President, Research*

Frederick G. Ruffner, Jr., *Publisher*

Copyright © 1996, Omnigraphics, Inc.

Library of Congress Cataloging-in-Publication Data

Cancer sourcebook for women : basic information about specific forms of cancer that affect women, featuring facts about breast cancer, cervical cancer, ovarian cancer, cancer of the uterus and uterine sarcoma, cancer of the vagina, and cancer of the vulva; statistical and demographic data; treatments, self-help management suggestions, and current research initiatives / edited by Alan R. Cook.
    p.   cm. — (Health reference series ; v. 10)
Includes bibliographical references and index.
ISBN 0-7808-0076-1 (lib. bdg. : alk. paper)
1. Generative organs, Female—Cancer. 2. Breast—Cancer. 3. Women—Diseases. I. Cook, Alan R. II. Series.
RC280.G5C34 1995   95-36875
616.99'4'0082—dc20   CIP

∞

This book is printed on acid-free paper meeting the ANSI Z39.48 Standard. The infinity symbol that appears above indicates that the paper in this book meets that standard.

Printed in the United States

Contents

Preface ix
Introduction: Cancer Today xiii

Part I: Major Cancers That Specifically Affect Women

Chapter 1—Women and Cancer 3
Chapter 2—Breast Cancer 7
Chapter 3—Early Stage Breast Cancer 29
Chapter 4—Inflammatory Breast Cancer 43
Chapter 5—Cancer of the Cervix 45
Chapter 6—Ovarian Epithelial Cancer 67
Chapter 7—Ovarian Germ Cell Cancer 87
Chapter 8—Cancer of the Uterus 95
Chapter 9—Uterine Sarcoma 111
Chapter 10—Gestational Trophoblastic Tumor 117
Chapter 11—Vaginal Cancer 123
Chapter 12—Vulvar Cancer 129

Part 2: The Road to Recovery: Treatments, Therapy and Coping

Chapter 13—Questions to Ask Your Doctor About
                Breast Cancer 137
Chapter 14—Progress Against Breast Cancer 149

Chapter 15—Breast Cancer: Understanding Treatment
    Options 167
Chapter 16—Questions and Answers About Breast Lumps 183
Chapter 17—Breast Biopsy: What You Should Know 195
Chapter 18—Mastectomy: A Treatment for Breast Cancer 203
Chapter 19—Breast Reconstruction: A Matter of Choice 219
Chapter 20—Survival Following Breast-Sparing Surgery
    Versus Mastectomy 237
Chapter 21—Breast Implants 239
Chapter 22—Breast Reconstruction Trials Using
    Saline-Filled Implants 277
Chapter 23—Radiation Therapy: A Treatment for Early
    Stage Breast Cancer 279
Chapter 24—Adjuvant Therapy: Facts For Women With
    Breast Cancer 295
Chapter 25—Delivering Cancer Fighting Drugs 301
Chapter 26—"The Queen of Neurosis": Gilda Radner's
    Experience With Ovarian Cancer 307
Chapter 27—When the Woman You Love Has Breast Cancer ... 319
Chapter 28—Cosmetic Help for Cancer Patients 335
Chapter 29—Ovarian Cancer: Screening, Treatment, and
    Follow-up 343

Part 3: Prevention

Chapter 30—Implementation of the Breast and Cervical
    Cancer Mortality Prevention Act 365
Chapter 31—Results from the National Breast and Cervical
    Cancer Early Detection Program 387
Chapter 32—Preventive Mastectomy 395
Chapter 33—Mammogram Facilities Must Meet Quality
    Standards 397
Chapter 34—Chances Are you Need a Mammogram: A Guide
    for Mid-life and Older Women 405
Chapter 35—Screening as Cancer Prevention 413
Chapter 36—Cancer Programs Make Good Business Sense 421
Chapter 37—Establishing Workplace Cancer Screening
    Programs 427
Chapter 38—The Papanicolaou Test: Routine Cancer
    Detection with the Pap Smear 443

Part 4: Risk Factors and Current Research

Chapter 39—Breast Cancer and Low-Fat Diets 455
Chapter 40—Life-time Probability of Breast Cancer in
    American Women 461
Chapter 41—Research to Improve Methods of Breast
    Cancer Detection 463
Chapter 42—Reducing the Risk of Mammography 467
Chapter 43—Oral Contraceptives and Breast Cancer 471
Chapter 44—Abortion and Possible Risk for Breast Cancer 477
Chapter 45—Fertility Drugs As a Risk for Ovarian Cancer 479
Chapter 46—Personal Use of Hair Coloring Products and
    Risk of Cancer 481
Chapter 47—Menopausal Hormone Replacement Therapy
    and Cancer Risk 487
Chapter 48—Inheritance of Proliferative Breast Disease in
    Families with Breast Cancer 491
Chapter 49—Scientists Nab Breast Cancer Gene 495

Part V: Glossary

Chapter 50—Glossary of Common Medical Terms 499

Index 517

Preface

About This Book

This book contains numerous publications produced by government and private agencies, including the National Institutes of Health (NIH), Department of Health and Human Services (DHHS), the Centers for Disease Control (CDC), National Cancer Institute (NCI), American Cancer Society and Y-ME Publications. The documents chosen present basic medical information for the interested layperson and for patients and their families coping with cancers and cancer treatments. Some articles include scientific and statistical data which can serve as a starting point for more intensive research.

The focus of this text is cancers that afflict women either exclusively or predominantly. Generally, cancers of the reproductive system fit this category. They include ovarian, cervical, uterine, vaginal and vulvar cancers. Breast cancer is by far the most important cancer striking as many as 1 in every 8 women, so information on this form comprises much of the text. Even though lung cancer is the most common form of cancer death for women, it is not covered in detail in this sourcebook. This is because the disease is not specific to women alone, and still strikes more men than women. For that reason, discussions of lung cancer are presented in Omnigraphics' *The New Cancer Sourcebook* (1996).

The companion text to this sourcebook, *The New Cancer Sourcebook*, examines other forms of cancer and provides detailed information on treatments, coping, diet, and current research in a more general format. Many of these topics may well be of interest to readers of this sourcebook.

How To Use This Book

Introduction: Cancer Today is itself a short primer on the subject of cancer. It gives a quick overview of the problem of cancer in the United States. Topics covered in this section include a few basic terms, some trends in cancer in general, and new directions in treatments and research. It also examines specific cancers important to women in particular with a series of "report cards," followed by two graphs and one table demonstrating the impact of specific cancers on women.

Part I: *Major Cancers That Specifically Affect Women* provides detailed information on specific cancers found predominantly or exclusively in women, their detection and treatment, and ways to control symptoms and discomfort. Reprinted articles from government sources examine specific cancers in alphabetic order. They present common symptoms, causes and risk factors, methods of diagnosis, treatments, and possible side effects of treatments.

Part II: *The Road to Recovery: Treatments, Therapy, and Coping* turns to the period after a positive diagnosis for cancer. It focusses on the main methods of treatment: surgery, radiation, chemotherapy, hormone therapy, and clinical trials. It presents some of the major decisions the cancer patient will be faced with and some of the options available. In addition, it examines the psychological damage caused by the disease and some ways of minimizing those effects on patient, family, and friends.

Part III: *Prevention* examines methods of preventing cancer and of detecting the disease early enough to make treatment regimens effective. The section presents some ways for women in high-risk categories to gain control over cancer by detecting the disease early and understanding what medical aid is necessary. It also presents some statistical data investigating the history and effectiveness of screening and prevention strategies.

Part IV: *Risk Factors and Current Research* describes some of the factors that can place a woman into the high-risk for cancer category as well as some current research initiatives.

Part V: *Glossary* provides a listing and short explanation of some important medical terms used throughout this volume.

Part VI: *Index* gives page references for key elements arising from the various treatments of the subject matter.

Acknowledgements

The editors wish to thank Y-ME Publications and the American Cancer Society for their permissions to reprint their useful and important articles, Margaret Mary Missar for her continuing search of medical libraries and government offices which resulted in the documents that make up this volume, Karen Bellenir for her technical assistance and advice, and Bruce the Scanman and special assistant Mike for their electronic magic.

Note from the Editor

This book is part of Omnigraphics' *Health Reference Series*. The series provides basic information about a broad range of medical concerns. It is not intended to serve as a tool for diagnosing illness, in prescribing treatments, or as a substitute for the physician/patient relationship. All persons concerned about medical symptoms or the possibility of disease are encouraged to seek professional care from an appropriate health care provider.

Introduction: Cancer Today

Cancer: Basic Facts

What is cancer?

Cancer is a group of diseases characterized by uncontrolled growth and spread of abnormal cells. If the spread is not controlled, it can result in death.

What causes cancer?

Cancer is caused by both external (chemicals, radiation, and viruses) and internal (hormones, immune conditions, and inherited mutations) factors. Causal factors may act together or in sequence to initiate or promote carcinogenesis. Ten or more years often pass between exposures or mutations and detectable cancer.

Can cancer be prevented?

Yes, since some external factors can be controlled. About 90 percent of the 800,000 skin cancers that will be diagnosed in 1995 could have been prevented by protection from the sun's rays. All cancers caused by cigarette smoking and heavy use of alcohol could be prevented completely. The American Cancer Society estimates that in

American Cancer Society *Cancer Facts & Figures-1995*. Used by permission.

1995, about 170,000 lives will be lost to cancer because of tobacco use. About 18,000 cancer deaths will be related to excessive alcohol use, frequently in combination with cigarette smoking.

Diets high in fruits, vegetables, and fiber may reduce the incidence of some types of cancers. Regular screening and self-exams can detect cancers of the breast, tongue, mouth, colon, rectum, cervix, prostate, testis, and melanoma at an early stage, when treatment is more likely to be successful. These sites include over half of all new cases. Of these cases, about two-thirds of all patients currently survive five years. With early detection, about 92 percent would survive. This means that of those persons diagnosed with these cancers in 1995, about 100,000 more would survive if their cancers had been detected in a localized stage and treated promptly.

How is a person's cancer treated?

By surgery, radiation, radioactive substances, chemicals, hormones, and immunotherapy.

Who gets cancer?

Anyone. Since incidence rises with age, most cases affect adults in mid-life or older. Among children ages 1-14, cancer causes more deaths in the United States than any other disease. In the 1980s, there were over 4.5 million cancer deaths, almost 9 million new cancer cases, and some 12 million people under medical care for cancer.

How many people alive today have ever had cancer?

Over 8 million Americans alive today have a history of cancer, 5 million diagnosed five or more years ago. Most of these 5 million can be considered cured, while others still have evidence of cancer. "Cured" means that a patient has no evidence of disease and has the same life expectancy as a person who never had cancer.

How many new cases will there be this year?

About 1,252,000 new cancer cases will be diagnosed. This estimate does not include carcinoma in situ and basal and squamous cell

Introduction: Cancer Today

skin cancers. The incidence of these skin cancers is estimated to be over 800,000 cases annually.

How many people will die?

This year about 547,000 will die of cancer. That is nearly 1,500 people a day. One out of every five deaths in the United States is from cancer.

What is the national cancer death rate?

There has been a steady rise in the cancer mortality rate in the United States in the last half-century. The age-adjusted rate in 1930 was 143 per 100,000 population. It rose to 157 in 1950, to 163 in 1970, and was 174 in 1990. The major cause of this increase has been lung cancer. Death rates for many major cancer sites have leveled off or declined over the past 50 years. If lung cancer deaths were excluded, cancer mortality would have declined 14 percent between 1950 and 1990.

How many people are surviving cancer?

In the early 1900s, few cancer patients had any hope of long-term survival. In the 1930s, less than one in five was alive five years after treatment. In the 1940s, it was one in four, and in the 1960s, it was one in three. About 500,000 Americans, or 4 of 10 patients who get cancer this year, will be alive 5 years after diagnosis. The gain from 1 in 3 in the 1960s to 4 in 10 now represents over 88,000 persons each year.

This 4 in 10, or about 40 percent is called the "observed" survival rate. When adjusted for normal life expectancy (factors such as dying of heart disease, accidents, and diseases of old age), a "relative" 5-year survival rate of 54 percent is seen for all cancers. The relative survival rate is commonly used to measure progress in the early detection and treatment of cancer.

What is the difference between *in situ* and invasive cancer?

In situ cancers are early localized tumors. Traditionally, *in situ* cancers are counted separately from invasive cancers because it is not certain they will become invasive. Also, the reporting of *in situ* cancers is not as reliable as it is for invasive cancers. For example, a physician may remove a patient's *in situ* skin cancer in his/her office and it won't be reported the same as cancers removed in a hospital.

Research, Prevention, Diagnosis, and Treatment

The vocabulary of cancer is ever increasing, as knowledge about the disease mounts. In the past decade, words such as oncogenes, retinoids, and growth factors have become standard. Indeed, our knowledge of the genetics of cancer has soared, and it is now possible to envision the day when the genetic basis of individual cancers will be known, along with mechanisms to correct the problem.

In addition to looking to the future, we can enjoy some successes now. Some cancers that only a few decades ago had a very poor outlook are often cured today: acute lymphocytic leukemia in children, Hodgkin's disease, Burkitt's lymphoma, Ewing's sarcoma (a form of bone cancer), Wilms' tumor (a kidney cancer in children), rhabdomyosarcoma (a cancer in certain muscle tissue), testicular cancer, and osteogenic (bone) sarcoma.

Oncogenes, which play a role in normal cell growth and differentiation, can mutate and cause the runaway cell growth associated with cancer. The *ras* oncogene is mutated in 50 percent of colon cancers and 90 percent of pancreatic cancers. The presence of certain oncogenes is being used to predict which tumors are likely to recur after surgery and/or to identify family members at risk.

Suppressor genes, which exist in normal cells to control cell growth, also play a role in cancer. Some cancers are caused when mutations occur in these genes, allowing uncontrolled cell growth. For example, the p53 suppressor gene is altered in more than 50 percent of cancers, including breast and lung. In one familial syndrome, where family members have high rates of cancer, about 90 percent of those who inherit the abnormal p53 gene get cancer by the age of 50. Family members can now be screened for this genetic abnormality before cancer develops.

Recent research has targeted a gene responsible for familial breast cancer and genes which cause susceptibility to colon cancer. These genes have tremendous potential for risk assessment and/or early detections.

Introduction: Cancer Today

Through genetic engineering, researchers may be able to correct or modify hereditary susceptibility to cancer by transplanting normal copies of genes into cells that have mutated copies of those genes. They also hope to counteract resistance to drugs.

Growth factors can be used to stimulate normal bone marrow cells to withstand very high doses of chemotherapeutic drugs.

A genetic fusing of cancer cells with normal cells can produce disease-fighting monoclonal antibodies (specific antibodies tailored to seek out chosen targets on cancer cells). Their potential in the diagnosis and treatment of cancer is under study, and they are showing promise for carrying cancer-killing radiation and drugs to a precise location.

Researchers are understanding how cancer cells spread to healthy tissues, a process called metastasis. A powerful enzyme inhibitor, TIMP-2 is showing promise for abolishing the metastatic potential of tumor cells. A metastasis suppressor gene, NM23, has also been identified.

Pain has been a significant problem for 50-70 percent of patients with cancer pain, but cancer pain can usually be relieved. The patient's own assessment of pain should be used to guide therapy, which may be given orally, by injection, or by infusion, and should include narcotics when needed.

Anti-nausea drugs have been developed to help with this side effect of chemotherapy.

Researchers are examining synthetic retinoids (cousins of vitamin A) and other substances to see if recurrences of certain cancers can be prevented and if these agents can reduce cancer in high-risk groups. The cancer prevention capabilities of many other compounds are also being researched.

Substances originally found in nature, such as taxol, are being synthesized in laboratories and tested on a variety of cancers. Other compounds derived from sea urchins, plants, etc. are rich resources for anticancer drugs.

New approaches to drug therapy use combinations of chemotherapeutic drugs, or chemotherapy plus surgery or radiation. New classes of agents are being tested for their effectiveness in treating patients whose disease is resistant to drug therapies now in use. Understanding the basis of drug resistance and developing solutions are major areas of research today.

Many patients with primary bone cancer now are treated successfully by removing and replacing a section of bone rather than by amputating the leg or arm. Drugs and radiation therapy are being used effectively after bone cancer surgery, resulting in dramatic improvement in survival.

New high-technology diagnostic imaging techniques have replaced exploratory surgery for some cancer patients. Magnetic resonance imaging (MRI) is one example of such technology. In MRI, an electromagnet is used to detect hidden tumors by mapping the vibrations of the various atoms in the body on a computer screen. Computerized tomography (CT) scanning uses x-rays to examine parts of the body. In both of these painless, non-invasive procedures, cross-section pictures can show a tumor's shape and location more accurately than is possible with conventional x-ray techniques. For patients undergoing radiation therapy, CT scanning may enable the therapist to pinpoint the tumor more precisely, and thus provide more accurate radiation dosage while sparing normal tissue. Positron emission tomography (PET) is another imaging technique. One of the advances in the area of imaging combines two or three different types of images (e.g., MRI and PET) in a computer to create a three-dimensional picture that can be rotated on the screen. This technology is currently used in some medical centers to help plan for surgery and radiation therapy in areas such as the brain.

Immunotherapy holds the hope of enhancing the body's own disease-fighting systems to help control cancer. Interferon (a naturally occurring body protein capable of killing cancer cells or stopping their growth), interleukin-2 (a growth factor that stimulates cells of the immune system to fight cancer), and other biologic response modifiers are under study. Recently, interferon was made available to all doctors as the treatment for hairy cell leukemia, a rare blood cancer of older Americans. Interleukin-2 is under active research in the treatment of kidney cancer and melanoma. Vaccines against several types of cancer are also being developed, with notable progress with malignant melanoma.

Many cancers develop in a two-stage process through exposure to substances known as initiators and promoters. Research scientists are exploring ways to interrupt this process as a means to prevent cancer.

Ongoing research into anticancer drug development will result in less toxicity to normal cells and more potency against tumor cells. For

Introduction: Cancer Today

example, by attaching antibodies, which can react with a receptor on a cancer cell, to the drug, scientists can increase the drug's ability to home in on that particular cell type. New ways of increasing the action of drugs is also being studied by developing drugs that combine with the cancer cells' DNA and makes the cell more susceptible to radiation. In addition, novel drug delivery systems are allowing more of the drug to reach cancer cells. Researchers have encapsulated drugs inside lipid capsules which, in essence, tricks the cancer cells into taking in the drug at a higher rate than normal cells, thus increasing the rate of cell killing.

New technologies have made it possible to use bone marrow transplantation as an important treatment option in select patients with leukemia and lymphoma. Bone marrow transplantation for breast cancers and other malignant tumors is under study. Because disruption of bone marrow function is a side effect of some cancer treatments, researchers are evaluating autologous bone marrow transplants, in which a portion of the patient's own marrow is removed before treatment, saved, and later restored. This procedure eliminates the problems of matching a donor with the recipient patient, and may make it possible for the patient to tolerate larger doses of anticancer drugs or radiation therapy.

Improvements in cancer treatment have made possible more conservative management of some early cancers. In early cancer of the larynx, many patients are now able to retain the larynx and voice; in colorectal cancer, fewer permanent colostomies are needed; in many cases, the surgery for breast cancer is often more limited; and special nerve-sparing surgery now commonly used for prostate cancer could enable men to maintain normal penile function.

Prostatic ultrasound (a rectal probe using ultrasonic waves to produce an image of the prostate) is currently being investigated as a potential means to increase the early detection of occult (not clinically suspected) prostate cancer. Recently, prostatic ultrasound has been combined with a blood test for prostate-specific antigen to aid in early detection of prostate cancer.

A large clinical trial is underway to evaluate the usefulness of an estrogen-blocking drug called tamoxifen. Commonly used to treat women when they have breast cancer, this large study hopes to see if tamoxifen can also be used to prevent breast cancer in women who are at high risk.

With medical progress producing longer survival periods for many cancer patients, clinical concerns are expanding to include not only patients' physical well-being, but also their psychosocial needs. The response of both patient and family to the disease, the patient's sexual concerns, employment and insurance needs, and ways to provide psychosocial support have emerged as important areas of research and clinical care.

Psychosocial and behavioral research is showing much promise as evidence mounts that lifestyle (tobacco, diet) and environmental factors influence a person's general health and chances of developing cancer, as well as the mental and emotional ability to cope with cancer if it occurs. Research on behavioral modification is having a significant impact on symptoms of cancer and its treatment, such as pain, nausea, and vomiting. Other research deals with stress during treatment and during recovery after surgery or radiation treatment. A number of investigations concentrate on breast cancer, specifically on how women can be motivated to make use of mammography screening, and how to adjust to surgery, if such intervention becomes necessary.

Report Cards on Selected Cancers

Lung Cancer

New Cancer Cases: An estimated 169,900 new cases in 1995. The incidence rate, which had been increasing steadily in men and women for several decades, has declined in men, from a high of 87 per 100,000 in 1984 to 80 in 1991. The incidence rate in women continues to increase to 42 per 100,000 in 1991.

Mortality: An estimated 157,400 deaths in 1995. Since 1987, more women have died of lung cancer than breast cancer, which, for over 40 years, was the major cause of cancer death in women.

Signs and Symptoms: Persistent cough, sputum streaked with blood, chest pain, recurring pneumonia or bronchitis.

Risk Factors: Cigarette smoking; exposure to certain industrial substances, such as arsenic, certain organic chemicals and asbestos, particularly for persons who smoke; radiation exposure from occupational, medical, and environmental sources. Radon exposure may increase risk, especially in cigarette smokers. Exposure to sidestream cigarette smoke increases the risk for non-smokers.

Introduction: Cancer Today

Early Detection: Because symptoms often don't appear until the disease is in advanced stages, early detection is very difficult. In smokers who stop smoking at the time of early precancerous cellular changes, damaged bronchial lining tissues often return to normal. Smokers who persist in smoking may form abnormal cell growth patterns that lead to cancer. Chest x-ray, analysis of the types of cells contained in sputum, and fiberoptic examination of the bronchial passages assist diagnosis.

Treatment: Determined by the type and stage of the cancer. Options include surgery, radiation therapy, and chemotherapy. For many localized cancers, surgery is usually the treatment of choice. Because the disease has usually spread by the time it is discovered, radiation therapy and chemotherapy are often needed in combination with surgery. In small cell cancer, chemotherapy alone or combined with radiation has replaced surgery as the treatment of choice; on this regimen, a large percentage of patients experience remission, which in some cases is long-lasting.

Survival: The 5-year relative survival rate is only 13 percent in all patients, regardless of stage at diagnosis. The rate is 47 percent for cases detected when the disease is still localized, but only 15 percent of lung cancers are discovered that early.

Breast Cancer

New Cancer Cases: An estimated 182,000 new invasive cases among women in the United States during 1995. About 1,400 new cases of breast cancer will be diagnosed in men in 1995. Breast cancer incidence rates for women have increased about 2 percent a year since 1980, but recently have leveled off at about 110 per 100,000. Most of the recent rise in rates is believed to be due to marked increases in mammography utilization, allowing the detection of early stage breast cancers, frequently before they would become clinically apparent. Other reasons for a longer-term increase in breast cancer are not yet understood.

Mortality: An estimated 46,240 deaths (46,000 women, 240 men) in 1995; in women, the second major cause of cancer death. Preliminary data for 1992 suggest that mortality is falling in white women, but not in blacks, perhaps because of early detection and improved treatment.

Signs and Symptoms: Pre-clinical radiographic signs seen on a mammogram. Breast changes, such as a lump, thickening, swelling, dimpling, skin irritation, distortion, retraction, scaliness, pain, tenderness of the nipple, or nipple discharge, may be symptoms of breast cancer and a physician should be consulted.

Risk Factors: The risk of breast cancer increases with age; personal or family history of breast cancer; early age at menarche, late age at menopause, lengthy exposure to cyclical estrogen, never had children or late age at first live birth, and higher education and socioeconomic status. International variability in cancer incidence rates correlate with variations in diet, especially fat intake, although a causal role for dietary factors has not been firmly established. A majority of women will have one or more risk factors for breast cancer. However, most risks are at such a low level that they only partly explain the high frequency of the disease in the population. Thus, breast cancer risk factors appear to be more useful in providing clues to the development of cancer than in identifying prevention strategies. Since adult women may not be able to alter their personal risk factors in any practical sense, the best current opportunity for reducing mortality is through early detection.

Early Detection: The American Cancer Society recommends that asymptomatic women have a screening mammogram by age 40; women 40 to 49 should have a mammogram every 1-2 years; women age 50 and over should have a mammogram every year. In addition, a clinical physical examination of the breast is recommended every three years for women 20 to 40, and every year for those over 40. The Society also recommends monthly breast self-examination as a routine good health habit for women 20 years or older. Most breast lumps are not cancer, but only a physician can make a diagnosis.

Mammography is recognized as a valuable diagnostic technique for women who have findings suggestive of breast cancer. When a suspicious area is identified on a mammogram, or when a woman has a suspicious lump, mammography can help determine if there are other lesions too small to be felt in the same or opposite breast. Since a small percentage of breast cancers may not be seen on a mammogram, all suspicious lumps should be biopsied for a definitive diagnosis, even when current or recent mammography findings are described as normal.

Treatment: Taking into account the medical situation and the patient's preferences, treatment may require lumpectomy (local re-

Introduction: Cancer Today

moval of the tumor), mastectomy (surgical removal of the breast), radiation therapy, chemotherapy, or hormone manipulation therapy. Often, two or more methods are used in combination.

Patients should discuss with their physicians possible options for the best management of their breast cancer.

New techniques in recent years have made breast reconstruction possible after mastectomy, and the cosmetic results usually are good. Reconstruction has become an important part of treatment and rehabilitation.

Survival: The 5-year survival rate (which includes all women living five years after diagnosis, whether the patient is in remission, disease-free, or under treatment) for localized breast cancer has risen from 78 percent in the 1940s to 94 percent today. If the cancer has spread regionally at the time of diagnosis, however, the 5-year survival rate is 73 percent, for persons with distant metastases at the time of diagnosis, the 5-year survival rate is 18 percent.

Unlike survival for many other cancers that tend to level off after five years, survival after a diagnosis of breast cancer continues to decline beyond the five years. According to the most currently available data, 63 percent of the women diagnosed with breast cancer survive 10 years and 56 percent survive 15 years.

Uterus (Cervix) Cancer

New Cancer Cases: An estimated 15,800 invasive and 65,000 carcinoma *in situ* cases will be diagnosed in 1995. The rate of invasive cervical cancer has decreased steadily over the last several decades, but has increased in recent years in women under 50. Cervical carcinoma *in situ*, a precancerous condition, is now more frequent than invasive cancer, especially in women under 50.

Mortality: An estimated 4,800 deaths from cervical cancer in 1995. The mortality rate is more than twice as high for black women as for white women.

Signs and Symptoms: Abnormal uterine bleeding or spotting; abnormal vaginal discharge. Pain and systemic symptoms are late manifestations of the disease.

Risk Factors: Early age at first intercourse, multiple sex partners, cigarette smoking, and infection with certain types of human papillomavirus.

Early Detection: The Pap test is a simple procedure that can be performed at appropriate intervals by health care professionals as part of a pelvic examination. A small sample of cells is swabbed from the cervix, transferred to a slide, and examined under a microscope. This test should be performed annually with a pelvic examination in women who are, or have been, sexually active or who have reached age 18 years. After three or more consecutive annual examinations with normal findings, the Pap test may be performed less frequently at the discretion of the physician.

Treatment: Cervix cancers generally are treated by surgery or radiation, or by a combination of the two. In precancerous (*in situ*) stages, changes in the cervix may be treated by cryotherapy (the destruction of cells by extreme cold), by electro-coagulation (the destruction of tissue through intense heat by electric current), or by local surgery.

Survival: The 5-year survival rate for cervical cancer patients is 67 percent. For women diagnosed with localized disease the survival rate is 90 percent.

Uterus (Endometrial) Cancer

New Cancer Cases: An estimated 32,800 cases of cancer of the corpus (body) of the uterus, usually of the endometrium (lining). Endometrial cancer is most frequently diagnosed in women over age 50.

Mortality: An estimated 5,900 deaths in 1995.

Signs and Symptoms: Abnormal uterine staining or bleeding, especially postmenopausal. Pain and weight loss occur late in the disease.

Risk Factors: Early menarche, late menopause, history of infertility, failure to ovulate, tamoxifen or unopposed estrogen therapy, obesity.

During menopause, the level of hormones (estrogens) normally produced by the ovaries declines. This causes symptoms such as "hot flashes" or painful sexual intercourse due to thinning of the vaginal lining. To control these symptoms, estrogen replacement therapy may be given to women during and after menopause. This therapy may increase the risk of endometrial cancer, therefore, the benefits and risks of such treatment should be discussed by the woman and her physician.

Introduction: Cancer Today

Early Detection: The Pap test, highly effective in detecting early cancer of the uterine cervix, is only partially effective in detecting endometrial cancer. Women 40 and over should have an annual pelvic exam by a health professional. Women at high risk of developing endometrial cancer should have an endometrial tissue sample evaluated at menopause.

Treatment: Uterine cancers are usually treated with surgery, radiation, hormones, and/or chemotherapy depending on the stage of disease.

Survival: The 5-year survival rate for endometrial cancer is 83 percent overall, 94 percent if discovered at an early stage, and 67 percent if diagnosed at a regional stage.

Ovary Cancer

New Cancer Cases: An estimated 26,600 new cases in the United States in 1995. It accounts for 5 percent of all cancers among women.

Mortality: An estimated 14,500 deaths in 1995. Although ovarian cancer ranks second in incidence among gynecologic cancers, it causes more deaths than any other cancer of the female reproductive system.

Signs and Symptoms: Ovarian cancer is often "silent," showing no obvious signs or symptoms until late in its development. The most common sign is enlargement of the abdomen, which is caused by the accumulation of fluid. Rarely will there be abnormal vaginal bleeding. In women over 40, vague digestive disturbances (stomach discomfort, gas, distention) that persist and cannot be explained by any other cause may indicate the need for a thorough evaluation for ovarian cancer.

Risk Factors: Risk for ovarian cancer increases with age. Women who have never had children are more likely to develop ovarian cancer than those who have. Increased number of pregnancies and the use of oral contraceptives, appear to be protective against ovarian cancer. Women who have had breast cancer or have a family history of ovarian cancer are at increased risk. Certain rare genetic disorders are associated with increased risk. With the exception of Japan, the highest incidence rates are reported from the more industrialized countries.

Early Detection: Periodic, thorough pelvic examinations are important. The Pap test, useful in detecting cervical cancer, does not reveal ovarian cancer. Women over the age of 40 should have a cancer-related checkup every year.

Treatment: Surgery, radiation therapy, and drug therapy are treatment options. Surgery usually includes the removal of one or both ovaries (oophorectomy), the uterus (hysterectomy), and the fallopian tubes (salpingectomy). In some very early tumors, only the involved ovary will be removed, especially in young women. In advanced disease, an attempt is made to remove all intra-abdominal disease, to enhance the effect of chemotherapy.

Survival: Overall, the 5-year survival rate for ovarian cancer is 42 percent. If diagnosed and treated early, the relative survival rate is 90 percent; however, only about 23 percent of all cases are detected at the localized stage. Survival rates for women with regional and distant disease are 41 percent and 21 percent, respectively.

Introduction: Cancer Today

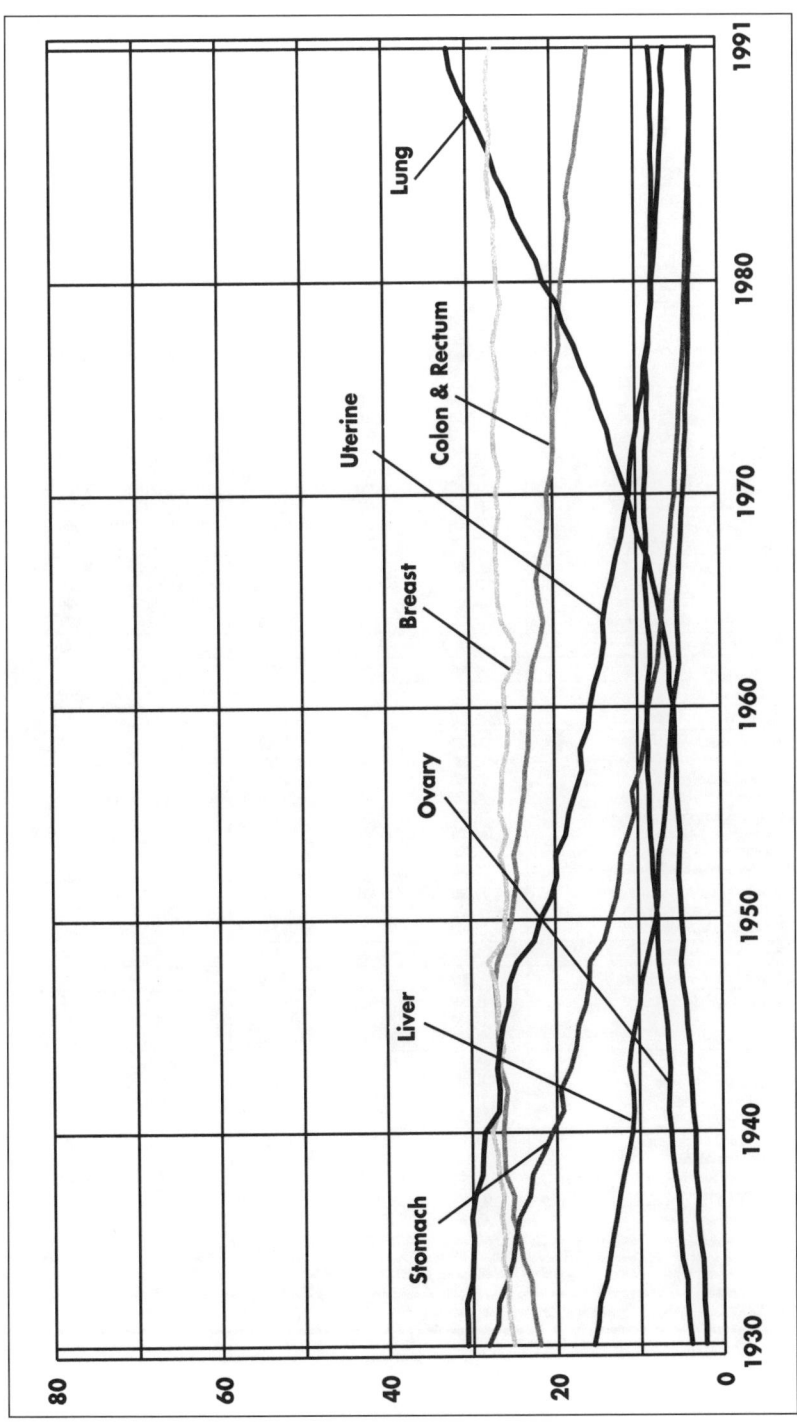

Cancer Death Rates by Site, Females, United States, 1930-91

Cancer Sourcebook for Women

Estimated New Cancer Cases and Deaths by Sex for All Sites, United States, 1995*

	Estimated New Cases			Estimated Deaths		
	Both Sexes	Male	Female	Both Sexes	Male	Female
All sites	1,252,000	677,000	575,000	547,000	289,000	258,000
Buccal cavity & pharynx (Oral)	28,150	18,800	9,350	8,370	5,480	2,890
Lip	2,500	1,900	600	100	80	20
Tongue	5,550	3,600	1,950	1,870	1,200	670
Mouth	11,000	6,900	4,100	2,300	1,300	1,000
Pharynx	9,100	6,400	2,700	4,100	2,900	1,200
Digestive organs	223,000	118,000	105,000	124,330	66,130	58,200
Esophagus	12,100	8,800	3,300	10,900	8,200	2,700
Stomach	22,800	14,000	8,800	14,700	8,800	5,900
Small intestine	4,600	2,400	2,200	1,120	590	530
Large intestine (Colon-Rectum)	100,000	49,000	51,000	47,500	23,000	24,500
Rectum	38,200	21,700	16,500	7,800	4,200	3,600
Liver and biliary passages	18,500	9,800	8,700	14,200	7,700	6,500
Pancreas	24,000	11,000	13,000	27,000	13,200	13,800
Other and unspecified digestive	2,800	1,300	1,500	1,110	440	670
Respiratory system	186,300	108,400	77,900	162,950	99,470	63,480
Larynx	11,600	9,000	2,600	4,090	3,200	890
Lung	169,900	96,000	73,900	157,400	95,400	62,000
Other & unspecified respiratory	4,800	3,400	1,400	1,460	870	590
Bone	2,070	1,100	970	1,280	750	530
Connective tissue	6,000	3,300	2,700	3,600	1,800	1,800
Melanoma of skin	34,100	18,700	15,400	7,200	4,500	2,700
Breast	183,400	1,400	182,000	46,240	240	46,000
Genital organs	333,100	252,200	80,900	67,380	40,980	26,400
Cervix uteri	15,800	—	15,800	4,800	—	4,800
Corpus & unspecified (Uterus)	32,800	—	32,800	5,900	—	5,900
Ovary	26,600	—	26,600	14,500	—	14,500
Other & unspecified genital, female	5,700	—	5,700	1,200	—	1,200
Prostate	244,000	244,000	—	40,400	40,400	—
Testis	7,100	7,100	—	370	370	—
Other & unspecified genital, male	1,100	1,100	—	210	210	—
Urinary organs	79,300	54,400	24,900	22,900	14,600	8,300
Bladder	50,500	37,300	13,200	11,200	7,500	3,700
Kidney & other urinary	28,800	17,100	11,700	11,700	7,100	4,600
Eye	1,870	1,000	870	240	130	110
Brain & central nervous system	17,200	9,700	7,500	13,300	7,300	6,000
Endocrine glands	15,380	3,900	11,480	1,780	760	1,020
Thyroid	13,900	3,200	10,700	1,120	440	680
Other endocrine	1,480	700	780	660	320	340
Leukemia	25,700	14,700	11,000	20,400	11,100	9,300
Lymphocytic leukemia	11,000	6,700	4,300	6,400	3,500	2,900
Granulocytic leukemia	11,100	5,900	5,200	8,400	4,600	3,800
Other & unspecified leukemia	3,600	2,100	1,500	5,600	3,000	2,600
Other blood & lymph tissues	71,200	41,100	30,100	34,450	18,120	16,330
Hodgkin's disease	7,800	4,500	3,300	1,450	820	630
Non-Hodgkin's lymphoma	50,900	29,500	21,400	22,700	12,000	10,700
Multiple myeloma	12,500	7,100	5,400	10,300	5,300	5,000
All other & unspecified sites	45,230	30,300	14,930	32,580	17,640	14,940

*Excludes basal and squamous cell skin cancers and in situ carcinomas except bladder. Carcinoma in situ of the uterine cervix accounts for about 65,000 new cases annually, carcinoma in situ of the female breast accounts for about 25,000 new cases annually, and melanoma carcinoma in situ accounts for about 10,000 new cases annually. Overall, about 120,000 new cases of carcinoma in situ of all sites of cancer are diagnosed each year.

Basal cell and squamous cell skin cancers account for more than 800,000 new cases annually. About 2,100 nonmelanoma skin cancer deaths will occur in 1995.

Incidence estimates are based on rates from NCI SEER program 1989-91.

Introduction: Cancer Today

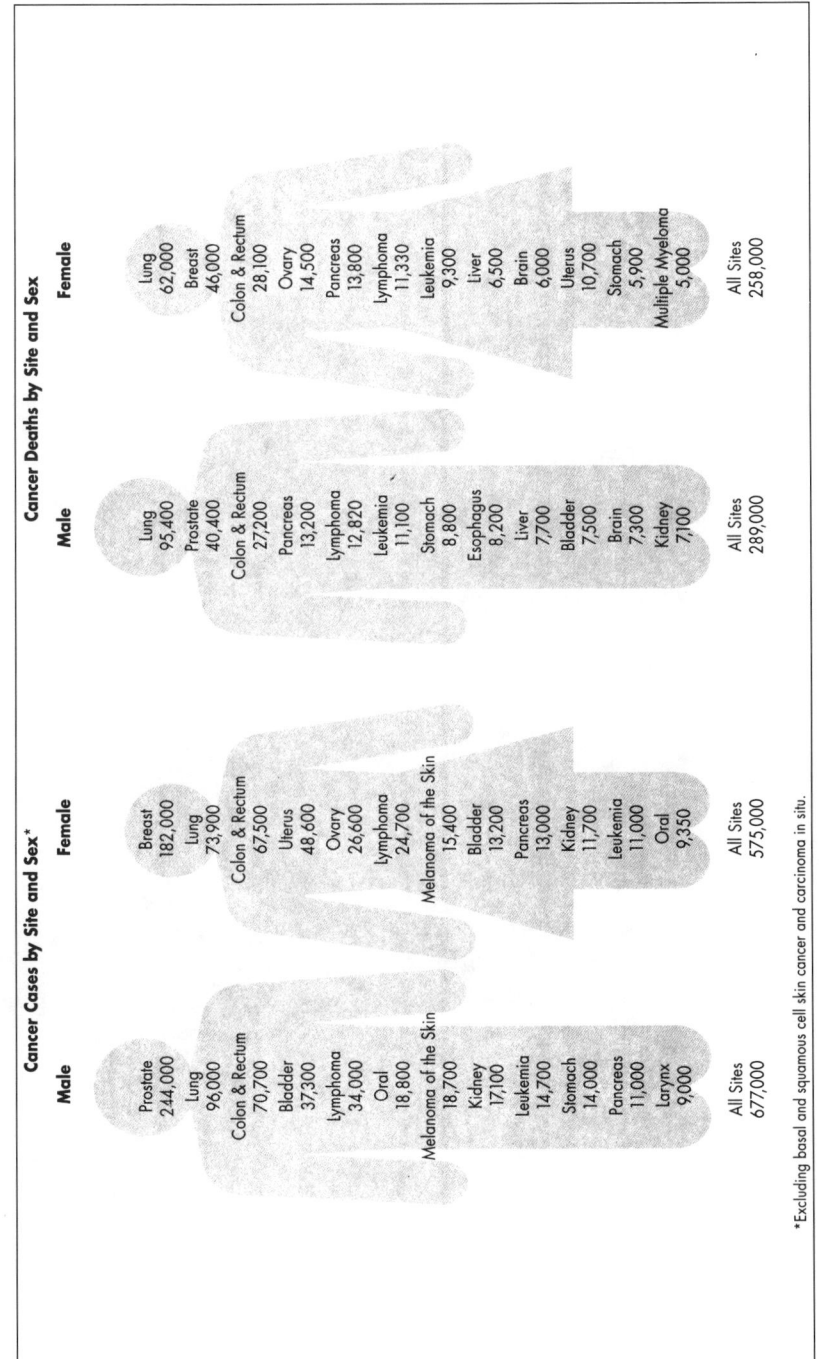

Leading Sites of New Cancer Cases and Deaths—1995 Estimates

Part One

Major Cancers that Specifically Affect Women

Chapter 1

Women and Cancer

Statistical Associations of Women to Specific Cancers

Breast Cancer

Breast cancer is a complex and devastating disease and the most frequently diagnosed cancer in women in the United States today. In 1995, there will be an estimated 182,000 new cases of breast cancer diagnosed and over 46,000 women will die from this disease in 1995.

Breast cancer incidence rates for women have increased about 2 percent per year since 1980, but recently have leveled off.

The death rate for breast cancer in American women declined 4.7 percent between 1989 and 1992, the largest such short-term decline in the United States for this disease since 1950. Death rates for white women declined 5.5 percent between 1989 and 1992, however, death rates for African-American women increased 2.6 percent during the same time.

In mid-September, 1994, researchers in Utah and North Carolina reported they isolated the BRCA-1 gene, a breast cancer susceptibility gene, located on chromosome 17. Days later, researchers isolated another breast cancer susceptibility gene, BRCA-2, mapped to chromosome 13.

NCI Cancerfax 208/400079.

Approximately 5 percent of all breast cancer cases are related to BRCA-1. Normally BRCA-1 helps to restrain tumor growth.

An estimated 25 percent of women who have early-onset breast cancer (diagnosed before 30 years of age) have this gene.

Increased risk of breast cancer has been observed in families with inherited syndromes, including the Li-Fraumeni syndrome, characterized by soft-tissue sarcoma, breast cancer and leukemia.

NCI has a major breast cancer prevention trial using tamoxifen as the active agent. The study is currently evaluating and enrolling patients. Sixteen thousand women ages 35 and older who have been determined by a complex matrix of factors to be at high risk for breast cancer are eligible for enrollment.

The Long Island Breast Cancer Study Project (LIBCSP), supported by the NCI and NIEHS, will use epidemiologic methods to examine a wide variety of environmental factors, including exposures to pesticides and other organochlorine toxins, contaminated drinking water, indoor air pollution, aircraft and auto emissions, electromagnetic fields, hazardous waste and municipal waste. Dietary factors, radiation, estrogen exposures, and occupational exposures are also being assessed.

Lung Cancer

The National Health Interview Survey reports that from 1974 to 1992, smoking among women decreased from 33 percent to 25 percent. Smoking prevalence is highest among people with incomes below the poverty level: 40 percent of men and 32 percent of women of that socioeconomic status are smokers.

Since 1987, more women have died of lung cancer than breast cancer, which, for 40 years, was the major cause of cancer death in women.

Of the 169,900 estimated new lung cancer cases in 1995, 73,900 will be women.

Because of the toll of smoking-related cancers, NCI places a major emphasis on smoking prevention and cessation. NCI supports the American Stop Smoking Intervention Study (ASSIST), a comprehensive tobacco control program designed to reach 20 million smokers in 17 states. ASSIST is a collaborative effort between the NCI, American Cancer Society, state and local health departments, and other voluntary organizations.

The Prostate, Lung, Colorectal and Ovarian Cancer Screening Trials (PLCO) is an NCI-supported randomized, controlled clinical trial designed to determine whether particular screening modalities will reduce the number of deaths through early detection of these cancers. Over the next eight years, 198,000 participants will be evaluated.

Colon and Rectum Cancer

An estimated 138,200 new cases of colon and rectum cancer will occur in 1995.

Mortality from colorectal cancer has fallen 29 percent for women and 7 percent for men over the last 30 years.

NCI-supported scientists have described genes associated with inherited forms of colon cancer. Mutations in two genes, hMSH2 and hMLH1, are associated with a high percentage of hereditary non-polyposis colorectal cancer cases. Such mutations account for roughly 15 percent of overall colon cancer cases and are also linked to cancers occurring within affected families—endometrial, stomach, bladder, ovarian, and possibly breast cancer.

Uterine Cancer

In 1995, an estimated 32,800 cases of cancer of the corpus (body) of the uterus will occur, usually of the endometrial (lining). Endometrial cancer is most frequently diagnosed in women over age 50.

Ovarian Cancer

An estimated 26,600 new cases of ovarian cancer will occur in 1995, accounting for 5 percent of all cancers among women.

NCI is evaluating the tumor marker CA-125 in the diagnosis of ovarian cancer in the Prostate, Lung, Colorectal, and Ovarian (PLC0) screening clinical trial.

In 1983, NCI began conducting clinical trials of the safety of Taxol (Paclitaxel) and its effectiveness against various types of cancer, including ovarian cancer. In December 1992, the Food and Drug Administration approved the use of the drug Taxol for refractory (treatment resistant) ovarian cancer.

The National Cancer Institute has a coordinated cancer research program that includes basic cancer research, research on better diagnostic technology, prevention, treatment, rehabilitation, and community outreach.

NCI's programs of information dissemination has made the best information about cancer and cancer treatment easily available to the public, patients and health care providers. Diffusion of research results and treatment advances are carried out through many professional meetings, workshops and via the Cancer Information Service (CIS) reached by its toll-free 1-800-4-CANCER telephone number. CIS information specialists have extensive training in providing up-to-date and understandable information about cancer.

Chapter 2

Breast Cancer

What Is Cancer?

Cancer is a group of diseases. It occurs when cells become abnormal and divide without control or order.

Every organ in the body is made up of various kinds of cells. Cells normally divide in an orderly way to produce more cells only when they are needed. This process helps keep the body healthy.

If cells divide when new cells are not needed, they form too much tissue. The mass of extra tissue, called a tumor, can be benign or malignant.

- Benign tumors are not cancer. They can usually be removed, and in most cases, they don't come back. Most important, the cells in benign tumors do not invade other tissues and do not spread to other parts of the body. Benign breast tumors are not a threat to life.

- Malignant tumors are cancer. They can invade and damage nearby tissues and organs. Also, cancer cells can break away from a malignant tumor and enter the bloodstream or lymphatic system. That is how breast cancer spreads and forms secondary tumors in other parts of the body. The spread of cancer is called metastasis.

NIH 94-1556.

The Breasts

Each breast has 15 to 20 sections, called lobes, that are arranged like the petals of a daisy. Each lobe has many smaller lobules, which end in dozens of tiny bulbs that can produce milk. The lobes, lobules, and bulbs are all linked by thin tubes called ducts. These ducts lead to the nipple in the center of a dark area of skin called the areola. Fat fills the spaces between lobules and ducts. There are no muscles in the breast, but muscles lie under each breast and cover the ribs.

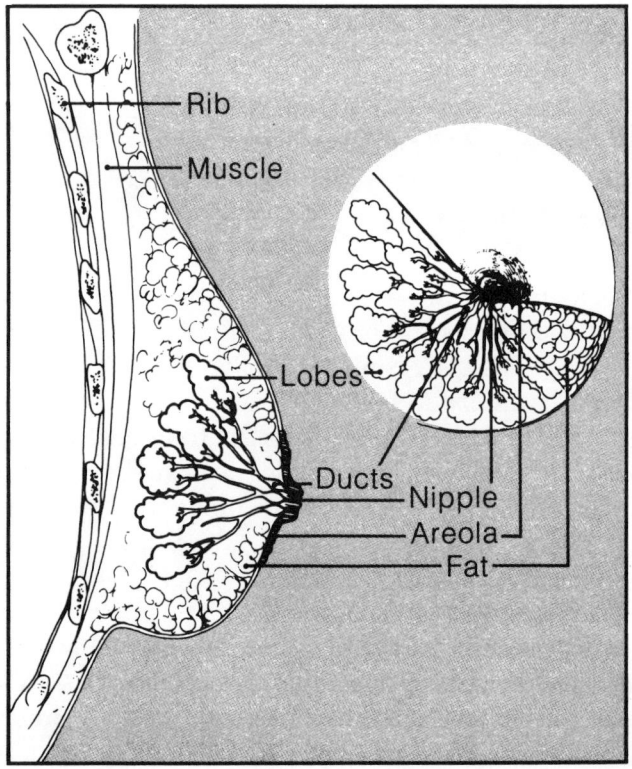

Figure 2.1. This diagram illustrates the parts of a breast.

Each breast also contains blood vessels and vessels that carry lymph. The lymph vessels lead to small bean-shaped organs called lymph nodes. Clusters of lymph nodes are found under the arm, above the collarbone, and in the chest. Lymph nodes are also found in many other parts of the body.

Types of Breast Cancer

There are more than 100 different types of cancer, including several types of breast cancer. The most common type of breast cancer begins in the lining of the ducts and is called ductal carcinoma. Another type, called lobular carcinoma, arises in the lobules. Cancers that begin in other tissues in the breast are rare and are not discussed in this chapter.

When breast cancer spreads outside the breast, cancer cells are often found in the lymph nodes under the arm. If the cancer has reached these nodes, it may mean that cancer cells have spread to other parts of the body, other lymph nodes and other organs, such as the bones, liver, or lungs.

Cancer that spreads is the same disease and has the same name as the original (primary) cancer. When breast cancer spreads, it is called metastatic breast cancer, even though the secondary tumor is in another organ. Doctors may call this problem "distant" disease.

Early Detection

When breast cancer is found and treated early, a woman has more treatment choices and a good chance of complete recovery. So it is important to detect breast cancer as early as possible. The National Cancer Institute encourages women to take an active part in early detection. They should talk with their doctor about this disease, the symptoms to watch for, and an appropriate schedule of checkups. The doctor's advice will be based on the woman's age, medical history, and other factors. Women should ask the doctor about:

- Mammograms (x-rays of the breast);
- Breast exams by a doctor or nurse; and
- Breast self-examination (BSE).

A mammogram is a special kind of x-ray. It is different from a chest x-ray or x-rays of other parts of the body.

Mammography involves two x-rays of each breast, one taken from the side and one from the top. The breast must be squeezed between two plates for the pictures to be clear. While this squeezing may be a bit uncomfortable, it lasts only a few seconds. In many cases, mammograms can show breast tumors before they cause symptoms or can be felt. A mammogram can also show small deposits of calcium in the breast. A cluster of very tiny specks of calcium (called microcalcifications) may be an early sign of cancer.

Mammography should be done only by specially trained people using machines designed just for taking x-rays of the breast. The pictures should be checked by a qualified radiologist. Women should talk with their doctor or call the Cancer Information Service for help in finding out where to get a mammogram.

Mammography is an excellent tool, but we know that it cannot find every abnormal area in the breast. So another important step in early detection is for women to have their breasts examined regularly by a doctor or nurse.

Between visits to the doctor, women should examine their breasts every month. (An easy-to-follow breast self-examination guide appears below.) It's important to remember that every woman's breasts are different. And each woman's breasts change because of age, the menstrual cycle, pregnancy, menopause, or taking birth control pills or other hormones. It is normal for the breasts to feel lumpy and uneven. Also, it's common for a woman's breasts to be swollen and tender right before or during her menstrual period. These are some of the reasons why many women are not certain what their breasts are supposed to feel like. By doing monthly BSE, a woman learns what is normal for her breasts, and she is more likely to detect a change. Any changes should be reported to the doctor.

Symptoms

Early breast cancer usually does not cause pain. In fact, when it first develops, breast cancer may cause no symptoms at all. But as the cancer grows, it can cause changes that women should watch for:

- A lump or thickening in or near the breast or in the underarm area;
- A change in the size or shape of the breast;
- A discharge from the nipple; or
- A change in the color or feel of the skin of the breast, areola, or nipple (dimpled, puckered, or scaly).

A woman should see her doctor if she notices any of these changes. Most often, they are not cancer, but only a doctor can tell for sure.

Diagnosis

An abnormal area on a mammogram, a lump, or other changes in the breast can be caused by cancer or by other, less serious problems. To find out the cause of any of these signs or symptoms, a woman's doctor does a careful physical exam and asks about her personal and family medical history. In addition to checking general signs of health, the doctor may do one or more of the breast exams described below to help make a diagnosis.

Palpation. The doctor can tell a lot about a lump by palpation (carefully feeling the lump and the tissue around it): its size, its texture, and whether it moves easily. Benign lumps often feel different from cancerous ones.

Mammography. X-rays of the breast can give the doctor important information about a breast lump. If an area on the mammogram looks suspicious or is not clear, additional views may be needed.

Ultrasonography. Sometimes the doctor orders ultrasonography, which can often show whether a lump is solid or filled with fluid. This exam uses high-frequency sound waves, which cannot be heard by humans. The sound waves enter the breast and bounce back. The pattern of their echoes produces a picture called a sonogram, which is displayed on a screen. This exam is often used along with mammography.

Based on these exams, the doctor may decide that no further tests are needed and no treatment is necessary. In such cases, the doctor may want to check the woman regularly to watch for any changes. Often, however, the doctor must remove fluid or tissue from the breast to make a diagnosis.

Aspiration or needle biopsy. The doctor uses a needle to remove fluid or a small amount of tissue from a breast lump. This procedure may show whether the lump is a fluid-filled cyst (not cancer) or a solid mass (which may or may not be cancer). The material removed in a needle biopsy goes to a lab to be checked for cancer cells.

Surgical biopsy. The doctor cuts out part or all of a lump or suspicious area. A pathologist examines the tissue under a microscope to check for cancer cells.

When a woman needs a biopsy, these are some questions she may want to ask her doctor:

- What type of biopsy will I have? Why?
- How long will the biopsy or aspiration take? Will I be awake? Will it hurt?
- How soon will I know the results?
- If I do have cancer, who will talk with me about treatment? When?

When Cancer Is Found

When cancer is present, the pathologist can tell what kind of cancer it is (whether it began in a duct or a lobule) and whether it is invasive (has invaded nearby tissues in the breast).

Special laboratory tests of the tissue help the doctor learn more about the cancer. For example, hormone receptor tests (estrogen and progesterone receptor tests) can show whether the cancer is sensitive to hormones. Positive test results mean hormones help the cancer grow and the cancer is likely to respond to hormone treatment. Other lab tests are sometimes done to help the doctor predict whether the cancer is likely to grow slowly or quickly. If the diagnosis is cancer, the patient may want to ask these questions:

- What kind of breast cancer do I have? Is it invasive?
- What did the hormone receptor test show? What other lab tests were done on the tumor tissue, and what did they show?
- How will this information help the doctor decide what type of treatment or further tests to recommend?

The patient's doctor may refer her to doctors who specialize in treating breast cancer. Treatment generally follows within a few weeks after the diagnosis. The woman will have time to talk with the doctor about her treatment choices, to consider getting a second opinion, and to prepare herself and her loved ones.

Treatment

Many treatment methods are used for breast cancer. Treatment depends on the size and location of the tumor in the breast, the results of lab tests (including hormone receptor tests) done on the cancer cells, and the stage (or extent) of the disease. The patient may have further tests to find out whether the cancer has spread. For example, the doctor usually orders x-rays of the lungs and blood tests to check the liver. In some cases, the doctor orders other special exams of the liver, lungs, or bones because breast cancer tends to spread to these areas. To develop a treatment plan to fit each patient's needs, the doctor also considers the woman's age and general health as well as her feelings about the treatment options. Women with breast cancer are likely to have many questions and concerns about their treatment plan. They want to learn all they can about their disease and their treatment choices so they can take an active part in decisions about their medical care. The doctor is the best person to answer questions about how the disease can be treated, how successful the treatment is expected to be, and how much it is likely to cost. Also, the patient may want to talk with her doctor about taking part in a research study of new treatment methods.

Many patients find it helps to make a list of questions before seeing the doctor. Taking notes during talks with the doctor can make it easier to remember what the doctor says. Some patients also find that it helps to have a family member or friend with them when they see the doctor, to take part in the discussion, to take notes, or just to listen.

Here are some questions a woman may want to ask the doctor before treatment begins:

- What is the stage of the disease?
- What are my treatment choices? Which do you recommend for me? Why?
- What are the expected benefits of each kind of treatment?
- What are the risks and possible side effects of each treatment?

- Would a clinical trial be appropriate for me?

Most patients also want to know how they will look after treatment and whether they will have to change their normal activities. There's a lot to learn about breast cancer and its treatment. Patients should not feel that they need to ask all their questions or understand all the answers at once. They will have many other chances to ask the doctor to explain things that are not clear and to ask for more information.

Planning Treatment

Before starting treatment, the patient might want a second opinion about the diagnosis and the treatment plan. It may take a week or two to arrange to see another doctor. Studies show that a brief delay between biopsy and treatment does not make breast cancer treatment less effective. There are a number of ways to find a doctor for a second opinion:

- The patient's doctor may refer her to a specialist. Specialists who treat breast cancer include surgeons. medical oncologists, and radiation oncologists. Sometimes these doctors work together at cancer centers or special centers for breast diseases.

- The Cancer Information Service, at 1-800-4-CANCER, can tell callers about cancer centers and other NCI-supported programs in their area.

- Patients can get the names of specialists from their local medical society, a nearby hospital, or a medical school.

Methods of Treatment

Methods of treatment for breast cancer are local or systemic. Local treatments are used to remove, destroy, or control the cancer cells in a specific area. Surgery and radiation therapy are local treatments. Systemic treatments are used to destroy or control cancer cells all over the body. Chemotherapy and hormone therapy are systemic treatments. A patient may have just one form of treatment or a combination, depending on her needs.

Surgery. Surgery is the most common treatment for breast cancer. An operation to remove the breast is a mastectomy; an operation to remove the cancer but not the breast is called breast-sparing surgery. Breast-sparing surgery usually is followed by radiation therapy to destroy any cancer cells that may remain in the area. In most cases, the surgeon also removes lymph nodes under the arm to help determine the stage of the disease.

Several types of surgery are used to treat breast cancer. The doctor can explain them in detail and can tell the patient how each will affect her appearance.

- In lumpectomy, the surgeon removes just the breast lump and a margin of normal tissue around it. In partial (segmental) mastectomy, the tumor, some of the normal breast tissue around it, and the lining over the chest muscles below the tumor are removed.

- In total (simple) mastectomy, the whole breast is removed.

- In modified radical mastectomy, the surgeon removes the breast, some of the lymph nodes under the arm, and the lining over the chest muscles. Sometimes the smaller of the two chest muscles is removed.

- In radical mastectomy (also called Halsted radical mastectomy), the surgeon removes the breast, the chest muscles, all of the lymph nodes under the arm, and some additional fat and skin. This operation was the standard one for many years, but it is seldom used now.

These are some questions a woman may want to ask her doctor before surgery:

- What kind of operation will it be?
- How will I feel after the operation? If I have pain, how will you help me?
- Where will the scars be? What will they look like?
- If I decide to have plastic surgery to rebuild my breast, when can that be done?

- Will I have to do special exercises?
- When can I get back to my normal activities?

Radiation Therapy or Radiotherapy. In radiation therapy (also called radiotherapy), high-energy rays are used to damage cancer cells and stop them from growing. Radiation may come from a machine outside the body (external radiation). It can also come from radioactive materials placed directly in the breast in thin plastic tubes (implant radiation). Sometimes the patient receives both kinds of radiation therapy.

Patients go to the hospital or clinic each day for external radiation treatments. When this therapy follows breast-sparing surgery, the treatments are given 5 days a week for 5 to 6 weeks. At the end of that time, an extra "boost" of radiation is often given to the tumor site. The boost may be either external or internal (using an implant). Patients stay in the hospital for a short time for implant radiation.

Before radiation therapy, a patient may want to ask her doctor these questions:

- Why do I need this treatment?
- When will the treatments begin? When will they end?
- How will I feel during therapy?
- What can I do to take care of myself during therapy?
- Can I continue my normal activities?
- How will my breast look afterward?

Chemotherapy. Chemotherapy is the use of drugs to kill cancer cells. In most cases, breast cancer is treated with a combination of drugs. The drugs may be given by mouth or by injection into a vein or muscle. Either way, chemotherapy is a systemic therapy, because the drugs enter the bloodstream and travel through the body. Chemotherapy is given in cycles: a treatment period followed by a recovery period, then another treatment, and so on. Most patients have chemotherapy in an outpatient part of the hospital, at the doctor's office, or at home. Depending on which drugs are given and the woman's general health, however, she may need to stay in the hospital during her treatment.

Hormone Therapy. Hormone therapy is used to keep cancer cells from getting the hormones they need to grow. This treatment may include the use of drugs that change the way hormones work or surgery to remove the ovaries, which make hormones. Like chemotherapy, hormone therapy is a systemic treatment; it can affect cancer cells throughout the body.

Patients may want to ask these questions about chemotherapy or hormone therapy:

- Why do I need this treatment?
- If I need hormone treatment, which would be better for me—drugs or an operation?
- What drugs will I be taking? What will they do?
- Will I have side effects? What can I do about them?
- How long will I be on this treatment?

Treatment Choices

Treatment decisions are complex. These decisions are affected by the experience and judgment of the doctor and by the desires of the patient. The choices available for a particular patient depend on a number of factors. These include the woman's age and menopausal status, her general health, the location of the tumor, and the size of her breast. Certain features of the cancer cells (such as whether they depend on hormones and how fast they are growing) are also considered. The most important factor is the stage of the cancer. The stage is based on the size of the tumor and whether the cancer is only in the breast or has spread to other organs. On the following pages are brief descriptions of the treatments most often used for each stage of breast cancer.

Carcinoma *in situ*. Carcinoma *in situ* is very early breast cancer. Cancer cells are found in only a few layers of cells. Because it has not invaded nearby tissue, the cancer is called non-invasive.

Patients with carcinoma *in situ* may have breast-sparing surgery or mastectomy. The type of surgery depends mainly on whether the cancer developed in a duct (intraductal carcinoma) or a lobule (lobular carcinoma *in situ*). In some cases, some of the underarm lymph nodes are removed, and radiation therapy may be recommended.

Stage I and Stage II Cancers. Stage I and stage II are early stages of breast cancer, but the cancer has invaded nearby tissue.

Stage I means that cancer cells have not spread beyond the breast and the tumor is no more than about an inch across. Stage II means that cancer has spread to underarm lymph nodes and/or the tumor in the breast is 1 to 2 inches across.

Women with early stage breast cancer may have breast-sparing surgery followed by radiation therapy as their primary local treatment, or they may have a mastectomy. These treatments are equally effective. With either approach, lymph nodes under the arm generally are removed.

In addition, some women with stage I and most with stage II breast cancer have chemotherapy and/or hormone therapy in addition to their local treatment. This added treatment is called adjuvant therapy. It is given to prevent the cancer from recurring by killing undetected cancer cells that may have begun to spread.

Stage III Cancers. Stage III means the tumor in the breast is more than 2 inches across, the cancer is more extensive in the underarm lymph nodes, or it has spread to other lymph node areas or to other tissues near the breast. This stage of breast cancer is also called locally advanced cancer.

Patients with stage III breast cancer usually have both local treatment to remove or destroy the cancer in the breast and systemic treatment to stop the disease from spreading. The local treatment may be mastectomy and/or radiation therapy to the breast; also, the lymph nodes under the arm may be removed or treated with radiation. The systemic treatment may be chemotherapy, hormone therapy, or both; it may be given before local treatment.

Stage IV or Metastatic Cancers. Stage IV is metastatic cancer. The cancer has spread from the breast to other organs of the body.

Women who have stage IV breast cancer receive chemotherapy and/or hormone therapy to shrink the tumor or destroy cancer cells. They may have surgery or radiation therapy to control the cancer in the breast. Radiation may also be useful to control tumors in other parts of the body.

Recurrent Cancers. Recurrent cancer means the disease has reappeared, even though the patient's treatment has seemed to be successful. Even when a tumor in the breast seems to have been completely removed or destroyed, the disease sometimes returns because

Breast Cancer

undetected cancer cells have remained in the area after treatment or because the disease had already spread before treatment.

When the cancer returns only in the breast area, it is called a local recurrence. If the disease returns in another part of the body, it is called metastatic breast cancer (or distant disease). The doctor will choose one type of treatment or a combination of treatments to meet the woman's needs.

Side Effects of Treatment

It is hard to limit the effects of cancer treatment so that only cancer cells are removed or destroyed. Because healthy cells and tissues may also be damaged, treatment often causes unpleasant side effects.

Removal of a breast can cause a woman's weight to shift and be out of balance, especially if she has large breasts. This imbalance can also cause discomfort in a woman's neck and back. Also, the skin in the breast area may be tight, and the muscles of the arm and shoulder may feel stiff. After a mastectomy, a few women have some permanent loss of strength in these muscles, but for most women, reduced strength and limited movement are temporary. The doctor, nurse, or physical therapist can recommend exercises to help a woman regain movement and strength in her arm and shoulder.

Because nerves are injured or cut during surgery, a woman may have numbness and tingling in the chest, underarm, shoulder, and arm. These feelings usually go away within a few weeks or months, but some numbness may be permanent.

Removing the lymph nodes under the arm slows the flow of lymph. In some women, lymph builds up in the arm and hand and causes swelling (lymphedema). Also, it is harder for the body to fight infection after the lymph nodes have been removed, so women need to protect the arm and hand on the treated side from injury, for the rest of their lives. They should ask the doctor how to handle any cuts, scratches, insect bites, or other injuries that may occur. Also, they should contact the doctor if an infection develops. The radiation oncologist will explain the possible side effects of radiation therapy for breast cancer, including uncommon side effects that may involve the heart, lungs, and ribs, before treatment begins. Some of the more common side effects are described here. For example, during radiation therapy, patients may become very tired, especially in the later weeks of treatment. Resting is important, but doctors usually advise their patients to try to stay reasonably active. Women should match their activities to their energy level. It's common for radiation to cause the skin in the treated area to become red and dry, tender, and itchy. Toward the end of treatment, the skin may become moist and "weepy." This area should be exposed to the air as much as possible. Patients should avoid wearing a bra or clothes that may rub; loose-fitting cotton clothes are usually best. Good skin care is important at this time, but patients should not use any lotions or creams without the doctor's advice, and they should not use any deodorant on the treated side. The effects of radiation therapy on the skin are temporary. The area will heal when the treatment is over.

Following radiation therapy, the treated breast may be firmer. Also, it may be larger (due to fluid buildup) or smaller (because of tissue changes) than before. For some women, the breast skin is more sensitive after radiation treatment; for others, it is less sensitive.

The side effects of chemotherapy depend mainly on the drugs the patient receives. In addition, as with other types of treatment, side effects vary from person to person. In general, anticancer drugs affect rapidly dividing cells. These include blood cells, which fight infection, cause the blood to clot, and carry oxygen to all parts of the body. When blood cells are affected by anticancer drugs, patients are more likely to get infections, bruise or bleed easily, and have less energy. Cells in hair follicles and cells that line the digestive tract also divide rapidly. As a result of chemotherapy, patients may lose their hair and may have other side effects, such as loss of appetite, nausea, vomiting, or mouth sores. These generally are short-term side effects. They gradually go away during the recovery part of the chemotherapy cycle or after the treatment is over.

Some anticancer drugs can damage the ovaries. If the ovaries fail to produce hormones, the woman may have symptoms of menopause, such as hot flashes and vaginal dryness. Her periods may become irregular or may stop, and she may not be able to become pregnant. In women over the age of 35 or 40, some of these effects, such as infertility, are likely to be permanent.

Hormone therapy can cause a number of side effects. They depend largely on the specific drug or type of treatment, and they vary from patient to patient. Tamoxifen is the most commonly used form of hormone treatment. This drug blocks the body's use of estrogen but does not stop estrogen production. Its side effects usually are not severe. Tamoxifen may cause hot flashes, vaginal discharge or irritation, and irregular periods, but it does not cause menopause or infertility. Young women whose ovaries are removed to deprive the cancer cells of estrogen experience menopause immediately. The side effects they have, including hot flashes and vaginal dryness, are likely to be more severe than those of natural menopause.

Loss of appetite can be a problem for cancer patients. They may not feel hungry when they are uncomfortable or tired. Also, some of the common side effects of cancer treatment, such as nausea and vomiting, can make it hard to eat. The doctor may suggest medicine to help with these problems because good nutrition is important. Patients who eat well often feel better and have more energy. They also may be better able to withstand the side effects of their treatment. Eating well means getting enough calories and protein to help prevent weight loss, regain strength, and rebuild normal tissues. Many patients find that eating several small meals and snacks during the day works better than trying to have three large meals.

The side effects of cancer treatment are different for each person, and they may even be different from one treatment to the next. Doctors try to plan treatment to keep problems to a minimum. They also watch patients carefully so they can help with any problems that occur. Doctors, nurses, and dietitians can explain the side effects of treatment and can suggest ways to deal with them. The NCI booklets *Radiation Therapy and You*, *Chemotherapy and You*, and *Eating Hints* have helpful information about cancer treatment and coping with side effects. *(These pamphlets are reproduced in* <u>The New Cancer Sourcebook</u>. *See the index or the table of contents for page references.)*

After Treatment

Rehabilitation is a very important part of breast cancer treatment. The medical team makes every effort to help women return to their normal activities as soon as possible. Recovery will be different for each woman, depending on the extent of the disease, the treatment she had, and other factors.

Exercising after surgery can help a woman regain motion and strength in her arm and shoulder. It can also reduce pain and stiffness in her neck and back. Carefully planned exercises should be started as soon as the doctor says the woman is ready, often within a day or so after surgery. Exercising begins slowly and gently and can even be done in bed. Gradually, exercising can be more active, and regular exercise should become part of a woman's normal routine. (Women who have a mastectomy and immediate breast reconstruction—plastic surgery to rebuild the breast—need special exercises, which the doctor or nurse will explain.)

Lymphedema after surgery can be reduced or prevented with certain exercises and by resting with the arm propped up on a pillow. If lymphedema occurs later on, the doctor may suggest exercises and other ways to deal with this problem. For example, some women with lymphedema wear an elastic sleeve or use an elastic cuff to improve lymph circulation. The doctor also may suggest other approaches, such as medication or use of a machine that compresses the arm.

After a mastectomy, some women decide to wear a breast form (prosthesis). Others prefer to have breast reconstruction, either at the same time as the mastectomy or later on. Each plan has its pros and cons, and what is right for one woman may not be right for another. What's important is that nearly every woman treated for breast cancer has a choice. It may be helpful to talk with a plastic surgeon before the mastectomy, but reconstruction is still possible years later.

Various procedures are used to reconstruct the breast. Some use artificial implants; others use tissue moved from another part of the woman's body. The woman should ask the plastic surgeon to explain the risks and benefits of each type of reconstruction. The Cancer Information Service can suggest sources of printed information about breast reconstruction and can tell callers about breast cancer support groups. Members of such groups are often willing to share their personal experiences with breast reconstruction.

Followup Care

Regular follow-up exams are very important after breast cancer treatment. The doctor will continue to check the woman closely to be sure that the cancer has not returned. Regular checkups usually include exams of the chest, underarm, and neck. From time to time, the woman has a complete physical exam, blood and urine tests, mammography, and a chest x-ray. The doctor sometimes orders scans (special x-rays) and other exams as well. A woman who has had cancer in one breast has a higher-than-average risk of developing cancer in her other breast. She should continue to practice breast self-examination, checking both the treated area and her other breast each month. She should report any changes to her doctor right away.

Also, a woman who has had breast cancer should tell her doctor about other physical problems if they come up, such as pain, loss of appetite or weight, changes in menstrual periods, or blurred vision. She should also report dizziness, coughing or hoarseness, headaches, or digestive problems that seem unusual or that don't go away. These symptoms may be a sign that the cancer has returned, but they can also be signs of many other problems. Only the doctor can tell for sure.

Living With Cancer

The diagnosis of breast cancer can change a woman's life and the lives of those close to her. These changes can be hard to handle. It's common for the woman and her family and friends to have many different and sometimes confusing emotions.

At times, patients and their loved ones may be frightened, angry, or depressed. These are normal reactions when people face a serious health problem. Most people find it helps to share their thoughts and feelings with loved ones. Sharing can help everyone feel more at ease and can open the way for others to show their concern and offer their support.

Sometimes women who have had breast cancer are afraid that changes to their body will affect not only how they look but how other people feel about them. They may be concerned that breast cancer and its treatment will affect their sexual relationships. Most couples find that talking about these concerns helps them find ways to express their love during and after treatment.

Cancer patients may worry about holding a job, caring for their families, or starting new relationships. Worries about tests, treatments, hospital stays, and medical bills are also common. Doctors, nurses, or other members of the health care team can help calm fears and ease confusion about treatment, working, or daily activities. Also, meeting with a nurse, social worker, counselor, or member of the clergy can be helpful to patients who want to talk about their feelings or discuss their concerns about the future or about personal relationships.

Members of the health care team can provide information and suggest other resources. In addition, the public library is a good source of books and articles on living with cancer.

Support for Breast Cancer Patients

Finding the strength to deal with the changes brought about by breast cancer can be easier for patients and those who love them when they have appropriate support services.

Many patients find it helpful to talk with others who are facing problems like theirs. Cancer patients often get together in self-help and support groups, where they can share what they have learned about cancer and its treatment and about coping with the disease. Often a social worker or nurse meets with the group.

The American Cancer Society's Reach to Recovery program offers special help for breast cancer patients. Trained volunteers, who have had breast cancer themselves, visit patients at the doctor's request and lend emotional support to women before and after treatment. They share their experiences with breast cancer treatment and rehabilitation and with breast reconstruction.

Friends and relatives, especially those who have had cancer themselves, can also be very supportive. It's important to keep in mind, however, that each patient is different. Treatments and ways of dealing with cancer that work for one person may not be right for another even if they both have the same kind of cancer. It is always a good idea to discuss the advice of friends and family members with the doctor.

Often, the doctor's staff or a social worker at the hospital or clinic can suggest local and national groups that can help with emotional support, rehabilitation, financial aid, transportation, or home care. Information about programs and services for breast cancer patients and their families is also available through the Cancer Information Service.

What the Future Holds

Researchers are finding better ways to detect and treat breast cancer, and the chances of recovery keep improving. Still, it is natural for patients to be concerned about their future.

Sometimes patients use statistics they have heard to try to figure out their own chances of being cured. It is important to remember, however, that statistics are averages based on large numbers of patients. They can't be used to predict what will happen to a particular woman because no two cancer patients are alike. The doctor who takes care of the patient and knows her medical history is in the best position to talk with her about the chance of recovery (prognosis). Women should feel free to ask the doctor about their prognosis, but they should keep in mind that not even the doctor knows exactly what will happen. Doctors often talk about surviving cancer, or they may use the term remission. Doctors use these terms because, although many breast cancer patients are cured, the disease can recur.

The Promise of Cancer Research

Scientists at hospitals and medical centers all across the country are studying breast cancer. They are trying to learn more about what causes this disease and how to prevent it. They are also looking for better ways to diagnose and treat it.

Causes and Prevention

Each year, more than 180,000 women in the United States find out they have breast cancer. Although this disease also occurs in about 1,000 men in this country each year, more than 99 percent of all breast cancer patients are women.

Scientists do not know what causes breast cancer, and doctors can seldom explain why one person gets this disease and another doesn't. It is clear, however, that breast cancer is not caused by bumping, bruising, or touching the breast. And this disease is not contagious; no one can "catch" breast cancer from another person.

By studying large numbers of women all over the world, researchers have found certain risk factors that increase a woman's chance of developing breast cancer. Women with these risk factors have a higher-than-average chance of getting this disease. However, studies also show that most women with these risk factors do not get breast cancer. And many women who get breast cancer have none of the risk factors we know about. The following are some of the known risk factors for this disease:

- **Age.** The risk of breast cancer increases as a woman gets older. Most breast cancers occur in women over the age of 50; the risk is especially high for women over 60. This disease is uncommon in women under the age of 35.

- **Family history.** The risk of getting breast cancer increases for a woman whose mother, sister, or daughter has had the disease. The woman's risk increases more if her relative's cancer developed before menopause or if it affected both breasts.

- **Personal history.** Women who have had breast cancer face an increased risk of getting breast cancer again. About 15 percent of women treated for breast cancer get a second breast cancer later on. The risk is greater for women who have had lobular carcinoma in situ.

Other risk factors for breast cancer include starting to menstruate at an early age (before 12) or having a late menopause (after 55). The risk is also greater in women who had their first child after the age of 30 and those who never had children. Because these factors are all related to a woman's natural hormones, many people are concerned about medicines that contain hormones (either for birth control or as estrogen replacement therapy to control symptoms of menopause), especially if women take them for many years. At this time, no one knows for sure whether taking hormones affects the risk of breast cancer.

Scientists hope to find the answer to this important question by studying a large number of women taking part in hormone-related research.

Research suggests that a person's diet may affect the chances of getting some types of cancer. Breast cancer appears to be more likely to develop in women whose diet is high in fat. Older women who are overweight also seem to have a greater risk. Although the possible link between diet and breast cancer is still under study, some scientists believe that choosing a low-fat diet, eating well-balanced meals with plenty of fruits and vegetables, and maintaining ideal weight can lower a woman's risk.

Some studies suggest a slightly higher risk of breast cancer among women who drink alcohol. The risk appears to go up with the amount of alcohol consumed, so women who drink should do so only in moderation.

Many women are concerned about benign breast conditions. For most women, the ordinary "lumpiness" they feel in their breasts does not increase their risk of breast cancer. However, women who have had breast biopsies that show certain benign changes in breast tissues, such as atypical hyperplasia, do have an increased risk of breast cancer.

Women who are at high risk for breast cancer are taking part in a study of the drug tamoxifen, which is often used to treat breast cancer patients. This nationwide study is designed to help doctors learn whether tamoxifen can prevent breast cancer in these women. The Cancer Information Service can provide information about this study.

Detection

When breast cancer is found early, patients have more treatment choices and their chance of complete recovery is better. Because breast cancer often occurs in women with none of the known risk factors, it is important for all women to ask their doctor about mammography, breast exams by a doctor or nurse, and breast self-examination.

Unfortunately, the tests we have now cannot reveal every breast cancer at an early stage. Scientists are trying to find better ways to detect breast cancers when they are very small. For example, they are looking for ways to make mammography more accurate. They are also exploring new techniques to produce detailed pictures of the tissues in the breast.

In addition, researchers are studying tumor markers, substances that may be present in abnormal amounts in the blood or urine of a woman who has breast cancer. Several markers have been studied, and this research is continuing. At this time, however, no blood or urine test is reliable enough to reveal early breast cancer.

Treatment

Researchers also are looking for more effective ways to treat breast cancer. In addition, they are exploring ways to reduce the side effects of treatment and improve the quality of patients' lives. When laboratory research shows that a new treatment method has promise, cancer patients receive the treatment in clinical trials. These trials are designed to answer scientific questions and to find out whether the new approach is both safe and effective. Often, clinical trials compare a new treatment with a standard approach. Patients who take part in clinical trials make an important contribution to medical science and may have the first chance to benefit from improved treatment methods.

Trials to study new treatments for patients with all stages of breast cancer are under way. Researchers are testing new treatment methods, new doses and treatment schedules, and new ways of combining treatments. They are working with various anticancer drugs and drug combinations as well as several types of hormone therapy. They are also exploring new ways to combine chemotherapy with hormone therapy and radiation therapy. Some trials include biological therapy, treatment with substances that boost the immune system's response to cancer.

In a number of trials, doctors are trying to learn whether very high doses of anticancer drugs are more effective than the usual doses in destroying breast cancer cells. Because these higher doses seriously damage the patient's bone marrow, where blood cells are formed, researchers are testing ways to replace the bone marrow or to help it recover. These new approaches (bone marrow transplantation, peripheral stem cell support, and the use of colony-stimulating factors) are described in the glossary at the end of this book.

The possible benefits and risks of treatment studies are examined in the section on Clinical Trials. Those who are interested in taking part in a trial should discuss this option with their doctor.

One way to learn about clinical trials is through PDQ, a computerized resource developed by NCI. PDQ contains information about cancer treatment and an up-to-date list of trials all over the country. Doctors can obtain an access code and use a personal computer to get PDQ information. Also, the Cancer Information Service can provide PDQ information to doctors, patients, and the public.

Chapter 3

Early Stage Breast Cancer

Introduction

Carcinoma of the breast is the most common malignancy in women in the United States. As a cause of cancer death in women, breast cancer is exceeded only by lung cancer. The incidence of breast cancer has been rising steadily over the past decade. In the 1990s, more than 1.5 million women will be newly diagnosed with this disease; nearly 30 percent of these women will ultimately die from breast cancer. The increased number of reported cases may be partially attributable to their detection following more widespread use of screening mammography. Most of the increase has been in patients with smaller primary breast tumors. In 1982, approximately 12,000 women were diagnosed with tumors less than 2 centimeters in diameter and negative axillary lymph nodes. That number had risen to 32,000 by 1986. For those patients with axillary node positive breast cancer, there has been a less dramatic increase in tumors less than 2 centimeters (3,000 in 1982 to 7,000 in 1986) while there has been a decrease in the number presenting with tumors larger than 5 centimeters. Of the 150,000 new patients diagnosed with invasive breast cancer in 1990, 75 to 80 percent will have clinical Stage I or II disease, and approximately two-thirds of these will have no involvement of the axillary lymph nodes.

NIH Consensus Statement, NIH Consensus Development Conference, June 18-21, 1990, Vol 8, Number 6.

Traditional concepts through most of the 20th century held that breast cancer was a local/regional disease best managed by radical mastectomy. Over the past 20 years, there have been several clinical trials worldwide that have compared less extensive breast resections with standard radical mastectomy. These have included comparisons of total mastectomy (with and without radiation therapy and axillary lymph node dissection) with radical mastectomy. Subsequent studies have compared different approaches to breast conservation surgery with total mastectomy. At present, breast conservation therapy is used in a minority of patients. The appropriate use of breast conservation involves a variety of clinical, biological, and psychosocial factors that merit public debate.

Adjuvant therapy has become the standard of care for the majority of breast cancer patients with axillary lymph node involvement. More recently, several randomized trials from North America and Europe have shown an improvement in disease-free survival for node negative breast cancer patients receiving adjuvant therapy.

Absence of metastasis to the axillary lymph nodes has traditionally been considered a favorable biologic condition for patients with invasive breast cancer. However, all patients with node negative breast cancer are at risk for disease recurrence. Intensive efforts to define an individual patient's risk of recurrence have produced a plethora of potential prognostic factors, from patient characteristics to histologic, biochemical, and molecular characteristics of the tumor. The importance of these various prognostic factors has been the subject of controversy.

To evaluate the developing results of breast conservation, adjuvant therapy of node negative breast cancer, and clinical prognostic factors, the National Cancer Institute and the Office of Medical Applications of Research of the National Institutes of Health convened a Consensus Development Conference on the Treatment of Early-Stage Breast Cancer on June 18-21, 1990.

After 2 days of presentations by experts and discussion by the audience, a consensus panel drawn from specialists and generalists from the medical profession and related scientific disciplines, clinical investigators, methodologists, and public representatives considered the evidence and agreed on answers to the following key questions:

- What are the roles of mastectomy versus breast conservation in the treatment of early-stage breast cancer?

- What are the optimal techniques for breast conservation?

- What is the role of adjuvant therapy for patients with node negative breast cancer?

- How should prognostic factors be used in the management of node negative breast cancer?

- What are the directions for future research?

What Are the Roles of Mastectomy Versus Breast Conservation in the Treatment of Early-Stage Breast Cancer?

- Breast conservation treatment is an appropriate method of primary therapy for the majority of women with Stage I and II breast cancer and is preferable because it provides survival equivalent to total mastectomy and axillary dissection while preserving the breast.

In general, primary therapy for Stage I and II breast cancer consists of breast conservation treatment or total mastectomy. Breast conservation treatment is defined as excision of the primary tumor and adjacent breast tissue (this procedure is also referred to as lumpectomy, segmental mastectomy, or partial mastectomy), followed by radiation therapy. Total mastectomy is an appropriate primary therapy when breast conservation treatment is not indicated or selected. Both surgical therapies are accompanied by axillary dissection, which provides important prognostic information.

Prospective randomized trials comparing breast conservation treatment with total mastectomy with maximum follow-up of 17 years have demonstrated equivalent results as measured by overall patient survival. Important considerations in the choice of therapy for women with Stage I and II breast cancer include clinical criteria, factors that influence local/regional tumor control, cosmetic results, psychosocial issues and patient preferences for treatment method.

Patient Selection

In the selection of women for breast conservation treatment or mastectomy, certain women are not candidates for breast conservation treatment:

- Women with multicentric breast malignancies, including those with gross multifocal disease or diffuse microcalcifications detected by mammography.

- Patients for whom breast conservation treatment would produce an unacceptable cosmetic result. Examples include women whose tumors are large relative to breast size and those with certain collagen vascular diseases.

- Certain pathologic and clinical factors may influence treatment selection because of their potentially adverse impact on local recurrence after breast conservation treatment. Controversy exists about these factors, examples of which include the presence of extensive intraductal carcinoma within and adjacent to the primary tumor, extensive lymphatic involvement and young age (under 35-39 years). Prospective studies comparing primary therapies have included women whose primary tumors were usually less than or equal to 4 centimeters in diameter.

Local Control

Local control is a major goal of breast conservation treatment. The incidence of local recurrence is low in appropriately selected patients receiving optimal breast conservation treatment. Results of randomized trials have suggested that the use of adjuvant chemotherapy or hormonal therapy further reduces the rate of local recurrence after breast conservation treatment.

Cosmetic Result

A goal of primary breast cancer treatment is to produce the best cosmetic result consistent with achievement of local/regional control. In clinical trials, the majority of patients achieve good to excellent cosmetic results after breast conservation treatment. Optimal long-term results require integration of careful surgical excision and precise radiotherapy techniques. When mastectomy is indicated or selected, breast reconstruction should be considered to improve the cosmetic result.

Psychosocial Factors

Women should be educated about treatment choices and clinical trial options in order to make an informed decision in consultation with their physicians. A variety of factors have a major influence on a woman's choice of primary therapy. These include logistic and emotional considerations, personal financial issues, and proximity and access to appropriate medical care. A woman's body image and her beliefs and concerns may determine her preference for breast conservation treatment or mastectomy.

What Are the Optimal Techniques for Breast Conservation?

The objective of breast conservation is to obtain a high probability of local control, with survival at least equivalent to that obtained with total mastectomy and axillary dissection, combined with maximal cosmetic results and maintenance of normal function. The most widely used treatment that achieves these goals is the combination of local surgical excision, axillary dissection, and postoperative radiation therapy. Although this treatment approach produces survival equivalent to mastectomy, with a high likelihood of good cosmesis and function, further studies are required to refine certain treatment details. The following recommendations define the treatment details deemed optimal based on the available data.

Surgical Recommendations

- The diagnosis should be established by fine needle aspiration cytology, limited incisional biopsy (particularly for larger lesions), or definitive wide local excision.

- The type and placement of incisions can influence greatly the quality of cosmesis. Arcuate incisions with thick flaps, centered over the lesion, are superior to radial incisions, particularly for upper quadrant lesions. Routine excision of overlying skin is unnecessary except for very superficial lesions. Careful hemostasis is essential and drains are rarely necessary. In most instances, suture reapproximation of mammary tissue should be avoided.

- It is appropriate to excise the primary lesion with a normal tissue margin of approximately 1 centimeter. The intent of this recommendation is to achieve a surgical margin that is grossly and microscopically uninvolved with tumor. To obtain adequate pathological evaluation, it is necessary to mark the specimen for proper orientation and to ink the resection margins. When margins are grossly involved with tumor, further resection is indicated. Available data are inadequate to determine whether focal microscopic involvement of a margin increases the risk of local failure after optimal radiation therapy. Because cosmetic result is related to the amount of tissue excised, unnecessarily wide margins (> 2 cm) should be avoided.

- Because nodal status is the most important available prognostic factor, a Level I-II axillary dissection should be routine both for staging and for prevention of axillary recurrence. Separate incisions should usually be employed for the primary tumor excision and the axillary dissection to enhance functional and cosmetic results.

Radiation Therapy Recommendations

- Mega-voltage radiation therapy to the whole breast to a dose of 4,500 to 5,000 cGy (180 to 200 cGy per fraction) should be routinely used. Boost irradiation has been used in the majority of trials to date. However, the precise indications are not well defined. In the reported trials, the patients with focal microscopic involvement of margins have been treated with boost irradiation or mastectomy. There are no current data to support lesser treatment for these patients. Treatment planning should be done to minimize radiation exposure to lung and heart and to achieve uniform dosage to the treatment volume. Boost irradiation should be delivered by electron beam or implantation to doses of 1,000 to 1,500 cGy. Higher doses produce a greater incidence of cosmetic impairment.

- If a Level I-II axillary dissection has been performed, axillary nodal irradiation is not routinely indicated.

- No data indicate any increased risk of secondary malignancies or contralateral breast cancers resulting from breast irradiation. Longer follow-up of this population is necessary to resolve this issue fully.

- Although local control can be obtained in some patients with local excision alone, no subgroups have been identified in which radiation therapy can be avoided.

- In patients receiving adjuvant chemotherapy, no precise recommendations regarding the sequence and timing of radiation therapy and chemotherapy can be made.

- A small percentage of patients will develop a local recurrence following breast conservation therapy. Total mastectomy is effective salvage therapy for a substantial percentage of these patients. This is in contrast to the poor prognosis associated with local chest wall recurrence following mastectomy. Hence, in patients treated with breast conservation, long-term careful breast monitoring with physical examination and mammography is essential for early detection and treatment of local recurrence.

What Is the Role of Adjuvant Therapy for Patients with Node Negative Breast Cancer?

- The majority of patients with node negative breast cancer are cured by breast conservation treatment or total mastectomy and axillary dissection.

- There is clear evidence that the rate of local and distant recurrence is decreased by both adjuvant combination cytotoxic chemotherapy and by adjuvant tamoxifen.

Data from the 10 randomized trials reviewed show that adjuvant systemic therapy reduces the rate of recurrence by approximately one-third, with a broad range. For example, among a group of women with a 30 percent risk of recurrence adjuvant therapy would decrease that risk to about 20 percent. The role of these treatments in improving overall survival and other important parameters such as quality of life is still being defined.

The completed studies are not large enough, nor is the follow-up long enough, to estimate with acceptable precision the interactions between menopausal status or steroid receptor positivity and the effects of adjuvant therapy in node negative patients. Although all patient subsets experience lower rates of recurrence, relatively few patients with estrogen receptor-negative tumors have been included in tamoxifen studies. At the present time, reduced mortality is seen in nearly all trials but is not statistically significant in most. However, the rate of death in node negative patients is low, so a clinically important reduction in mortality may require a long follow-up to achieve statistical significance. For chemotherapy, more benefit is seen in trials in which antimetabolites (methotrexate and 5-fluorouracil) are administered intravenously than in trials in which they are given orally. For tamoxifen, studies using the drug for more than 2 years (usually 5 years) seem to result in greater reductions in the rate of recurrence than studies using shorter courses.

In prospective studies in node negative patients, tamoxifen reduces the clinical incidence of contralateral primary breast cancer. The overall benefits from tamoxifen in post-menopausal patients clearly outweigh any toxicities currently described. In pre-menopausal patients, the administration of tamoxifen may cause endocrine abnormalities with uncertain long-term consequences. Although there does not appear to be an excess number of cases of endometrial carcinoma in tamoxifen-treated pre-menopausal patients, the follow-up durations are too short to predict confidently whether or not this will occur. The influence of tamoxifen on the developing fetus is unknown. There are no data now available concerning the effects of combination chemotherapy plus tamoxifen in node negative patients. Trials addressing this issue are under way.

Recommendations

- The many unanswered questions in the adjuvant systemic

treatment of node negative breast cancer make it imperative that all patients who are candidates for clinical trials be offered the opportunity to participate.

The following recommendations apply only to patients who are not candidates for such trials or who refuse participation.

- All node negative patients should be made aware of the benefits and risks of adjuvant systemic therapy. The decision to use adjuvant treatment should follow a thorough discussion with the patient regarding the likely risk of recurrence without adjuvant therapy, the expected reduction in risk with adjuvant therapy, toxicities of therapy and its impact on quality of life. Some degrees of improvement may be so small that they are outweighed by the disadvantages of therapy.

- Adjuvant therapy should consist of either combination chemotherapy or tamoxifen (20 mg/day for at least 2 years).

No completed studies have directly compared tamoxifen with chemotherapy (with or without tamoxifen) in node negative patients. Tamoxifen has less acute toxicity than chemotherapy, but no statement is possible regarding chronic toxicity or comparative efficacy. The results of current and future trials concerning the safety of tamoxifen in pre-menopausal patients must be followed carefully.

How Should Prognostic Factors Be Used in the Management of Node Negative Breast Cancer?

Prognostic factors should be used to provide an estimate of risk of recurrence in women with early-stage breast cancer. Although no individual patient can be assured that she has no risk of recurrence, the majority of women will be cured with local/regional therapy.

A useful prognostic factor has the following characteristics:

- It has significant and independent predictive value that has been validated by clinical testing.

- Its determination must be feasible, reproducible, and widely available, with quality control.

- It must be readily interpretable by the clinician and have therapeutic implications.

Prognostic Factors

Tumor Size. There is a strong correlation between tumor size and risk of recurrence. Even within the T_1 category, there is variation in risk. Tumors less than or equal to 1 centimeter have a particularly good prognosis (e.g., < 10 percent recurrence at 10 years) relative to tumors 1.1 to 2 centimeters in diameter. In general, the risk of recurrence increases with increasing tumor size. The pathologist should perform a careful gross examination with documentation of tumor size.

Estrogen and Progesterone Receptor Status. Patients with receptor-positive tumors have a better prognosis than those with receptor-negative tumors. However, the difference in recurrence rates at 5 years is only 8 to 10 percent.

Nuclear Grade. This is a well-documented factor. When determined by experienced pathologists, it discriminates favorable and unfavorable prognostic groups. High nuclear grade is associated with a higher rate of recurrence. Nuclear grade is not currently part of the routine pathologic review of breast cancer specimens. The pathology community should adopt a uniform grading system and routinely use this discriminant.

Histologic Type. Several well-characterized histologic subtypes impart a favorable prognosis, although they are a distinct minority of all breast cancer cases. These subtypes include tubular, colloid (mucinous), and papillary types.

Proliferative Rate. Measurements of cellular proliferation in breast cancer specimens using a variety of techniques have shown a strong correlation with outcome. DNA flow cytometry has become widely available for the determination of S-phase fraction as well as ploidy status. S-phase fraction does correlate with prognosis, but ploidy status alone is not of clear prognostic value. Up to 25 percent of specimens are not evaluable by flow cytometry because of methodologic problems. Because of the complexity of the technology, quality control is especially critical. Although S-phase fraction has been shown to be an independent prognostic factor in some studies, its clinical value is being defined.

Other Factors. High levels of the protease cathepsin D are associated with an unfavorable prognosis. Data for HER-2/neu, epidermal growth factor receptor, and stress-response (heat shock) proteins are of interest, but further investigation is required before reaching any conclusions about their clinical value.

Estimating Individual Risk

Currently available prognostic factors are associated with a broad range of risk of recurrence in node negative breast cancer patients. There are extremes of high and low risk where it is possible to make recommendations about adjuvant systemic therapy. For example, outside of clinical trials, it is reasonable not to treat patients with tumors less than or equal to 1 cm in diameter because their chance of recurrence is less than 10 percent at 10 years. With increasing tumor diameter, other prognostic factors should be weighed in the decision to use adjuvant treatment. A major goal is the development of risk profile systems with sufficient accuracy and reproducibility to estimate prognosis in the individual patient.

What Are the Directions for Future Research?

To refine existing prognostic factors by:

- reassessing the predictive value of the tumor categories in the American Joint Committee on Cancer Tumor/ Node/ Metastasis staging system.

- standardizing a nuclear grading system.

- exploring relationships between individual prognostic factors and resistance to systemic therapy.

- developing and using new and existing tissue and clinical data banks for the study of prognostic factors.

To develop risk factor profile systems with sufficient accuracy and reproducibility to allow identification of subgroups that:

- may be treated with surgical excision without irradiation.
- do not require axillary node dissection.
- do not require systemic therapy.

To improve systemic chemotherapy regimens through:

- investigation of dose intensity, timing, and duration.
- introduction of new agents.
- evaluation of chemotherapy and hormonal therapy combinations.
- evaluation of preoperative (neo-adjuvant) chemotherapy.

To gather further data concerning tamoxifen, including:

- safety of prolonged use in premenopausal patients.
- optimal duration of therapy.
- efficacy in Patients with steroid receptor-negative tumors.
- comparison and combination with gonadotropin-releasing hormone agonists.

To assess quality-of-life parameters in future clinical trials.

To determine the optimal margin for local primary excision in the presence and absence of extensive intraductal cancer.

To determine whether boost irradiation is required in patients with pathologically negative margins and whether boost irradiation produces a high probability of local control in patients with microscopic involvement of margins.

To determine the optimal sequence and timing for radiation therapy and systemic adjuvant therapy.

Early Stage Breast Cancer

Conclusions and Recommendations

Breast conservation treatment is an appropriate method of primary therapy for the majority of women with Stage I and II breast cancer and is preferable because it provides survival equivalent to total mastectomy and axillary dissection while preserving the breast.

The recommended technique for breast conservation treatment includes:

- local excision of primary tumor with clear margins
- Level I-II axillary node dissection
- breast irradiation to 4,500-5,000 cGy with or without a boost

The many unanswered questions in the adjuvant systemic treatment of node negative breast cancer make it imperative that all patients who are candidates for clinical trials be offered the opportunity to participate.

The majority of patients with node negative breast cancer are cured by breast conservation treatment or total mastectomy and axillary dissection.

The rate of local and distant recurrence following local therapy for node negative breast cancer is decreased by both adjuvant combination cytotoxic chemotherapy and by adjuvant tamoxifen. The decision to use adjuvant treatment should follow a thorough discussion with the patient regarding the likely risk of recurrence without adjuvant therapy, the expected reduction in risk with adjuvant therapy, toxicities of therapy, and its impact on quality of life.

While all node negative patients have some risk for recurrence, patients with tumors less than or equal to 1 centimeter have an excellent prognosis and do not require adjuvant systemic therapy outside of clinical trials.

Chapter 4

Inflammatory Breast Cancer

Inflammatory breast cancer is an uncommon type of breast cancer that accounts for 1 to 4 percent of all cases of the disease. The average age of patients with this disease is 52 years, and approximately one-third of patients are premenopausal.

Inflammatory breast cancer invades the lymph vessels of the skin of the breast and blocks these vessels, resulting in a reddened appearance of the skin. Symptoms may include a lump in the breast, feelings of breast enlargement or thickness, pain in the breast or nipple, warmth, redness, and swelling. Ridges may appear on the skin, or the breast may appear pitted, like the skin of an orange (called "peau d'orange"). A small number of women with this type of cancer will have a discharge from the nipple, and the nipple may also be pulled back. A surgical biopsy is usually done to confirm the diagnosis.

Inflammatory breast cancer is generally rapid-growing and often the breast cancer cells metastasize (spread) to other sites. At present, some combination of chemotherapy, surgery, radiation therapy, and hormone therapy is used to treat this disease. Chemotherapy is often given first to help control the disease in the breast and to treat cancer cells that may have spread throughout the body. Surgery is generally done after chemotherapy to remove the breast (mastectomy). Radiation therapy to the tumor and nearby lymph nodes can help control the local growth of the cancer and is done either before or after surgery.

NCI Cancerfax 208/6000062.

Researchers are studying the effectiveness of high doses of anticancer drugs in improving the outcome of patients with inflammatory breast cancer. Some patients whose cancer cells depend on the female hormone estrogen for their growth may receive hormone therapy, which interferes with estrogen's effect, following chemotherapy.

Patients with inflammatory breast cancer should consider participating in one of the clinical treatment trials (research studies) in progress to improve treatment for this disease.

Chapter 5

Cancer of the Cervix

This chapter is about cancer of the cervix. If you have more questions about this disease, call the Cancer Information Service to talk with someone. The staff can talk with you in English or Spanish.

The number is 1-800-422-6237 (1-800-4-CANCER). The call is free.

Este folleto es acerca de cancer del cuello del utero. Usted podria tener preguntas acerca de esta enfermedad. Llame al Servicio de Informacion sobre el Cancer para hablar con alguien acerca del cancer del cuello del utero. Este servicio tiene personal que habla espanol.

El numero a llamar es el 1-800-422-6237 (1-800-4-CANCER). La llamada es gratis.

The Cervix

The cervix is the lower, narrow part of the uterus (womb). The uterus, a hollow, pear-shaped organ, is located in a woman's lower abdomen, between the bladder and the rectum. The cervix forms a canal that opens into the vagina, which leads to the outside of the body.

NIH 95-2047; NCI Cancerfax 208/00103

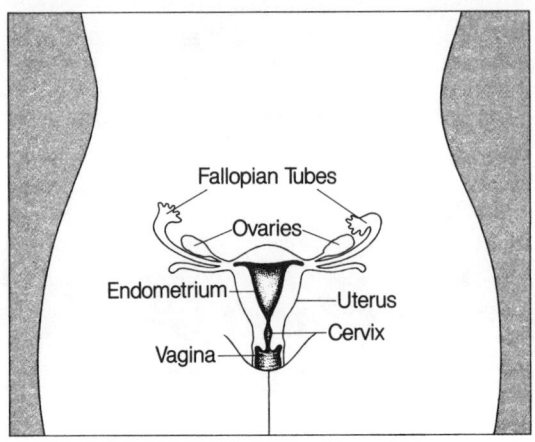

Figure 5.1. *This picture shows the uterus, cervix, and other parts of a woman's reproductive system.*

What Is Cancer?

Cancer is a group of more than 100 different diseases. They all affect the body's basic unit, the cell. Cancer occurs when cells become abnormal and divide without control or order.

Like all other organs of the body, the cervix is made up of many types of cells. Normally, cells divide to produce more cells only when the body needs them. This orderly process helps keep us healthy.

If cells keep dividing when new cells are not needed, a mass of tissue forms. This mass of extra tissue, called a growth or tumor, can be benign or malignant.

- Benign tumors are not cancer. They can usually be removed and, in most cases, they do not come back. Most important, cells from benign tumors do not spread to other parts of the body. Benign tumors are not a threat to life. Polyps, cysts, and genital warts are types of benign growths of the cervix.

- Malignant tumors are cancer. Cancer cells can invade and damage tissues and organs near the tumor. Cancer cells also can break away from a malignant tumor and enter the lymphatic system or the bloodstream. This is how cancer of the

Cancer of the Cervix

cervix can spread to other parts of the body, such as nearby lymph nodes, the rectum, the bladder, the bones of the spine, and the lungs. The spread of cancer is called metastasis.

Cancer of the cervix also may be called cervical cancer. Like most cancers, it is named for the part of the body in which it begins. Cancer of the cervix is different from cancer that begins in other parts of the uterus and requires different treatment. The most common type of cancer of the uterus begins in the endometrium, the lining of this organ. Endometrial cancer is discussed in the chapter on cancer of the Uterus. Cancers of the cervix also are named for the type of cell in which they begin. Most cervical cancers are squamous cell carcinomas. Squamous cells are thin, flat cells that form the surface of the cervix.

When cancer spreads to another part of the body, the new tumor has the same kind of abnormal cells and the same name as the original (primary) cancer. For example, if cervical cancer spreads to the bones, the cancer cells in the bones are cervical cancer cells. The disease is called metastatic cervical cancer (it is not bone cancer).

Pre-cancerous Conditions and Cancer of the Cervix

Cells on the surface of the cervix sometimes appear abnormal but not cancerous. Scientists believe that some abnormal changes in cells on the cervix are the first step in a series of slow changes that can lead to cancer years later. That is, some abnormal changes are pre-cancerous; they may become cancerous with time.

Over the years, doctors have used different terms to refer to abnormal changes in the cells on the surface of the cervix. One term now used is squamous intraepithelial lesion (SIL). (The word lesion refers to an area of abnormal tissue; intraepithelial means that the abnormal cells are present only in the surface layer of cells.) Changes in these cells can be divided into two categories:

- Low-grade SIL refers to early changes in the size, shape, and number of cells that form the surface of the cervix. Some low-grade lesions go away on their own. However, with time, others may grow larger or become more abnormal, forming a high-grade lesion. Pre-cancerous low-grade lesions also may be called mild dysplasia or cervical intraepithelial neoplasia 1 (CIN 1). Such early changes in the cervix most often occur in women between the ages of 25 and 35 but can appear in other age groups as well.

- High-grade SIL means there are a large number of pre-cancerous cells; they look very different from normal cells. Like low-grade SIL, these pre-cancerous changes involve only cells on the surface of the cervix. The cells will not become cancerous and invade deeper layers of the cervix for many months, perhaps years. High-grade lesions also may be called moderate or severe dysplasia, CIN 2 or 3, or carcinoma in situ. They develop most often in women between the ages of 30 and 40 but can occur at other ages as well.

If abnormal cells spread deeper into the cervix or to other tissues or organs, the disease is then called cervical cancer, or invasive cervical cancer. It occurs most often in women over the age of 40.

Early Detection

If all women had pelvic exams and Pap tests regularly, most pre-cancerous conditions would be detected and treated before cancer develops. That way, most invasive cancers could be prevented. Any invasive cancer that does occur would likely be found at an early, curable stage.

In a pelvic exam, the doctor checks the uterus, vagina, ovaries, fallopian tubes, bladder, and rectum. The doctor feels these organs for any abnormality in their shape or size. A speculum is used to widen the vagina so that the doctor can see the upper part of the vagina and the cervix.

The Pap test is a simple, painless test to detect abnormal cells in and around the cervix. A woman should have this test when she is not menstruating; the best time is between 10 and 20 days after the first day of her menstrual period. For about 2 days before a Pap test, she should avoid douching or using spermicidal foams, creams, or jellies or vaginal medicines (except as directed by a physician), which may wash away or hide any abnormal cells.

A Pap test can be done in a doctor's office or a health clinic. A wooden scraper (spatula) and/or a small brush is used to collect a sample of cells from the cervix and upper vagina. The cells are placed

Cancer of the Cervix

on a glass slide and sent to a medical laboratory to be checked for abnormal changes.

The way of describing Pap test results is changing. The newest method is the Bethesda System. Changes are described as low-grade or high-grade SIL. Many doctors believe that the Bethesda System provides more useful information than an older system, which uses numbers ranging from class 1 to class 5. (In class 1, the cells in the sample are normal, while class 5 refers to invasive cancer.) Women should ask their doctor to explain the system used for their Pap test.

Women should have regular checkups, including a pelvic exam and a Pap test, if they are or have been sexually active or if they are age 18 or older. Those who are at increased risk of developing cancer of the cervix should be especially careful to follow their doctor's advice about checkups. Women who have had a hysterectomy (surgery to remove the uterus, including the cervix) should ask their doctor's advice about having pelvic exams and Pap tests.

Symptoms

Pre-cancerous changes of the cervix usually do not cause pain. In fact, they generally do not cause any symptoms and are not detected unless a woman has a pelvic exam and a Pap test.

Symptoms usually do not appear until abnormal cervical cells become cancerous and invade nearby tissue. When this happens, the most common symptom is abnormal bleeding. Bleeding may start and stop between regular menstrual periods, or it may occur after sexual intercourse, douching, or a pelvic exam. Menstrual bleeding may last longer and be heavier than usual. Bleeding after menopause also may be a symptom of cervical cancer. Increased vaginal discharge is another symptom of cervical cancer.

These symptoms may be caused by cancer or by other health problems. Only a doctor can tell for sure. It is important for a woman to see her doctor if she is having any of these symptoms.

Diagnosis

The pelvic exam and Pap test allow the doctor to detect abnormal changes in the cervix. If these exams show that an infection is present, the doctor treats the infection and then repeats the Pap test at a later time. If the exam or Pap test suggests something other than an infection, the doctor may repeat the Pap test and do other tests to find out what the problem is.

Colposcopy is a widely used method to check the cervix for abnormal areas. The doctor applies a vinegar-like solution to the cervix and then uses an instrument much like a microscope (called a colposcope) to look closely at the cervix. The doctor may then coat the cervix with an iodine solution (a procedure called the Schiller test). Healthy cells turn brown; abnormal cells turn white or yellow. These procedures may be done in the doctor's office.

The doctor may remove a small amount of cervical tissue for examination by a pathologist. This procedure is called a biopsy. In one type of biopsy, the doctor uses an instrument to pinch off small pieces of cervical tissue. Another method used to do a biopsy is called loop electro-surgical excision procedure (LEEP). In this procedure, the doctor uses an electric wire loop to slice off a thin, round piece of tissue. These types of biopsies may be done in the doctor's office using local anesthesia. The doctor also may want to check inside the opening of the cervix, an area that cannot be seen during colposcopy. In a procedure called endocervical curettage (ECC), the doctor uses a curette (a small, spoon-shaped instrument) to scrape tissue from inside the cervical opening.

These procedures for removing tissue may cause some bleeding or other discharge. However, healing usually occurs quickly. Women also often experience some pain similar to menstrual cramping, which can be relieved with medicine.

These tests may not show for sure whether the abnormal cells are present only on the surface of the cervix. In that case, the doctor will then remove a larger, cone-shaped sample of tissue. This procedure, called conization or cone biopsy, allows the pathologist to see whether the abnormal cells have invaded tissue beneath the surface of the cervix. Conization also may be used as treatment for a pre-cancerous lesion if the entire abnormal area can be removed. This procedure requires either local or general anesthesia and may be done in the doctor's office or in the hospital.

In a few cases, it may not be clear whether an abnormal Pap test or a woman's symptoms are caused by problems in the cervix or in the endometrium (the lining of the uterus). In this situation, the doctor may do dilatation and curettage (D and C). The doctor stretches the cervical opening and uses a curette to scrape tissue from the lining of the uterus as well as from the cervical canal. Like conization, this procedure requires local or general anesthesia and may be done in the doctor's office or in the hospital.

Treating Pre-cancerous Conditions

Treatment for a pre-cancerous lesion of the cervix depends on a number of factors. These factors include whether the lesion is low or high grade, whether the woman wants to have children in the future, the woman's age and general health, and the preference of the woman and her doctor. A woman with a low-grade lesion may not need further treatment, especially if the abnormal area was completely removed during biopsy, but she should have a Pap test and pelvic exam regularly. When a pre-cancerous lesion requires treatment, the doctor may use cryosurgery (freezing), cauterization (burning, also called diathermy), or laser surgery to destroy the abnormal area without harming nearby healthy tissue. The doctor also can remove the abnormal tissue by LEEP or conization. Treatment for pre-cancerous lesions may cause cramping or other pain, bleeding, or a watery discharge.

In some cases, a woman may have a hysterectomy, particularly if abnormal cells are found inside the opening of the cervix. This surgery is more likely to be done when the woman does not want to have children in the future.

Treating Cancer of the Cervix

Staging

The choice of treatment for cervical cancer depends on the location and size of the tumor, the stage (extent) of the disease, the woman's age and general health, and other factors. Staging is a careful attempt to find out whether the cancer has spread and, if so, what parts of the body are affected. Blood and urine tests usually are done. The doctor also may do a thorough pelvic exam in the operating room with the patient under anesthesia. During this exam, the doctor may do procedures called cystoscopy and proctosigmoidoscopy. In cystoscopy, the doctor looks inside the bladder with a thin, lighted instrument. Proctosigmoidoscopy is a procedure in which a lighted instrument is used to check the rectum and the lower part of the large intestine. Because cervical cancer may spread to the bladder, rectum, lymph nodes, or lungs, the doctor also may order x-rays or tests to check these areas. For example, the woman may have a series of x-rays of the kidneys and bladder, called an intravenous pyelogram. The doctor also may check the intestines and rectum using a barium enema. To look for lymph nodes that may be enlarged because they contain cancer cells, the doctor may order a CT or CAT scan, a series of x-rays put together by a computer to make detailed pictures of areas inside the body. Other procedures that may be used to check organs inside the body are ultrasonography and MRI.

Your doctor needs to know the stage of your disease to plan treatment. The following stages are used for cancer of the cervix:

- **Stage 0 or carcinoma in situ.** Stage 0 cervical cancer is very early cancer. The cancer is found only in the first layer of cells of the lining of the cervix.

- **Stage I.** Cancer is found throughout the cervix, but has not spread nearby.
- **Stage IA.** A very small amount of cancer is found deeper in the tissues of the cervix.
- **Stage IB.** A larger amount of cancer is in the tissues of the cervix.

- **Stage II.** Cancer has spread to nearby areas, but is still inside the pelvic area.
- **Stage IIA.** Cancer has spread beyond the cervix to the upper two-thirds of the vagina.
- **Stage IIB.** Cancer has spread to the tissue around the cervix.

- **Stage III.** Cancer has spread throughout the pelvic area. Cancer cells may have spread to the bones of the pelvis and/or gone into the lower part of the vagina. The cells also may have spread to block the tubes that connect the kidneys to the bladder (the ureters).

- **Stage IV.** Cancer has spread to other parts of the body.
- **Stage IVA.** Cancer has spread to the bladder or rectum (organs close to the cervix).
- **Stage IVB.** Cancer has spread to faraway organs such as the lungs.

- **Recurrent.** Recurrent disease means that the cancer has come back (recurred) after it has been treated. It may come back in the cervix or in another place.

Getting a Second Opinion

Before starting treatment, the patient may want a second pathologist to review the diagnosis and another specialist to review the treatment plan. Some insurance companies require a second opinion; others may cover a second opinion if the patient requests it. It may take a week or two to arrange for a second opinion. This short delay will not reduce the chance that treatment will be successful. There are a number of ways to find a doctor who can give a second opinion:

- The woman's doctor may be able to suggest pathologists and specialists to consult.
- The Cancer Information Service, at 1-800-4-CANCER, can tell callers about treatment facilities, including cancer centers and other programs supported by the National Cancer Institute.
- Women can get the names of specialists from their local medical society, a nearby hospital, or a medical school.

Preparing for Treatment

Most women with cervical cancer want to learn all they can about their disease and treatment choices so they can take an active part in decisions about their medical care. Doctors and others on the medical team can help women learn what they need to know.

Here are some questions a woman with cervical cancer may want to ask the doctor before her treatment begins:

- What is the stage (extent) of my disease?
- What are my treatment choices? Which do you recommend for me? Why?
- What are the chances that the treatment will be successful?
- Would a clinical trial be appropriate for me?
- What are the risks and possible side effects of each treatment?
- How long will treatment last?

- Will it affect my normal activities?
- What is the treatment likely to cost?
- What is likely to happen without treatment?
- How often will I need to have checkups?

When a person is diagnosed with cancer, shock and stress are natural reactions. These feelings may make it difficult for patients to think of everything they want to ask the doctor. Often it helps to make a list of questions. Also, to help remember what the doctor says, patients may take notes or ask whether they may use a tape recorder. Some people also want to have a family member or friend with them when they talk to the doctor-to take part in the discussion, to take notes, or just to listen.

Patients should not feel they need to ask all their questions or remember all the answers at one time. They will have other chances to ask the doctor to explain things and to get more information.

Methods of Treatment

Most often, treatment for cervical cancer involves surgery and radiation therapy. Sometimes, chemotherapy or biological therapy is used. Patients are often treated by a team of specialists. The team may include gynecologic oncologists and radiation oncologists. The doctors may decide to use one treatment method or a combination of methods. Some patients take part in a clinical trial (research study) using new treatment methods. Such studies are designed to improve cancer treatment.

Surgery. Surgery is local therapy to remove abnormal tissue in or near the cervix. If the cancer is only on the surface of the cervix, the doctor may destroy the cancerous cells in ways similar to the methods used to treat pre-cancerous lesions. If the disease has invaded deeper layers of the cervix but has not spread beyond the cervix, the doctor may perform an operation to remove the tumor but leave the uterus and the ovaries. In other cases, however, a woman may need to have a hysterectomy or may choose to have this surgery, especially if she is not planning to have children in the future. In this procedure, the doctor removes the entire uterus, including the cervix; sometimes the ovaries and fallopian tubes also are removed. In addition, the doctor may remove lymph nodes near the uterus to learn whether the cancer has

Cancer of the Cervix

spread to these organs. Here are some questions a woman may want to ask the doctor before surgery:

- What kind of operation will it be?
- How will I feel after the operation?
- If I have pain, how will you help me?
- When can I return to my normal activities?
- How will this treatment affect my sex life?

Radiation therapy. Radiation therapy (also called radiotherapy) uses high-energy rays to damage cancer cells and stop them from growing. Like surgery, radiation therapy is local therapy; the radiation can affect cancer cells only in the treated area. The radiation may come from a large machine (external radiation) or from radioactive materials placed directly into the cervix (implant radiation). Some patients receive both types of radiation therapy.

A woman receiving external radiation therapy goes to the hospital or clinic each day for treatment. Usually treatments are given 5 days a week for 5 to 6 weeks. At the end of that time, the tumor site very often gets an extra "boost" of radiation.

For internal or implant radiation, a capsule containing radioactive material is placed directly in the cervix. The implant puts cancer-killing rays close to the tumor while sparing most of the healthy tissue around it. It is usually left in place for 1 to 3 days, and the treatment may be repeated several times over the course of 1 to 2 weeks. The patient stays in the hospital while the implants are in place.

The National Cancer Institute booklet *Radiation Therapy and You* contains more information about this form of treatment. *(This pamphlet is reproduced in The New Cancer Sourcebook. See the index or the table of contents for the page reference.)* Here are some questions a woman may want to ask the doctor before radiation therapy:

- What is the goal of this treatment?
- How will the radiation be given?
- How long will treatment last?
- How will I feel during therapy?
- What can I do to take care of myself during therapy?
- Can I continue my normal activities?
- How will this treatment affect my sex life?

Chemotherapy. Chemotherapy is the use of drugs to kill cancer cells. It is most often used when cervical cancer has spread to other parts of the body. The doctor may use just one drug or a combination of drugs.

Anticancer drugs used to treat cervical cancer may be given by injection into a vein or by mouth. Either way, chemotherapy is systemic treatment, meaning that the drugs flow through the body in the bloodstream.

Chemotherapy is given in cycles: a treatment period followed by a recovery period, then another treatment period, and so on. Most patients have chemotherapy as an outpatient (at the hospital, at the doctor's office, or at home). Depending on which drugs are given and the woman's general health, however, she may need to stay in the hospital during her treatment. Here are some questions a woman may want to ask the doctor before chemotherapy begins:

- What is the goal of this treatment?
- What drugs will I be taking?
- Do the drugs have side effects? What can I do about them?
- How long will I need to take this treatment?

Biological therapy. Biological therapy is treatment using substances to improve the way the body's immune system fights disease. It may be used to treat cancer that has spread from the cervix to other parts of the body. Interferon is the most common form of biological therapy for this disease; it may be used in combination with chemotherapy. Most patients who receive interferon are treated as outpatients.

Clinical Trials. Some women with cervical cancer are treated in clinical trials. Doctors conduct clinical trials to find out whether a new treatment is both safe and effective and to answer scientific questions. Patients who take part in these studies may be the first to receive treatments that have shown promise in laboratory research. Some patients may receive the new treatment while others receive the standard approach. In this way, doctors can compare different therapies. Patients who take part in a trial make an important contribution to medical science and may have the first chance to benefit from improved treatment methods. Clinical trials of new treatments for cervical cancer are under way. Doctors are studying new types and

Cancer of the Cervix

schedules of radiation therapy. They also are looking for new drugs, drug combinations, and ways to combine various types of treatment.

Women with cervical cancer may want to read the National Cancer Institute booklet called *What Are Clinical Trials All About?*, which explains the possible benefits and risks of treatment studies. *(This pamphlet is reproduced in The New Cancer Sourcebook. See the index or the table of contents for the page reference.)* Those who are interested in taking part in a trial should talk with their doctor.

One way to learn about clinical trials is through PDQ, a computerized resource developed by the National Cancer Institute. This resource contains information about cancer treatment and about clinical trials in progress all over the country. The Cancer Information Service can provide PDQ information to doctors, patients, and the public.

Treatment by Stage

Treatments for cancer of the cervix depend on the stage of your disease, the size of your tumor, your age, your overall condition, and your desire to have children.

Treatment for cervical cancer during pregnancy may be delayed depending on the stage of your cancer and how many months you have been pregnant.

You may receive treatment that is considered standard based on its effectiveness in a number of patients in past studies, or you may choose to go into a clinical trial. Not all patients are cured with standard therapy and some standard treatments may have more side effects than are desired. For these reasons, clinical trials are designed to find better ways to treat cancer patients and are based on the most up-to-date information. Clinical trials are going on in most parts of the country for most stages of cancer of the cervix. If you wish to know more about clinical trials, call the Cancer Information Service at 1-800-4-CANCER (1-800-422-6237).

Stage 0 Cervical Cancer. Your treatment may be one of the following:

- Diathermy.
- Laser surgery.
- Conization.
- Cryosurgery.

- Surgery to remove the cancer, cervix, and uterus (total abdominal or vaginal hysterectomy) for those women who cannot or no longer want to have children.

Stage I Cervical Cancer. Treatment may be one of the following depending on how deep the tumor cells have invaded into the normal tissue:

For stage IA cancer:

- Surgery to remove the cancer, uterus, and cervix (total abdominal hysterectomy). The ovaries may also be taken out (bilateral salpingo-oophorectomy), but are usually not removed in younger women.
- Conization.
- For tumors with deeper invasion (3-5 mm): Surgery to remove the cancer, the uterus and cervix, ovaries and part of the vagina (radical hysterectomy) along with the lymph nodes in the pelvic area (lymph node dissection).
- Internal radiation therapy.

For stage IB cancer:

- Internal and external radiation therapy combined.
- Surgery to remove the cancer, the uterus and cervix, ovaries, and part of the vagina (radical hysterectomy) along with the lymph nodes in the pelvic area (lymph node dissection).
- Radical hysterectomy and lymph node dissection followed by radiation therapy.

Stage II Cervical Cancer. Your treatment may be one of the following:

For stage IIA cancer:

- Internal and external radiation therapy combined.
- Surgery to remove the cancer, the uterus and cervix, ovaries, and part of the vagina (radical hysterectomy) along with the lymph nodes in the pelvic area (lymph node dissection).

Cancer of the Cervix

- Radical hysterectomy and lymph node dissection followed by radiation therapy.

For stage IIB cancer:

- Internal and external radiation therapy combined.
- Clinical trials of radiation therapy plus chemotherapy.
- Clinical trials of surgery to determine your stage of disease with removal of lymph nodes thought to contain cancer followed by external radiation therapy.

Stage III Cervical Cancer. Your treatment may be one of the following:

- Internal and external radiation therapy combined.
- Radiation therapy plus chemotherapy.
- Clinical trials of surgery to determine your stage of disease with removal of lymph nodes thought to contain cancer followed by external radiation therapy.

Stage IV Cervical Cancer. Your treatment may be one of the following:

For stage IVA cancer:

- Internal and external radiation therapy combined.
- Surgery to take out the lower colon, rectum, or bladder (depending on where the cancer has spread) along with the cervix, uterus, and vagina (exenteration).
- Radiation therapy plus chemotherapy.
- Clinical trials of surgery to determine your stage of disease followed by external radiation therapy.

For stage IVB cancer:

- Radiation therapy to relieve symptoms such as pain.
- Systemic chemotherapy.

Recurrent Cervical Cancer. If the cancer has come back (recurred) in the pelvis, your treatment may be one of the following:

- Surgery to take out the lower colon, rectum, or bladder (depending on where the cancer has spread) along with the cervix, uterus, and vagina (exenteration).
- Radiation therapy and chemotherapy.

If the cancer has come back outside of the pelvis, you may choose to go into a clinical trial of systemic chemotherapy.

Side Effects of Treatment

It is hard to limit the effects of therapy so that only cancer cells are removed or destroyed. Because treatment also damages healthy cells and tissues, it often causes unpleasant side effects.

The side effects of cancer treatment depend mainly on the type and extent of the treatment. Also, each patient reacts differently. Doctors and nurses can explain the possible side effects of treatment, and they can help relieve symptoms that may occur during and after treatment. It is important to let the doctor know if any side effects occur. The booklets *Radiation Therapy and You* and *Chemotherapy and You* also have helpful information about cancer treatment and coping with side effects. *(These pamphlets are reproduced in The New Cancer Sourcebook. See the index or the table of contents for page references.)*

Surgery. Methods for removing or destroying small cancers on the surface of the cervix are similar to those used to treat pre-cancerous lesions. Treatment may cause cramping or other pain, bleeding, or a watery discharge.

Hysterectomy is major surgery. For a few days after the operation, the woman may have pain in her lower abdomen. The doctor can order medicine to control the pain. A woman may have difficulty emptying her bladder and may need to have a catheter inserted into the bladder to drain the urine for a few days after surgery. She also may have trouble having normal bowel movements. For a period of time after the surgery, the woman's activities should be limited to allow healing to take place. Normal activities, including sexual intercourse, usually can be resumed in 4 to 8 weeks.

Cancer of the Cervix

Women who have had their uterus removed no longer have menstrual periods. However, sexual desire and the ability to have intercourse usually are not affected by hysterectomy. On the other hand, many women have an emotionally difficult time after this surgery. A woman's view of her own sexuality may change, and she may feel an emotional loss because she is no longer able to have children. An understanding partner is important at this time. Women may want to discuss these issues with their doctor, nurse, medical social worker, or member of the clergy. They also may find it helpful to read the National Cancer Institute booklet called **Taking Time.** *(This pamphlet is reproduced in <u>The New Cancer Sourcebook</u>. See the index or the table of contents for the page reference.)*

Radiation Therapy. Patients are likely to become very tired during radiation therapy especially in the later weeks of treatment. Resting is important, but doctors usually advise patients to try to stay as active as they can.

With external radiation, it is common to lose hair in the treated area and for the skin to become red, dry, tender, and itchy. There may be permanent darkening or "bronzing" of the skin in the treated area. This area should be exposed to the air when possible but protected from the sun, and patients should avoid wearing clothes that rub the treated area. Patients will be shown how to keep the area clean. They should not use any lotion or cream on their skin without the doctor's advice.

Usually, women are told not to have intercourse during radiation therapy or while an implant is in place. However, most women can have sexual relations within a few weeks after treatment ends. Sometimes, after radiation treatment, the vagina becomes narrower and less flexible, and intercourse may be painful. Patients may be taught how to use a dilator as well as a water-based lubricant to help minimize these problems.

Patients who receive external or internal radiation therapy also may have diarrhea and frequent, uncomfortable urination. The doctor can make suggestions or order medicines to control these problems.

Chemotherapy. The side effects of chemotherapy depend mainly on the drugs and the doses the patient receives. In addition, as with other types of treatment, side effects vary from person to person.

Generally, anticancer drugs affect cells that divide rapidly. These include blood cells, which fight infection, help the blood to clot, or carry oxygen to all parts of the body. When blood cells are affected by anticancer drugs, patients are more likely to get infections, may bruise or bleed easily, and may have less energy. Cells in hair roots and cells that line the digestive tract also divide rapidly. When chemotherapy affects these cells, patients may lose their hair and may have other side effects, such as poor appetite, nausea, vomiting, or mouth sores. The doctor may be able to give medicine to help with side effects. Side effects gradually go away during the recovery periods between treatments or after treatment is over.

Biological Therapy. The side effects caused by biological therapies vary with the type of treatment the patient receives. These treatments may cause flu-like symptoms such as chills, fever, muscle aches, weakness, loss of appetite, nausea, vomiting, and diarrhea. Sometimes patients get a rash, and they may bleed or bruise easily. These problems can be severe, but they gradually go away after the treatment stops.

Nutrition for Cancer Patients

Some patients find it hard to eat well during cancer treatment. They may lose their appetite. In addition to loss of appetite, the common side effects of treatment, such as nausea, vomiting, or mouth sores, can make eating difficult. For some patients, foods taste different. Also, people may not feel like eating when they are uncomfortable or tired.

Eating well during cancer treatment means getting enough calories and protein to help prevent weight loss and regain strength. Patients who eat well often feel better and have more energy. In addition, they may be better able to handle the side effects of treatment.

Doctors, nurses, and dietitians can offer advice for healthy eating during cancer treatment. Patients and their families also may want to read the National Cancer Institute booklet *Eating Hints for Cancer Patients*, which contains many useful suggestions. *(This pamphlet is reproduced in* The New Cancer Sourcebook. *See the index or the table of contents for the page reference.)*

Follow-up Care

Regular follow-up exams, including a pelvic exam, a Pap test, and other laboratory tests, are very important for any woman who has been treated for pre-cancerous changes or for cancer of the cervix. The doctor will do these tests and exams frequently for several years to check for any sign that the condition has returned. Cancer treatment may cause side effects many years later. For this reason, patients should continue to have regular checkups and should report any health problems that appear.

Support for Cancer Patients

Living with a serious disease is not easy. Cancer patients and those who care about them face many problems and challenges. Coping with these problems is often easier when people have helpful information and support services. Several useful booklets, including the National Cancer Institute booklet *Taking Time*, are available from the Cancer Information Service. *(This pamphlet is reproduced in The New Cancer Sourcebook. See the index or the table of contents for the page reference.)*

Cancer patients may worry about holding their job, caring for their family, keeping up with daily activities, or starting a new relationship. Worries about tests, treatments, hospital stays, and medical bills are common. Doctors, nurses, and other members of the health care team can answer questions about treatment, working, or other activities. Also, meeting with a social worker, counselor, or member of the clergy can be helpful to patients who want to talk about their feelings or discuss their concerns.

Friends and relatives can be very supportive. Also, it helps many patients to discuss their concerns with others who have cancer. Cancer patients often get together in support groups, where they can share what they have learned about coping with cancer and the effects of treatment. It is important to keep in mind, however, that each patient is different. Treatments and ways of dealing with cancer that work for one person may not be right for another, even if they both have the same kind of cancer. It is always a good idea to discuss the advice of friends and family members with the doctor.

Often, a social worker at the hospital or clinic can suggest groups that can help with rehabilitation, emotional support, financial aid, transportation, or home care. For example, the American Cancer Society has many services for patients and their families. They also offer many free booklets, including one on sexuality and cancer. Local offices of the American Cancer Society are listed in the white pages of the telephone directory.

In addition, the public library has many books and articles on living with cancer. The Cancer Information Service also has information on local resources.

What the Future Holds

The outlook for women with pre-cancerous changes of the cervix or very early cancer of the cervix is excellent; nearly all patients with these conditions can be cured. Researchers continue to look for new and better ways to treat invasive cervical cancer.

Patients and their families are naturally concerned about what the future holds. Sometimes patients use statistics to try to figure out their chances of being cured. It is important to remember, however, that statistics are averages based on large numbers of patients. They cannot be used to predict what will happen to a particular woman because no two patients are alike; treatments and responses vary greatly. The doctor who takes care of the patient and knows her medical history is in the best position to talk with her about her chance of recovery (prognosis). Doctors often talk about surviving cancer, or they may use the term remission rather than cure. Although many women with cervical cancer recover completely, doctors use these terms because the disease can recur. (The return of cancer is called a recurrence.)

Cause and Prevention

By studying large numbers of women all over the world, researchers have identified certain risk factors that increase the chance that cells in the cervix will become abnormal or cancerous. They believe that, in many cases, cervical cancer develops when two or more risk factors act together.

Cancer of the Cervix

Research has shown that women who began having sexual intercourse before age 18 and women who have had many sexual partners have an increased risk of developing cervical cancer. Women also are at increased risk if their partners began having sexual intercourse at a young age, have had many sexual partners, or were previously married to women who had cervical cancer.

Scientists do not know exactly why the sexual practices of women and their partners affect the risk of developing cervical cancer. However, research suggests that some sexually transmitted viruses can cause cells in the cervix to begin the series of changes that can lead to cancer. Women who have had many sexual partners or whose partners have had many sexual partners may have an increased risk for cervical cancer at least in part because they are more likely to get a sexually transmitted virus.

Scientists are studying the effects of sexually transmitted human papilloma viruses (HPVs). Some sexually transmitted HPVs cause genital warts (condylomata acuminata). In addition, scientists believe that some of these viruses may cause the growth of abnormal cells in the cervix and may play a role in cancer development. They have found that women who have HPV or whose partners have HPV have a higher-than-average risk of developing cervical cancer. However, most women who are infected with HPV do not develop cervical cancer, and the virus is not present in all women who have this disease. For these reasons, scientists believe that other factors act together with HPVs. For example, the genital herpes virus also may play a role. Further research is needed to learn the exact role of these viruses and how they act together with other factors in the development of cervical cancer.

Smoking also increases the risk of cancer of the cervix, although it is not clear exactly how or why. The risk appears to increase with the number of cigarettes a woman smokes each day and with the number of years she has smoked.

Women whose mothers were given the drug diethylstilbestrol (DES) during pregnancy to prevent miscarriage also are at increased risk. (This drug was used for this purpose from about 1940 to 1970.) A rare type of vaginal and cervical cancer has been found in a small number of women whose mothers used DES.

Several reports suggest that women whose immune system is weakened are more likely than others to develop cervical cancer. For example, women who have the human immunodeficiency virus (HIV), which causes AIDS, are at increased risk. Also, organ transplant patients, who receive drugs that suppress the immune system to prevent rejection of the new organ, are more likely than others to develop pre-cancerous lesions.

Some researchers believe that there is an increased risk of cervical cancer in women who use oral contraceptives (the pill). However, scientists have not found that the pill directly causes cancer of the cervix. This relationship is hard to prove because the two main risk factors for cervical cancer–intercourse at an early age and multiple sex partners-may be more common among women who use the pill than among those who do not. Still, oral contraceptive labels warn of this possible risk and advise women who use them to have yearly Pap tests.

Some research has shown that vitamin A may play a role in stopping or preventing cancerous changes in cells like those on the surface of the cervix. Further research with forms of vitamin A may help scientists learn more about preventing cancer of the cervix.

At present, early detection and treatment of pre-cancerous tissue remain the most effective ways of preventing cervical cancer. Women should talk with their doctor about an appropriate schedule of checkups. The doctor's advice will be based on such factors as the women's age, medical history, and risk factors.

Chapter 6

Ovarian Epithelial Cancer

The Ovaries

The ovaries are a pair of female-reproductive organs. They are located in the pelvis, one on each side of the uterus. Each ovary is about the size and shape of an almond. The ovaries have two functions: they produce eggs and female hormones.

Each month, during the menstrual cycle, an egg is released from one ovary. The egg travels from the ovary through a fallopian tube to the uterus.

The ovaries are the main source of female hormones (estrogen and progesterone). These hormones control the development of female body characteristics, such as the breasts, body shape, and body hair. They also regulate the menstrual cycle and pregnancy.

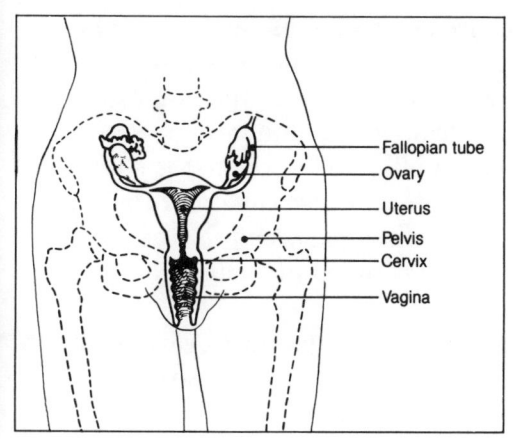

Figure 6.1.

NIH 94-1561; NCI Cancerfax 208/00950.

What Is Cancer?

Cancer is a group of more than 100 different diseases. They all affect the body's basic unit, the cell. Cancer occurs when cells become abnormal and keep dividing and forming more cells without control or order.

Like all other organs of the body, the ovaries are made up of many types of cells. Normally, cells divide to produce more cells only when the body needs them. This orderly process helps keep us healthy.

If cells keep dividing when new cells are not needed, a mass of tissue forms. This mass of extra tissue, called a growth, or tumor, can be benign or malignant:

- Benign tumors are not cancer. They can usually be removed and, in most cases, they do not come back. Most important, cells from benign tumors do not invade nearby tissues and do not spread to other parts of the body. Benign tumors are rarely life threatening.

  In women under age 30, most ovarian growths are benign, fluid-filled sacs called cysts. Cysts may occur during a woman's monthly cycle and often go away without any treatment. If a cyst does not go away, the doctor may suggest removing it, especially if it is causing problems or seems to be changing. In some cases, the doctor may decide to wait and watch for changes with ultrasonography or other tests.

- Malignant tumors are cancer. Cancer cells can invade and damage tissues and organs near the tumor. Also, cancer cells can break away from a malignant tumor in the ovary and spread to other organs in the abdomen and form new tumors. Ovarian cancer spreads most often to the colon, the stomach, and the diaphragm. The cancer cells also can enter the lymphatic system or the bloodstream and spread to other parts of the body. The spread of cancer is called metastasis.

There are several types of ovarian cancer. Most ovarian cancers are epithelial carcinomas, which begin in the lining of the ovary. Other types of ovarian cancer are rare.

When cancer spreads, the new tumor has the same kind of abnormal cells and the same name as the original (primary) tumor. For ex-

Ovarian Epithelial Cancer

ample, ovarian cancer that spreads to the colon is metastatic ovarian cancer. It is not colon cancer, even though the new tumor is in the colon.

Symptoms

Ovarian cancer is hard to find early. Often there are no symptoms in the early stages and, in many cases, the cancer has spread by the time it is found. The cancer may grow for some time before it causes pressure, pain, or other problems. Even when symptoms appear, they may be so vague that they are ignored.

As the tumor grows, the woman may feel swollen or bloated, or may have general discomfort in the lower abdomen. The disease may cause a loss of appetite or a feeling of fullness, even after a light meal. Other symptoms may include gas, indigestion, nausea, and weight loss. A large tumor may press on nearby organs, such as the bowel or bladder, causing diarrhea or constipation, or frequent urination. Less often, bleeding from the vagina is a symptom of ovarian cancer.

Ovarian cancer may cause swelling due to a buildup of fluid in the abdomen (ascites). Fluid also may collect around the lungs, causing shortness of breath.

These symptoms may be caused by cancer or by other, less serious conditions. Only a doctor can tell for sure.

Diagnosis and Staging

To find the cause of any of these symptoms, the doctor asks about the woman's medical history and does a careful physical exam, including a pelvic exam. The doctor feels the vagina, rectum, and lower abdomen for masses or growths. A Pap smear (a common test for cancer of the cervix) is often part of the pelvic exam, but it is not a reliable way to find or diagnose ovarian cancer. The doctor may also order other tests:

- Ultrasonography is the use of high-frequency sound waves. These waves, which cannot be heard by humans, are aimed at the ovaries. The pattern of the echoes they produce creates a picture called a sonogram. Healthy tissues, fluid-filled cysts, and tumors produce different echoes.

- CT (or CAT) scan is a series of x-rays put together by a computer.

- A lower GI series, or barium enema, is a series of x-rays of the colon and rectum. The pictures are taken after the patient is given an enema with a white, chalky solution containing barium. The barium outlines the colon and rectum on the x-ray, which helps the doctor see tumors or other abnormal areas.

- An intravenous pyelogram (IVP) is an x-ray of the kidneys and ureters, taken after the injection of a dye.

Often, the doctor orders a blood test to measure a substance in the blood called CA-125. This substance, called a tumor marker, can be produced by ovarian cancer cells. However, CA-125 is not always present in women with ovarian cancer, and it may be present in women who have benign ovarian conditions. Thus, this blood test cannot be used alone to diagnose cancer.

The only sure way to know if cancer is present is for a pathologist to examine a sample of tissue under the microscope. Removing tissue from the body for this examination is called a biopsy. To obtain the tissue, the surgeon does an operation called a laparotomy. If cancer is suspected, the surgeon removes the entire ovary (oophorectomy). This is important because, if the problem is cancer, cutting through the outer layer of the ovary could allow cancer cells to escape and cause the disease to spread. If cancer is found at this time, the surgeon proceeds with surgery.

During surgery, the surgeon removes nearby lymph nodes, and takes samples of tissue from the diaphragm and other organs in the abdomen. The surgeon also collects fluid from the abdomen. All of these samples are examined by a pathologist to check for cancer cells. This process, called surgical staging, is needed to find out whether the cancer has spread. Staging is important in the planning of follow-up treatment.

Stages of Cancer of the Ovary

Once cancer of the ovary has been found, more tests will be done to find out if the cancer has spread to other parts of the body (staging).

Ovarian Epithelial Cancer

Unless your doctor is sure the cancer has spread from the ovaries to other parts of the body, an operation called a laparotomy will be done to help stage your cancer. Your doctor must cut into your abdomen and carefully look at all the organs to see if they contain cancer. During the operation your doctor will cut out small pieces of tissue (biopsy) so they can be looked at under a microscope to see whether they contain cancer. Usually your doctor will remove the cancer and other organs that contain cancer during the laparotomy. Your doctor needs to know the stage of your disease to plan further treatment. The following stages are used for cancer of the ovary:

- **Stage I**—Cancer is found only in one or both of the ovaries.

- **Stage II**—Cancer is found in one or both ovaries and/or has spread to the uterus, and/or the fallopian tubes (the pathway used by the egg to get from the ovary to the uterus), and/or other body parts within the pelvis.

- **Stage III**—Cancer is found in one or both ovaries and has spread to lymph nodes or to other body parts inside the abdomen, such as the surface of the liver or intestine. (Lymph nodes are small bean-shaped structures that are found throughout the body. They produce and store infection-fighting cells.)

- **Stage IV**—Cancer is found in one or both ovaries and has spread outside the abdomen or has spread to the inside of the liver.

- **Recurrent or refractory**—Recurrent disease means that the cancer has come back (recurred) after it has been treated. It may come back in the ovary that is left or in another place. Refractory disease means the cancer did not respond to the initial therapy.

Treatment

Treatment for ovarian cancer depends on a number of individual factors, including the stage of the disease and the woman's age and general health. Treatment for ovarian cancer is best planned by doctors who specialize in the diagnosis and treatment of this disease.

Most people with cancer want to learn all they can about their disease and their treatment choices so they can take an active part in decisions about their medical care. The doctor is the best person to answer their questions. When talking about treatment choices, the patient may want to ask the doctor about taking part in a research study. Such studies, called clinical trials, are designed to improve cancer treatment.

When a person is diagnosed with cancer, shock and stress are natural reactions. These feelings may make it difficult to think of every question to ask the doctor. Also, patients may find it hard to remember everything the doctor says. But they do not need to ask all their questions or remember all the answers at one time. They will have other chances for the doctor to explain things that are not clear and to ask for more information.

Often it helps to make a list of questions to ask the doctor. Also, to help remember what the doctor says, patients may take notes or ask the doctor whether they may use a tape recorder. Some patients also want to have a family member or friend with them to take part in the discussion, to take notes, or just to listen.

Here are some questions a woman may want to ask her doctor before treatment begins:

- What is the stage of the disease?
- What are my treatment choices? Which do you recommend for me? Why?
- Would a clinical trial be appropriate for me?
- What are the expected benefits of each kind of treatment?
- What are the risks and possible side effects of each treatment?

Getting a Second Opinion

Treatment decisions are complex. Sometimes, it is helpful for patients to have more than one doctor's advice about the diagnosis and treatment plan. There are several ways to find a doctor who can give a second opinion:

Ovarian Epithelial Cancer

- The patient's doctor may refer her to a gynecologic oncologist, who specializes in treating cancer of the female reproductive organs.

- The Cancer Information Service, at 1-800-4-CANCER, can tell callers about treatment facilities, including cancer centers and other programs that are supported by the National Cancer Institute.

- A woman can get the names of specialists from a local medical society or a nearby hospital or medical school.

Methods of Treatment

Ovarian cancer may be treated with surgery, chemotherapy, or radiation therapy. The doctor may use just one method or combine them.

- Surgery is the initial treatment for almost every woman with ovarian cancer.

- Chemotherapy may be used following surgery as adjuvant therapy, to kill any cancer cells that may remain in the body. It may also be used at a later time if there are signs that the cancer has recurred.

- Radiation therapy may be used in a small number of patients to kill cancer cells that may remain in the pelvic area after surgery.

Surgery for ovarian cancer usually involves removal of the ovaries, the uterus, and the fallopian tubes. This operation is called hysterectomy with bilateral salpingo-oophorectomy. (If a woman has a very early, slow-growing tumor and wants to remain able to have a child, the doctor may remove only the affected ovary.) If the cancer has spread, the surgeon removes as much of the cancer as possible in a procedure called tumor debulking. Tumor debulking reduces the amount of cancer to be treated with chemotherapy or radiation therapy.

Here are some questions a woman may want to ask her doctor before surgery:

- What kind of operation will I have?
- How will I feel after the operation?
- If I have pain, how will you help me?
- When can I get back to my normal activities?

Chemotherapy for ovarian cancer often involves a combination of drugs. Anticancer drugs are usually given by injection into a vein or by mouth. Either way, chemotherapy is called systemic therapy because the drugs travel all through the body in the bloodstream.

Chemotherapy is usually given in cycles: a treatment period followed by a recovery period, then another treatment period, and so on. A woman may receive chemotherapy as an outpatient at the hospital, at the doctor's office, or at home. Depending on which drugs are used, how they are given, and her general health, a woman may need to stay in the hospital while receiving chemotherapy.

Doctors are studying another way of giving anticancer drugs called intraperitoneal chemotherapy. In this approach, the drugs are put directly into the abdomen through a catheter. In this way, drugs reach the cancer directly. This treatment is given in the hospital.

Here are some questions a patient may want to ask the doctor before chemotherapy:

- What is the goal of this treatment?
- What drugs will I be taking? What should I expect?
- What can be done to help with side effects?
- How will we know if the drugs are working?
- How often will I receive treatment? How long will I be on the treatment?
- Where will I receive this treatment?
- Can I continue my regular activities?

Radiation therapy (also called radiotherapy) is the use of high-energy rays to damage cancer cells and stop them from growing. Radiation may come from a machine (external radiation) or from radioactive material placed into or near the tumor (internal radiation). Like surgery, radiation therapy is local therapy; it affects cancer cells only in the treated area.

For external radiation therapy, the patient goes to the hospital or clinic each day. Usually, the treatments are given 5 days a week for about 5 weeks.

Some women receive a type of internal radiation called intraperitoneal irradiation. Radioactive liquid is put into the abdomen through a catheter. A short hospital stay may be necessary for this treatment.

Here are some questions the patient may want to ask her doctor before radiation therapy:

- What is the goal of this treatment?
- How will the radiation be given?
- When will the treatments begin? When will they end?
- What can be done to help with side effects?
- How will we know if the radiation therapy is working?
- Can I continue my regular activities?

Clinical Trials

Many patients with ovarian cancer are treated in clinical trials (treatment studies). Doctors conduct clinical trials to find out whether a new treatment is both safe and effective and to answer scientific questions. Patients who take part in these studies may be among the first to receive treatments that have shown promise in laboratory research.

Some patients may receive the new treatment while others receive a standard approach. In this way, doctors can compare different therapies. Patients who take part in a trial make an important contribution to medical science and may have the first chance to benefit from improved treatment methods.

Various trials for ovarian cancer patients are under way. Doctors are studying new drugs, new drug combinations, and different treatment schedules. They also are exploring drugs designed to make radiation therapy more effective, and other ways of combining different types of treatment. Biological therapy, the use of substances that boost the immune system's response to cancer or protect the body from some of the side effects of treatment, is under study in patients with recurrent or advanced ovarian cancer.

A woman with ovarian cancer who is interested in participating in a trial should talk with her doctor. The National Cancer Institute booklet *What Are Clinical Trials All About?* explains the possible benefits and risks of treatment studies. *(This pamphlet is reproduced in The New Cancer Sourcebook. See the index or the table of contents for the page reference.)*

One way to learn about clinical trials is through PDQ, a computerized cancer information resource developed by the National Cancer Institute. PDQ contains information about cancer treatment and about clinical trials in progress all over the country. The Cancer Information Service can provide information from PDQ to doctors, patients, and the public.

Treatment by Stage

Treatment for cancer of the ovary depends on the stage of your disease, the type of disease, your age, and your overall condition.

You may receive treatment that is considered standard based on its effectiveness in a number of patients in past studies, or you may choose to go into a clinical trial. Not all patients are cured with standard therapy and some standard treatments may have more side effects than are desired. For these reasons, clinical trials are designed to find better ways to treat cancer patients and are based on the most up-to-date information. Clinical trials are going on in most parts of the country for most stages of cancer of the ovary. If you want more information, call the Cancer Information Service at 1-800-4-CANCER (1-800-422-6237).

Stage I Ovarian Epithelial Cancer. Your treatment may be one of the following:

- Surgery to remove the cancer, both ovaries, the fallopian tubes, uterus, and part of the tissue that stretches from the stomach to nearby organs in the abdomen (omentun). This is called a total abdominal hysterectomy and bilateral salpingo-oophorectomy with omentectomy. During surgery, samples of lymph nodes and other tissues in the pelvis and abdomen are cut out (biopsied) and checked for cancer.

- Surgery to remove the ovary in which the cancer is found and the fallopian tube on the same side of the body (unilateral salpingo-oophorectomy), in selected patients who wish to have

Ovarian Epithelial Cancer

children at a later time. Lymph nodes and other tissues in the pelvis and abdomen are biopsied during surgery.

- Total abdominal hysterectomy and bilateral salpingo-oophorectomy with omentectomy and biopsy of lymph nodes and other tissues in the pelvis and abdomen, followed by intraperitoneal radiation therapy.

- Total abdominal hysterectomy and bilateral salpingo-oophorectomy with omentectomy and biopsy of lymph nodes and other tissues in the pelvis and abdomen, followed by systemic chemotherapy.

- Total abdominal hysterectomy and bilateral salpingo-oophorectomy with omentectomy and biopsy of lymph nodes and other tissues in the pelvis and abdomen, followed by external beam radiation therapy to the abdomen and pelvis.

Stage II Ovarian Epithelial Cancer. Your treatment will probably be surgery to remove both ovaries, both fallopian tubes, the uterus, and as much of the cancer as possible (total abdominal hysterectomy and bilateral salpingo-oophorectomy with tumor debulking). During the surgery, samples of lymph nodes and other tissues in the pelvis and abdomen are cut out (biopsied) and checked for cancer. After the operation, your treatment may be one of the following:

- Systemic chemotherapy. Clinical trials are testing new drugs and combinations of drugs.

- External beam radiation therapy to the abdomen and pelvis.

- Intraperitoneal radiation therapy when only a small amount of tumor is found.

Stage III Ovarian Epithelial Cancer. Your treatment will probably be surgery to remove both ovaries, both fallopian tubes, the uterus, and as much of the cancer as possible (total abdominal hysterectomy and bilateral salpingo-oophorectomy with tumor debulking). During the surgery, samples of lymph nodes and other tissues in the pelvis and abdomen are cut out (biopsied) and checked for cancer. After the operation, your treatment may be one of the following:

- Systemic chemotherapy. Clinical trials are testing new drugs and combinations of drugs.

- External beam radiation therapy to the abdomen and pelvis.

- Clinical trials of intraperitoneal chemotherapy. Your doctor may operate again to look for any remaining cancer.

Stage IV Ovarian Epithelial Cancer. Your treatment will probably be surgery to remove as much of the cancer as possible (tumor debulking), followed by one of the following:

- Systemic chemotherapy. Clinical trials are testing new drugs and combinations of drugs.

- Clinical trials of intraperitoneal chemotherapy if the cancer has not spread outside the abdomen.

Recurrent Ovarian Epithelial Cancer. If the cancer comes back, your treatment may be one of the following:

- Systemic chemotherapy. Clinical trials are testing new drugs and combinations of drugs.

- Surgery to relieve symptoms.

- Clinical trials of intraperitoneal chemotherapy.

Side Effects of Treatment

It is hard to limit the effects of therapy so that only cancer cells are destroyed. Because treatment often damages healthy cells and tissues, it can cause unpleasant side effects.

The side effects of cancer treatment vary, depending on the type of treatment. Also, each woman reacts differently. Doctors try to keep side effects to a minimum, but problems may occur. The National Cancer Institute booklets *Radiation Therapy and You* and *Chemotherapy and You* have helpful information about cancer treatment and coping with side effects. *(These pamphlets are reproduced in <u>The New Cancer Sourcebook</u>. See the index or the table of contents for page references.)*

Surgery

Surgery for ovarian cancer is a major operation. For several days after surgery, the patient may have difficulty emptying her bladder and having normal bowel movements. Drugs may be given to relieve pain and to prevent or treat infection. A woman should ask the doctor or nurse for medicine to relieve pain. For a period of time after the surgery, some of the woman's normal activities are limited to let healing take place.

In younger women, when the ovaries are removed, the body's natural source of estrogen is lost and menopause starts. Symptoms of menopause are likely to appear soon after the surgery. Hormone replacement therapy is commonly used to ease such symptoms as hot flashes and vaginal dryness in menopausal women. However, the use of hormone replacement therapy has not been studied in women who have had ovarian cancer. Deciding whether to use it is an individual matter; ovarian cancer patients should discuss the possible risks and benefits of hormone replacement therapy with their doctor.

Chemotherapy

The side effects of chemotherapy depend mainly on which drugs the patient receives. In addition, side effects vary from patient to patient. In general, anticancer drugs affect rapidly dividing cells. These include blood cells, which fight infection, cause the blood to clot, and carry oxygen to all parts of the body. When blood cells are affected by anticancer drugs, women are more likely to get infections, bruise or bleed easily, and have less energy. Cells in hair roots and cells that line the digestive tract also divide rapidly. As a result, women may lose their hair and may have other side effects, such as nausea, vomiting, or mouth sores. Usually the doctor can suggest diet changes or medications to ease these problems. Most side effects of chemotherapy gradually go away during the recovery period or after treatment stops.

Certain drugs used in the treatment of ovarian cancer can cause kidney damage. To help protect the kidneys while taking these drugs, patients are given large amounts of fluid. These drugs also may cause tingling in the fingers or toes, ringing in the ears, or difficulty hearing. These problems may continue after treatment stops.

Radiation Therapy

Patients are likely to become very tired during radiation therapy, especially in the later weeks of treatment. Resting is important, but doctors usually advise patients to try to stay as active as they can.

It is also common for the skin in the treated area to become red, dry, tender, and itchy. There may be permanent darkening or "bronzing" of the skin in the treated area. This area should be exposed to the air as much as possible, but protected from sunlight. Patients should avoid wearing clothes that rub the treated area. The radiation therapist or nurse will give advice about keeping the skin clean. Patients should not use any lotion or cream on their skin without checking with the doctor or nurse.

Radiation treatment to the lower abdomen may cause nausea, vomiting, diarrhea, or urinary discomfort. Usually the doctor can suggest diet changes or medicines to ease these problems.

Radiation therapy for ovarian cancer also can cause vaginal dryness and interfere with intercourse. Women may be advised not to have intercourse during treatment. However most women are able to resume sexual activity a few weeks after radiation treatment ends.

Biological Therapy

The side effects caused by biological therapy vary with the type of treatment. Often, these treatments cause flu-like symptoms, such as chills, fever, muscle aches, weakness, nausea, vomiting, and diarrhea. Sometimes patients get a rash, and they may bleed or bruise easily or have bone pain. These problems can be severe, and patients may need to stay in the hospital during treatment.

Nutrition for Cancer Patients

Some patients find it hard to eat well. In addition to loss of appetite, the common side effects of therapy, such as nausea, vomiting, or mouth sores, can make eating difficult. For some patients, food tastes different. Also, people may not feel like eating when they are uncomfortable or tired.

Eating well means getting enough calories and protein to help prevent weight loss and regain strength. Patients who eat well during cancer treatment often feel better and have more energy. In addition, they may be better able to handle the side effects of treatment.

Doctors, nurses, and dietitians can offer advice for healthy eating during cancer treatment. Patients and their families also may want to read the National Cancer Institute booklet *Eating Hints*, which contains many useful suggestions.

Follow-up Care

In some cases, doctors recommend "second-look" surgery after chemotherapy is complete. This allows the doctor to examine the abdomen directly and take fluid and tissue samples to see whether the treatment has been successful. If cancer is found, additional treatment is needed.

When treatment is over, regular checkups generally include a physical exam, as well as a pelvic exam and Pap smear. Sometimes doctors also order chest x-rays, a CT scan of the abdomen, and laboratory tests such as urinalysis, a complete blood count, and the CA-125 assay. Often the CA-125 level in a patient's blood is high before surgery and returns to normal within several weeks after the tumor has been removed. If the CA-125 level begins to rise again, it may mean the cancer has come back.

Depending on the drugs she has received, a woman treated for ovarian cancer with chemotherapy may have an increased risk of developing leukemia later in life. However, it is important to keep in mind that the benefits of receiving treatment for ovarian cancer far outweigh the risks of future disease.

Women should carefully follow their doctor's advice on health care and checkups, and should report any problem to the doctor as soon as it appears.

Support for Cancer Patients

Living with a serious disease is not easy. Cancer patients and those who care about them face many problems and challenges. Coping with these difficulties is easier when people have helpful information and support services. Several useful booklets, including *Taking*

Time: Support for People With Cancer and the People Who Care About Them, are available from the Cancer Information Service. *(This pamphlet is reproduced in The New Cancer Sourcebook.)*

Cancer patients may worry about holding their job, caring for their family, or keeping up with daily activities. Concerns about tests, treatments, hospital stays, and medical bills are also common. Doctors, nurses, and other members of the health care team can answer questions about treatment, working, or other activities. Meeting with a nurse, social worker, counselor, or member of the clergy can be helpful to patients who want to talk about their feelings or discuss their concerns about the future or about personal relationships.

Friends and relatives can be very supportive. Also, many patients find it helps to discuss their concerns with others who have cancer. Cancer patients often get together in support groups, where they can share what they have learned about coping with cancer and the effects of treatment. It is important to keep in mind, however, that each patient is different. Treatments and ways of dealing with cancer that work for one person may not be right for another—even if they both have the same kind of cancer. It is always a good idea to discuss the advice of friends and family members with the doctor.

Often, a social worker at the hospital or clinic can suggest groups that can help with rehabilitation, emotional support, financial aid, transportation, or home care. For example, the American Cancer Society has many services for patients and their families. Local offices of the American Cancer Society are listed in the white pages of the telephone directory. Information about other programs and services is available through the Cancer Information Service. The toll-free number is 1-800-4-CANCER.

The public library has many books and articles on living with cancer.

What the Future Holds

Patients and their families are naturally concerned about what the future holds. Sometimes they use statistics to try to figure out whether the patient will be cured or how long she will live. It is important to remember, however, that statistics are averages based on large numbers of patients. They cannot be used to predict what will happen to a particular patient because no two cancer patients are alike; treatments and responses vary greatly. Patients should talk with the doctor about their chance of recovery (prognosis). When doctors talk about surviving cancer, they may use the term remission rather than cure. Even though ovarian cancer can be cured, doctors use these terms because the disease can return. (The return of cancer is called a recurrence.)

The Promise of Cancer Research

Scientists at hospitals and medical centers all across the country are studying ovarian cancer. They are trying to learn more about what causes this disease and how to prevent it. They are also looking for ways to detect it earlier and to treat it more effectively.

Cause and Prevention

About 1 in every 70 women in the United States will develop ovarian cancer during her lifetime. Most cases occur in women over the age of 50, but it can also affect younger women. The disease is more common in white women than in black women, but doctors do not know why.

Scientists do not know what causes ovarian cancer. It is clear, however, that this disease is not contagious; no one can "catch" ovarian cancer from another person.

By studying large numbers of women all over the world, researchers have found certain risk factors that increase a woman's chance of developing ovarian cancer. However, studies also show that most women with these risk factors do not get ovarian cancer, and many women who do get the disease have none of the risk factors we know about.

The following are some of the known risk factors for ovarian cancer:

- **Family medical history.** The risk of getting ovarian cancer increases for a woman whose close relative (mother, sister, daughter) has had the disease. The risk is especially high if two or more close relatives have had the disease. The risk is not quite as high for women with other relatives (grandmother, aunt, or cousin) who have had ovarian cancer.

- **Childbearing.** Women who have never been pregnant are more likely to develop ovarian cancer than are women who have had children. In fact, the more times a woman has been pregnant, the less likely she is to develop ovarian cancer. Also, women who use oral contraceptives (birth control pills) are less likely to develop ovarian cancer than are women who do not. A possible reason is that the pill creates hormone levels in the body that are similar to those during pregnancy.

  Recent research raises the question of whether infertile women who take fertility drugs and do not become pregnant may be at increased risk of developing ovarian cancer. But this possible link has not been proven. Further research is under way to see whether ovarian cancer is related to infertility and/or to the use of fertility drugs.

- **Age.** The risk of developing ovarian cancer increases as a woman gets older. Most ovarian cancers occur in women over the age of 50; the risk is especially high for women over 60.

- **Personal medical history.** Women who have had breast cancer are twice as likely to develop ovarian cancer as are women who have not had breast cancer.

Women who think they may be at risk for developing ovarian cancer should discuss this concern with their doctor, who can plan an appropriate schedule of checkups.

Early Detection

Most health problems respond best to treatment when they are found early. Women who have regular pelvic exams increase the chance that, if ovarian cancer occurs, it will be found before the disease causes symptoms. However, pelvic exams often cannot find ovarian cancer at an early stage. Scientists are trying to find better ways to detect ovarian cancer earlier, when treatment may be more successful. For example, they are exploring the usefulness of measuring the level of CA-125 in the blood. Other ways of detecting the disease, such as new ultrasound techniques, also are under study.

Women over age 60 are taking part in a nationwide study of CA-125 and transvaginal ultrasound. In this study, scientists are trying to learn whether these tests can detect early ovarian cancer (in women who have no symptoms of the disease) and reduce the number of deaths from this disease. The Cancer Information Service can provide information about this study.

Chapter 7

Ovarian Germ Cell Tumor

What Is Ovarian Germ Cell Tumor?

Ovarian germ cell tumor, an uncommon cancer in women, is a disease in which cancer (malignant) cells are found in egg-making cells in the ovary. The ovary is the small sac that holds the eggs that can develop into a baby. There are two ovaries: one located on the left side of the uterus (the hollow, pear-shaped organ where a baby grows) and one located on the right. Ovarian germ cell tumors usually occur in teenage girls or young women. Ovarian germ cell tumor is different from cancer that occurs in the lining (epithelium) of the ovary (see the chapter on cancer of the ovary for treatment of cancer of the ovary).

Ovarian germ cell tumor can be difficult to find (diagnose) early. Often there are no symptoms in the early stages, but sometimes it can be found when it is very small if you go to the doctor for regular checkups. You should see your doctor if you have swelling of your abdomen without gaining weight in other places or bleeding from your vagina after you have gone through the time when you stop having your menstrual periods (menopause).

Your doctor may use several tests to see if you have cancer, usually beginning with an internal (pelvic) exam. During the exam, your doctor will feel for any lumps or changes in the shape of the pelvic organs. Blood and urine tests and an ultrasound exam may be done.

NCI Cancerfax 208/03125.

During the ultrasound exam, sound waves are used to find tumors. You may also have a CT scan, which is a special type of x-ray.

Your chance of recovery (prognosis) and choice of treatment depend on the type of tumor and stage of your cancer (whether it is just in one part of the ovary, the whole ovary, or has spread to other places) and your general state of health.

Stages of Ovarian Germ Cell Tumor

Once ovarian germ cell tumor has been found, more tests will be done to find out if the cancer has spread from the ovary to other parts of the body (staging). Unless your doctor is sure the cancer has spread from the ovaries to other parts of the body, surgery is required to determine your stage of cancer in an operation called a laparotomy. During this operation, your doctor must cut into your abdomen and carefully look at all the organs to see if they contain cancer. During the operation, your doctor will cut out small pieces of tissue (biopsy) and look at them under a microscope to see whether they contain cancer. Usually your doctor will remove the cancer and other organs that contain cancer during the laparotomy (see section on How Ovarian Germ Cell Tumor is Treated).

Your doctor needs to know the stage of your disease to plan further treatment. Your doctor also needs to know what cell type your cancer is, based on how the cells look under the microscope. Germ cell tumors called dysgerminoma are often treated differently than other germ cell tumors (endodermal sinus tumors, embryonal carcinoma, teratoma, polyembryoma). The following stages are used for ovarian germ cell tumor:

- **Stage I**—Cancer is found only in one or both of the ovaries.

- **Stage II**—Cancer is found in one or both ovaries and/or has spread to the uterus, and/or the fallopian tubes (the pathway used by egg cells to get from the ovary to the uterus), and/or other body parts within the pelvis.

- **Stage III**—Cancer is found in one or both ovaries and has spread to lymph nodes or to other body parts inside the abdomen, such as the surface of the liver or intestine. (Lymph

Ovarian Germ Cell Tumor

nodes are small, bean-shaped structures that are found throughout the body; they produce and store infection-fighting cells).

- **Stage IV**—Cancer is found in one or both ovaries and has spread outside the abdomen or has spread to the inside of the liver.

- **Recurrent**—Recurrent disease means that the cancer has come back (recurred) after it has been treated. It may come back in the ovary that is left or in another place.

How Ovarian Germ Cell Tumor Is Treated

There are treatments for all patients with ovarian germ cell tumor. Three kinds of treatment are used: surgery (taking out the cancer in an operation) radiation therapy (using high-dose x-rays or other high-energy rays to kill cancer cells and shrink tumors) chemotherapy (using drugs to kill cancer cells).

Surgery is the most common treatment for ovarian germ cell tumor. Your doctor may take out the cancer (often during the staging laparotomy) using one of the following operations:

- **Unilateral salpingo-oophorectomy**—taking out the ovary with the cancer and the fallopian tube on the same side.

- **Total abdominal hysterectomy and bilateral salpingo-oophorectomy**—removing both ovaries and fallopian tubes and the uterus.

- **Tumor debulking**—taking out as much of the cancer as possible.

Radiation therapy uses x-rays or other high-energy rays to kill cancer cells and shrink tumors. Radiation for ovarian germ cell tumors usually comes from a machine outside the body (external radiation).

Chemotherapy uses drugs to kill cancer cells. Chemotherapy may be taken by pill, or it may be put into the body by a needle in the vein or muscle. Chemotherapy is called a systemic treatment because the drug enters the bloodstream, travels through the body, and can kill cancer cells outside the ovary.

Following radiation or chemotherapy, sometimes an operation called a second-look laparotomy is done. This is similar to the laparotomy that is done to determine the stage of the cancer. During the second-look operation, your doctor will take samples of lymph nodes and other tissues in the abdomen to see if any cancer is left.

Treatment by Stage

Treatment of ovarian germ cell tumor depends on the stage and cell type of your disease, your age, and your overall condition. You may receive treatment that is considered standard based on its effectiveness in a number of patients in past studies, or you may choose to go into a clinical trial. Not all patients are cured with standard therapy and some standard treatments may have more side effects than are desired. For these reasons, clinical trials are designed to find better ways to treat cancer patients and are based on the most up-to-date information. Clinical trials are going on in many parts of the country for patients with ovarian germ cell tumor. If you want more information, call the Cancer Information Service at 1-800-4-CANCER (1-800-422-6237).

Stage I Ovarian Germ Cell Tumor. Your treatment depends on how the cancer cells look under a microscope (cell type). If you have a tumor called a dysgerminoma, your treatment may be one of the following:

1. Surgery to remove the ovary where the cancer is found and the fallopian tube on the same side as the involved ovary (unilateral salpingo-oophorectomy) followed by radiation therapy.

2. Unilateral salpingo-oophorectomy followed by chemotherapy if you wish to have children in the future.

3. Unilateral salpingo-oophorectomy alone (in selected patients).

If you have another type of germ cell tumor, your treatment may be one of the following:

1. Unilateral salpingo-oophorectomy followed by chemotherapy. Clinical trials are testing new combinations of chemotherapy drugs.

2. Unilateral salpingo-oophorectomy alone (in selected patients).

Stage II Ovarian Germ Cell Tumor. Your treatment depends on how the cancer cells look under a microscope (cell type). If you have a tumor called a dysgerminoma, your treatment may be one of the following:

1. Surgery to remove the uterus and both ovaries and fallopian tubes (total abdominal hysterectomy and bilateral salpingo-oophorectomy) followed by radiation therapy.

2. If your cancer is found only in the ovary and the fallopian tube on the same side and you want to have children in the future, surgery to remove the ovary where cancer is found and the fallopian tube on the same side as the involved ovary (unilateral salpingo-oophorectomy) can be done. Chemotherapy is given following surgery.

If you have another type of germ cell tumor, your treatment may be one of the following:

1. Total abdominal hysterectomy and bilateral salpingo-oophorectomy. If the cancer cannot be totally removed, as much of the cancer as possible will be taken out (tumor debulking). Surgery is followed by chemotherapy.

2. If your cancer is found only in the ovary and the fallopian tube on the same side and you want to have children in the future, a unilateral salpingo-oophorectomy can be done. Chemotherapy is given following surgery.

3. Total abdominal hysterectomy and bilateral salpingo-oophorectomy, and removal of as much of the cancer as possible (tumor debulking), followed by chemotherapy. If the cancer remains following chemotherapy, another operation may be done to remove as much remaining tumor as possible.

Stage III Ovarian Germ Cell Tumor. Your treatment depends on how the cancer cells look under a microscope (cell type). If you have a tumor called a dysgerminoma, your treatment may be one of the following:

1. Surgery to remove the uterus and both ovaries and fallopian tubes (total abdominal hysterectomy and bilateral salpingo-oophorectomy) and removal of as much of the cancer as possible (tumor debulking). If the cancer left after surgery is very small, external radiation therapy is given to your abdomen following surgery.

2. Total abdominal hysterectomy and bilateral salpingo-oophorectomy and tumor debulking. If the cancer left after surgery is large, systemic chemotherapy is given following surgery.

3. If you want to have children in the future, surgery can be done to remove only the ovary where cancer is found and the fallopian tube on the same side (unilateral salpingo-oophorectomy). Chemotherapy is given following surgery.

If you have another type of germ cell tumor, your treatment may be one of the following:

1. Total abdominal hysterectomy and bilateral salpingo-oophorectomy and tumor debulking, followed by systemic chemotherapy. If the cancer remains following surgery, another operation may be done in some cases.

2. Systemic chemotherapy followed by total abdominal hysterectomy and bilateral salpingo-oophorectomy and tumor debulking. Following this operation, you may receive more chemotherapy.

3. If your cancer is found only in the ovary and the fallopian tube on the same side and you want to have children in the future, a unilateral salpingo-oophorectomy can be done. Chemotherapy is given following surgery.

Stage IV Ovarian Germ Cell Tumor. Your treatment depends on how the cancer cells look under the microscope (cell type). If you have a tumor called a dysgerminoma, your treatment may be one of the following:

1. Surgery to remove the uterus, both ovaries, and the fallopian tubes (total abdominal hysterectomy and bilateral salpingo-oophorectomy) and removal of as much of the cancer as possible (tumor debulking). Chemotherapy is given after surgery. If cancer remains following chemotherapy, additional chemotherapy with different drugs may be needed.

2. If your cancer is found only in one ovary and the fallopian tube on the same side and you want to have children in the future, surgery can be done to remove only the ovary where cancer is found and the fallopian tube on the same side (unilateral salpingo-oophorectomy). Chemotherapy is given following surgery.

If you have another type of germ cell tumor, your treatment may be one of the following:

1. Total abdominal hysterectomy and bilateral salpingo-oophorectomy and tumor debulking. Chemotherapy is given after surgery. If the cancer remains following chemotherapy, another operation may be done to remove as much remaining tumor as possible. Following this operation, you may receive more chemotherapy if there is still active disease.

2. Systemic chemotherapy followed by total abdominal hysterectomy and bilateral salpingo-oophorectomy and tumor debulking. Depending on the results of this operation, you may need more chemotherapy.

3. If your cancer is found only in the ovary and the fallopian tube on the same side and you want to have children in the future, unilateral salpingo-oophorectomy can be done. Chemotherapy is given following surgery.

Recurrent Ovarian Germ Cell Tumor. Your treatment depends on how the cancer cells look under a microscope (cell type). If you have a tumor called dysgerminoma, your treatment will probably be systemic chemotherapy with or without radiation therapy. If you have another type of germ cell tumor, your treatment will probably be systemic chemotherapy.

Chapter 8

Cancer of the Uterus

The Uterus

The uterus (womb) is a hollow, pear-shaped organ located in a woman's lower abdomen between the bladder and the rectum. The narrow, lower portion of the uterus is the cervix; the broader, upper part is the corpus. The corpus is made up of two layers of tissue.

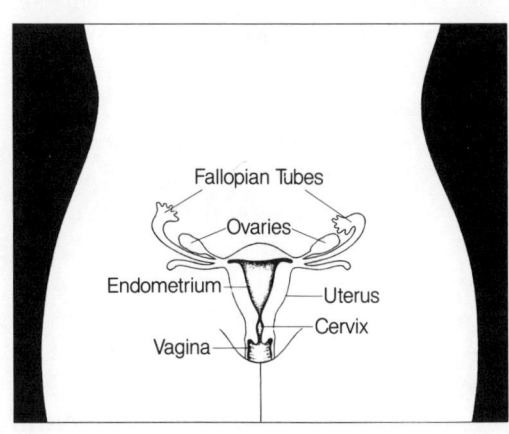

Figure 8.1.

In women of childbearing age, the inner layer of the uterus (endometrium) goes through a series of monthly changes known as the menstrual cycle. Each month, endometrial tissue grows and thickens in preparation to receive a fertilized egg. Menstruation occurs when this tissue is not used and passes out through the vagina. The outer layer of the corpus (myometrium) is a

NIH 93-1562 and NCI Cancerfax 208/01176.

muscle that expands during pregnancy to hold the growing fetus. Because most uterine cancer develops in the endometrium, cancer of the uterus also is called endometrial cancer.

What Is Cancer?

Cancer is a group of more than 100 diseases. Cancer occurs when cells become abnormal and divide without control or order.

The organs of the body are made up of many kinds of cells. Cells normally divide in an orderly way to produce more cells only when they are needed. This process helps keep the body healthy.

If cells divide when new cells are not needed, they form too much tissue. The mass of extra tissue, called a tumors can be benign or malignant.

Benign Tumors

Benign tumors are not cancer. They do not spread to other parts of the body and are seldom a threat to life. Several types of benign tumors occur in the uterus. In some cases, these growths do not need to be treated. Sometimes, however, benign tumors must be removed by surgery. Once removed, these tumors are not likely to return.

Fibroids are benign tumors in the uterus that are found most often in women over 35 years of age. Although single fibroid tumors do occur, multiple tumors are more common. Symptoms of fibroids depend on the size and location of the tumors and may include irregular bleeding, vaginal discharge, and frequent urination. When fibroids press against nearby organs and cause pain, surgery may be recommended. Often, however, fibroids do not cause symptoms and do not need to be treated, although they should be checked often. When a woman stops having menstrual periods (menopause), fibroids may become smaller, and sometimes they disappear. Another benign condition of the uterus is endometriosis. In this condition, tissue that looks and acts like endometrial tissue begins to grow in unusual places, such as on the surface of the ovaries, on the outside of the uterus, and in other tissues in the abdomen. Endometriosis is most common in women in their thirties and forties. This condition causes painful menstrual periods and abnormal bleeding; sometimes, it causes infertility. Some patients with endometriosis are treated with medication, and some are treated with surgery.

Cancer of the Uterus

Hyperplasia is an increase in the number of normal cells lining the uterus. Although this condition is not cancer, it may develop into cancer in some women. The most common symptoms of hyperplasia are heavy menstrual periods and bleeding between periods. Treatment depends on the extent of the condition (mild, moderate, or severe) and on the age of the patient. Young women usually are treated with female hormones, and the endometrial tissue is checked often. Hyperplasia in women near or after menopause may be treated with hormones if the condition is not severe. Surgery to remove the uterus is the usual treatment for severe cases.

Malignant Tumors

Malignant tumors are cancer. They invade and destroy nearby healthy tissues and organs. Cancer cells also can metastasize, or spread, to other parts of the body and form new tumors. When cancer of the uterus spreads, it may travel through the bloodstream or lymphatic system. Cancer cells can be carried along by blood or lymph, an almost colorless fluid discharged by tissues into the lymphatic system. Lymph nodes scattered along this system filter bacteria and abnormal substances such as cancer cells. For this reason, surgeons often remove pelvic lymph nodes to learn whether they contain cancer cells.

Because uterine cancer can spread, it is important for the doctor to find out as early as possible if a tumor is present and whether it is benign or malignant. As soon as a diagnosis is made, the doctor can begin treatment.

Symptoms

Abnormal bleeding after menopause is the most common symptom of cancer of the uterus. Bleeding may begin as a watery, blood-streaked discharge. Later, the discharge may contain more blood.

Cancer of the uterus does not often occur before menopause, but it does occur around the time menopause begins. The reappearance of bleeding should not be considered simply part of menopause; it should always be checked by a doctor.

Abnormal bleeding is not always a sign of cancer. It is important for a woman to see her doctor, however, because that is the only way to find out what the problem is. Any illness should be diagnosed and treated as soon as possible, but early diagnosis is especially important for cancer of the uterus.

Diagnosing Cancer of the Uterus

When symptoms suggest uterine cancer, the doctor asks a woman about her medical history and conducts a thorough exam. In addition to checking general signs of health (temperature, pulse, blood pressure, and so on), the doctor usually performs one or more of the following exams:

- **Pelvic exam.** The doctor thoroughly examines the uterus, vagina, ovaries, bladder, and rectum (pelvic exam). The doctor feels these organs for any abnormality in their shape or size. A speculum is used to widen the opening of the vagina so that the doctor can look at the upper portion of the vagina and the cervix.

- **Biopsy.** For a biopsy, the doctor surgically removes a small amount of uterine tissue, which is examined under a microscope by a pathologist.

- **D and C.** In a D and C, the doctor dilates (widens) the cervix and inserts a curette (a small spoon-shaped instrument) to remove pieces of the lining of the uterus. A sample of the uterine lining also can be removed by applying suction through a slender tube (called suction curettage). The tissue is examined for evidence of cancer.

- **Pap smear.** The Pap smear is often used to detect cancer of the cervix. While it is sometimes done for cancer of the uterus, it is not a reliable test for uterine cancer because it cannot always detect abnormal cells from the endometrium.

If cancer cells are found, doctors use other tests to find out whether the disease has spread from the uterus to other parts of the body. These procedures include blood tests and a chest x-ray. For some patients, special x-rays are needed. For example, computed tomography (also called CT or CAT scan) is used to take a series of x-rays of various sections of the abdomen. Doctors may also use ultra-

Cancer of the Uterus

sound to view organs inside the body. In this procedure, high-frequency sound waves are bounced off internal organs, and the echoes can be seen on a screen that resembles a television. Patients also may have special exams of the bladder, colon, and rectum.

Treating Cancer of the Uterus

The doctor considers a number of factors to determine the best treatment for cancer of the uterus. Among these factors are the stage of the disease, the growth rate of the cancer, and the age and general health of the woman.

Planning Treatment

Decisions about treatment for uterine cancer are complex. Before starting treatment, the patient might want a second opinion about the diagnosis and the treatment plan. It may take a week or two to arrange to see another doctor. This short delay will not make treatment less effective. There are a number of ways to find a doctor for a second opinion:

- The patient's doctor may refer her to a specialist who treats uterine cancer.

- The Cancer Information Service, at 1-800-4-CANCER, can tell callers about cancer centers and other NCI-supported programs in their area.

- Patients can get the names of doctors from their local medical society, a nearby hospital, or a medical school.

Methods of Treating Uterine Cancer

Surgery, radiation therapy, hormone therapy, or chemotherapy may be used to treat uterine cancer.

Radiation therapy (also called x-ray therapy, radiotherapy, or irradiation) uses high-energy rays to kill cancer cells. Radiation may be given from a machine located outside the body (external radiation therapy), or radioactive material may be placed inside the body (internal radiation therapy). In **hormone therapy**, female hormones are used to stop the growth of cancer cells. **Chemotherapy** is the use of drugs to treat cancer. Often, a combination of these methods is used. In some cases, the patient is referred to specialists in the different kinds of cancer treatment.

In its early stage, cancer of the uterus usually is treated with surgery. The uterus and cervix are removed (hysterectomy), as well as the fallopian tubes and ovaries (salpingo-oophorectomy). Some doctors recommend radiation therapy before surgery to shrink the cancer. Others prefer to evaluate the patient carefully during surgery and recommend radiation therapy after surgery for patients whose tumors appear likely to recur. A combination of external and internal radiation therapy often is used. If the cancer has spread extensively or has recurred after treatment, the doctor may recommend a female hormone (progesterone) or chemotherapy.

Stages of Cancer of the Uterus

Once cancer of the endometrium has been found, more tests will be done to find out if the cancer has spread from the endometrium to other parts of the body (staging). Your doctor needs to know the stage of your disease to plan treatment. The following stages are used for cancer of the endometrium:

- **Stage 0 or carcinoma in situ.** Stage 0 cancer of the endometrium is very early cancer. The cancer is found inside the uterus only and is in only the surface layer of the endometrium.

- **Stage I.** Cancer is found only in the main part of the uterus (it is not found in the cervix).

- **Stage II.** Cancer cells have spread to the cervix.

- **Stage III.** Cancer cells have spread outside the uterus but have not spread outside the pelvis.

- **Stage IV.** Cancer cells have spread beyond the pelvis, to other body parts, or into the lining of the bladder (the sac which holds urine) or rectum.

Cancer of the Uterus

- **Recurrent.** Recurrent disease means the cancer has come back (recurred) after it has been treated.

Treatment by Stage

Treatment for cancer of the endometrium depends on the stage of your disease, the type of disease, your age, and your overall condition.

You may receive treatment that is considered standard based on its effectiveness in a number of patients in past studies, or you may choose to go into a clinical trial. Not all patients are cured with standard therapy and some standard treatments may have more side effects than are desired. For these reasons, clinical trials are designed to find better ways to treat cancer patients and are based on the most up-to-date information.

Stage 0. Your treatment may be one of the following:

- Dilation and curettage (D & C) followed by hormone therapy. Your doctor may tell you not to take any more medicine that contains estrogen.

- Hysterectomy.

Stage I.

- Surgery to remove the uterus and both ovaries and fallopian tubes (total abdominal hysterectomy and bilateral salpingo-oophorectomy) with removal of some of the lymph nodes in the pelvis and abdomen to see if they contain cancer.

- Total abdominal hysterectomy and bilateral salpingo-oophorectomy with removal of some of the lymph nodes in the pelvis and abdomen to see if they contain cancer, followed by radiation therapy to the pelvis.

- Clinical trials of radiation and/or chemotherapy following surgery.

- Radiation therapy alone for selected patients.

Stage II.

- Abdominal hysterectomy, bilateral salpingo-oophorectomy, and removal of some of the lymph nodes in the pelvis and abdomen to see if they contain cancer, followed by radiation therapy.

- Internal and external beam radiation therapy followed by surgery to remove the uterus and both ovaries and fallopian tubes (total abdominal hysterectomy and bilateral salpingo-oophorectomy). Some of the lymph nodes in the pelvis and abdomen are also removed to see if they contain cancer.

- Surgery to remove the cervix, uterus, fallopian tubes, ovaries, and part of the vagina (radical hysterectomy). Lymph nodes in the area may also be taken out (lymph node dissection).

Stage III.

- Surgery to remove the cervix, uterus, fallopian tubes, ovaries, and part of the vagina (radical hysterectomy). Lymph nodes in the area may also be taken out (lymph node dissection). Surgery is usually followed by radiation therapy.

- Internal and external beam radiation therapy.

- Hormone therapy.

Stage IV.

- Internal and external beam radiation therapy.

- Hormone therapy.

- Clinical trials of chemotherapy.

Recurrent Endometrial Cancer. If your cancer has come back, your treatment may be one of the following:

Cancer of the Uterus

- Radiation therapy to relieve symptoms, such as pain, nausea, and abnormal bowel functions.

- Hormone therapy.

- Clinical trials of chemotherapy.

Side Effects of Treatment

It is rarely possible to limit the effects of cancer treatment so that only cancer cells are destroyed. Normal, healthy cells may be damaged at the same time. That's why the treatment often causes side effects.

Hysterectomy is major surgery. After the operation, the hospital stay usually lasts about 1 week. For several days after surgery, patients may have problems emptying their bladder and having normal bowel movements. The lower abdomen will be sore. Normal activities, including sexual intercourse, usually can be resumed in 4 to 8 weeks.

Women who have their uterus removed no longer have menstrual periods. When the ovaries are not removed, women do not have symptoms of menopause (change of life) because their ovaries still produce hormones. If the ovaries are removed or damaged by radiation therapy, menopause occurs. Hot flashes or other symptoms of menopause caused by treatment may be more severe than those of natural menopause.

Sexual desire and the ability to have intercourse usually are not affected by hysterectomy. However, many women have an emotionally difficult time after a hysterectomy. They may have feelings of deep emotional loss because they are no longer able to become pregnant.

Radiation therapy destroys the ability of cells to grow and divide. Both normal and diseased cells are affected, but most normal cells are able to recover quickly. Patients usually receive external radiation therapy as an outpatient. Treatments are given 5 days a week for several weeks. This schedule helps to protect healthy tissues by spreading out the total dose of radiation.

Internal radiation therapy puts the radiation as close as possible to the site of the cancer, while sparing most of the healthy tissues around it. This type of radiation therapy requires a short hospital stay. A radiation implant, a capsule containing radioactive material, is inserted through the vagina into the uterus. The implant usually is left in place 2 or 3 days.

During radiation therapy, patients may notice a number of side effects, which usually disappear when treatment is completed. Patients may have skin reactions (redness or dryness) in the area being treated, and they may be unusually tired. Some may have diarrhea and frequent and uncomfortable urination. Treatment can also cause dryness, itching, and burning in the vagina. Intercourse may be painful, and some women are advised not to have intercourse at this time. Most women can resume sexual activity within a few weeks after treatment ends.

Hormones occur naturally in the body; their purpose is to regulate the growth of specific cells or organs. In cancer treatment, hormones are sometimes used to stop the growth of cancer cells. Hormones travel through the bloodstream to all parts of the body, affecting cancer cells far from the original tumor. Hormone therapy usually causes few side effects.

Anticancer drugs also travel through the bloodstream to almost every area of the body. Drugs used to treat cancer may be given in different ways: some are given by mouth; others are injected into a muscle, a vein, or an artery. Chemotherapy is most often given in cycles-a treatment period, followed by a recovery period, then another treatment period, and so on.

Depending on the drugs that the doctor orders, the patient may need to stay in the hospital for a few days so that the effects of the drugs can be watched. Often, the patient receives treatment as an outpatient at the hospital, at a clinic, at the doctor's office, or at home.

The side effects of chemotherapy depend on the drugs given and the individual response of the patient. Chemotherapy commonly affects hair cells, blood-forming cells, and cells lining the digestive tract. As a result, patients may have side effects such as hair loss, lowered blood counts, nausea, or vomiting. Most side effects go away during the recovery period or after treatment is over.

Loss of appetite can be a serious problem for patients receiving radiation therapy or chemotherapy. Researchers are learning that patients who eat well are often better able to withstand the side effects of treatment. Therefore, nutrition is important. Eating well means getting enough calories to prevent weight loss and having enough protein in the diet to build and repair skin, hair, muscles, and organs. Many patients find that eating several small meals throughout the day is easier than eating three large meals.

Cancer of the Uterus

The side effects that patients have during cancer therapy vary from person to person and may even be different from one treatment to the next. Doctors try to plan treatment to keep problems to a minimum, and fortunately, most side effects are temporary. Doctors, nurses, and dietitians can explain the side effects of cancer treatment and suggest ways to deal with them.

Follow-up Care

Regular follow-up exams are very important for any woman who has been treated for cancer of the uterus. The doctor will want to watch the patient closely for several years to be sure that the cancer has not returned. In general, follow-up examinations include a pelvic exam, a chest x-ray, and laboratory tests.

Adjusting to the Disease

When people have cancer, life can change for them and for the people who care about them. These changes in daily life can be difficult to handle. When a woman finds out she has uterine cancer, a number of different and sometimes confusing emotions may appear.

At times, patients and family members may feel depressed, angry, or frightened. At other times, feelings may vary from hope to despair or from courage to fear. Patients usually are better able to cope with their emotions if they can talk openly about their illness and their feelings with family members and friends.

Concerns about the future, as well as about medical tests, treatments, hospital stays, and medical bills, often arise. Talking to doctors, nurses, or other members of the health care team may help to ease fear and confusion. Patients can ask questions about their disease and its treatment and can take an active part in decisions about their medical care. Patients and family members often find it helpful to write down questions for the doctor as they think of them. Taking notes during visits to the doctor also can help patients remember what was said. Patients should ask the doctor to repeat or explain more fully anything that is not clear.

Patients have many important questions to ask about cancer, and their doctor is the best person to provide answers. Most people ask what kind of cancer they have, how it can be treated, and how successful the treatment is likely to be. The following are some other questions that patients might want to ask the doctor:

- What are the expected benefits of treatment?
- What are the risks and side effects of treatment?
- Will changes in my normal activities be required?
- Is it possible to keep working?
- How often are checkups needed?

Many women become concerned, especially after surgery and radiation therapy, that the changes to their bodies will affect how other people feel about them. They may worry about working, caring for their family, or about how cancer and its treatment will affect their sex life. Usually, as the patient recovers, the changes to her body become more accepted. With love and support, patients gradually feel reassured that they are just as appreciated as before.

The patient's doctor is the best person to give advice about working or other activities, but it may be hard to talk to the doctor about feelings and other very personal matters. Many patients find it helpful to talk with others who are facing similar problems. This kind of help is available through cancer-related support groups, such as those described in the next section. If the emotional problems of the patient or family become too hard to handle, a mental health counselor may be able to help.

Living with any serious disease is a difficult challenge. The public library is a good source of books and articles on living with cancer.

Support for Cancer Patients

Adapting to the changes brought about by having cancer is easier for both patients and their families when they get helpful information and support services. Often, the hospital or clinic social service office can suggest local and national agencies that will help with rehabilitation, emotional support, financial aid, transportation, or home care. The American Cancer Society (ACS), for example, is a nonprofit organization that offers a variety of services to patients and their families. Local offices of the ACS are listed in the telephone book.

Information about other resources and services is available through the Cancer Information Service at 1-800-4-CANCER.

What the Future Holds

There are more than 8 million Americans living today who have had some type of cancer. Many are women who have had cancer of the uterus. The outlook for women with very early cancer of the uterus is excellent; nearly all patients with this condition can be cured. The chances of controlling advanced disease are improving as researchers continue to look for better ways to treat this disease.

Doctors often talk about "surviving" cancer, or they may use the word "remission" rather than "cure." Even though many patients recover completely, doctors use these terms because cancer of the uterus may show up again at a later time. Patients are naturally concerned about their future and often try to use statistics they have read or heard about to figure out their own chances of being cured. It is important to remember that statistics describe an average of large numbers of people, and no two cancer patients are alike. The outlook for a particular patient depends on the type and stage of her disease, her age and general health, her response to treatment and other variables.

The Promise of Cancer Research

Scientists at hospitals and medical centers throughout the country are studying the possible causes of uterine cancer and how the disease might be prevented. In addition, they are researching new methods of treatment.

Cause and Prevention

Researchers study patterns of cancer in the population to discover which people are more likely to get certain cancers and what aspects of our surroundings and lifestyles may cause cancer.

Cancer of the uterus occurs most often in women between the ages of 55 and 70. This disease accounts for about 6 percent of all cancers in women. Research shows that some women are more likely than others to develop cancer of the uterus. These women are said to be "at risk." Obese women, women who have few or no children, women who began menstruating at a young age, those who had a late menopause, and women of high socioeconomic status are at increased risk of developing this disease. It appears that most of the risk factors for cancer of the uterus are related to hormones, especially excess estrogen.

Studies have shown that women taking estrogen replacement therapy (ERT) for menopausal symptoms have two to eight times greater risk of developing uterine cancer than women who do not take estrogens. The risk increases after 2 to 4 years of use and seems to be greatest when large doses are taken for long periods of time. A woman who takes ERT after her uterus has been removed is in no danger of developing uterine cancer. Many doctors now believe that using a combination of estrogen and progestin (another female hormone) for replacement therapy decreases the risk of cancer of the uterus. It is especially important for all women taking replacement therapy to be checked regularly for any signs of cancer. Unusual bleeding should be reported to the doctor at once.

Recent evidence shows that the use of birth control pills may decrease the risk of developing uterine cancer. Women who use a combination pill (containing both estrogen and progestin in each pill) for at least 1 year have only half the risk of endometrial cancer as women who use other types of birth control pills or none. The longer a woman takes the combination pill, the more this protection increases.

Treatment

Scientists continue to study new treatments for cancer of the uterus, including new drugs, drug combinations, and combinations of radiation therapy and chemotherapy. Scientists are studying these methods closely to learn whether they can be of value in future treatment.

When laboratory research shows that a new treatment method has promise, the method is used to treat cancer patients in clinical trials. These trials are designed to answer scientific questions and to find out if a promising new treatment is both safe and effective. They are done with the cooperation of cancer patients. Patients who take part in clinical trials make an important contribution to medical science and may have the first chance to benefit from improved treatment methods. Any woman with uterine cancer may consider participating in a trial and should discuss her interest with her doctor.

One way to learn about clinical trials is through PDQ, a computerized resource of information about cancer. Developed by NCI, PDQ contains an up-to-date list of trials all over the country. Doctors can

Cancer of the Uterus

obtain an access code and use a personal computer to get PDQ information, or they can use the services of a medical library. Also, the Cancer Information Service, at 1-800-4-CANCER, can provide PDQ information to doctors, patients, and the public.

Chapter 9

Uterine Sarcoma

What Is Sarcoma of the Uterus?

Sarcoma of the uterus, a very rare kind of cancer in women, is a disease in which cancer (malignant) cells start growing in the muscles or other supporting tissues of the uterus. The uterus is the hollow, pear-shaped organ where a baby grows. Sarcoma of the uterus is different from cancer of the endometrium, a disease in which cancer cells start growing in the lining of the uterus (see the section on endometrial cancer for information on that disease).

Women who have received therapy with high-dose x-rays (external beam radiation therapy) to their pelvis are at a higher risk to develop sarcoma of the uterus. These x-rays are sometimes given to women to stop bleeding from the uterus.

Like most cancers, sarcoma of the uterus is best treated when it is found (diagnosed) early. You should see your doctor if you have bleeding after menopause (the time when you no longer have menstrual periods) or bleeding that is not part of your periods (menstruation). Sarcoma of the uterus usually begins after menopause.

If you have signs of cancer, your doctor will do certain tests to check for Cancer, usually beginning with an internal (pelvic) exam. During the exam, your doctor will feel for any lumps or changes in the shapes of the pelvic organs. Your doctor may then do a Pap test, using

---

NCI Cancerfax 208/003371.

a piece of cotton, a small wooden stick, or brush to scrape gently the outside of the cervix (the opening of the uterus) and the vagina to pick up cells. Because sarcoma of the uterus begins inside, this cancer will not usually show up on the Pap test. Your doctor may also do a dilation and curettage (D & C) by stretching the cervix and inserting a small, spoon-shaped instrument into the uterus to remove pieces of the lining of the uterus. This tissue is then checked under a microscope for cancer cells.

Your prognosis (chance of recovery) and choice of treatment depend on the stage of your sarcoma (whether it is just in the uterus or has spread to other places), how fast your tumor cells are growing, and your general state of health.

Stages of Sarcoma of the Uterus

Once sarcoma of the uterus has been found, more tests will be done to find out if the cancer has spread from the uterus to other parts of the body (staging). Your doctor needs to know the stage of your disease to plan treatment. The following stages are used for sarcoma of the uterus:

Stage I. Cancer is found only in the main part of the uterus (it is not found in the cervix).

Stage II. Cancer cells have spread to the cervix.

Stage III. Cancer cells have spread outside the uterus but have not spread outside the pelvis.

Stage IV. Cancer cells have spread beyond the pelvis, to other body parts, or into the lining of the bladder (the sac that holds urine) or rectum.

Recurrent disease. The cancer has come back (recurred) after it has been treated.

How Sarcoma of the Uterus is Treated

There are treatments for all patients with sarcoma of the uterus.

Four kinds of treatment are used:

- Surgery (taking out the cancer in an operation)
- Radiation therapy (using high-dose x-rays or other high-energy rays to kill cancer cells and shrink tumors)
- Chemotherapy (using drugs to kill cancer cells)
- Hormone therapy (using female hormones to kill cancer cells).

Surgery is the most common treatment for sarcoma of the uterus. Your doctor may take out the cancer in an operation to remove the uterus, fallopian tubes and the ovaries, along with some lymph nodes in the pelvis and around the aorta (the main vessel in which blood passes away from the heart). The operation is called a total abdominal hysterectomy, bilateral salpingo-oophorectomy, and lymphadenectomy. (The lymph nodes are small bean-shape structures that are found throughout the body. They produce and store infection-fighting cells, but may contain cancer cells.)

Radiation therapy uses x-rays or other high-energy rays to kill cancer cells and shrink tumors. Radiation therapy for sarcoma of the uterus usually comes from a machine outside the body (external radiation). Radiation may be used alone or in addition to surgery.

Chemotherapy uses drugs to kill cancer cells. Chemotherapy may be taken by pill, or it may be put into the body by a needle in a vein or a muscle. Chemotherapy is called a systemic treatment because the drugs enter the bloodstream, travel through the body, and can kill cancer cells outside the uterus.

Hormone therapy uses female hormones, usually taken by pill, to kill cancer cells.

Treatment by Stage

Treatment for sarcoma of the uterus depends on the stage and cell type of your disease, your age, and your overall condition. You may receive treatment that is considered standard based on its effectiveness in a number of patients in past studies, or you may choose to go into a clinical trial. Not all patients are cured with standard therapy and some standard treatments may have more side effects than are desired. For these reasons, clinical trials are designed to find better ways to treat cancer patients and are based on the most up-to-date information. Clinical trials are going on in most parts of the country for most stages of sarcoma of the uterus. If you want more information, call the Cancer Information Service at 1-800-4-CANCER (1-800-422-6237).

Stage I Uterine Sarcoma. Your treatment may be one of the following:

- Surgery to remove the uterus, fallopian tubes and the ovaries, and some of the lymph nodes in the pelvis and abdomen (total abdominal hysterectomy, bilateral salpingo-oophorectomy, and lymph node dissection).

- Total abdominal hysterectomy, bilateral salpingo-oophorectomy, and lymph node dissection, followed by radiation therapy to the pelvis.

- Clinical trials of surgery followed by chemotherapy.

Stage II Uterine Sarcoma. Your treatment may be one of the following:

- Surgery to remove the uterus, fallopian tubes and the ovaries, and some of the lymph nodes in the pelvis and abdomen (total abdominal hysterectomy, bilateral salpingo-oophorectomy, and lymph node dissection).

- Total abdominal hysterectomy, bilateral salpingo-oophorectomy, and lymph node dissection, followed by radiation therapy to the pelvis.

- Clinical trials of surgery followed by chemotherapy.

Stage III Uterine Sarcoma. Your treatment may be one of the following:

- Surgery to remove the uterus, fallopian tubes and the ovaries, and some of the lymph nodes in the pelvis and abdomen (total abdominal hysterectomy bilateral salpingo-oophorectomy, and lymph node dissection). Your doctor will also try to remove as much of the cancer that has spread to nearby tissues as possible.

- Total abdominal hysterectomy, bilateral salpingo-oophorectory, and lymph node dissection, followed by radiation therapy to the pelvis.

- Clinical trials of surgery followed by chemotherapy.

Stage IV Uterine Sarcoma. Your treatment will usually be a clinical trial using chemotherapy.

Recurrent Uterine Sarcoma. If the cancer has come back (recurred), your treatment may be one of the following:

- Clinical trials of chemotherapy or hormone therapy.

- External radiation therapy to relieve symptoms such as pain, nausea, or abnormal bowel functions.

Chapter 10

Gestational Trophoblastic Tumor

What Is Gestational Trophoblastic Tumor?

Gestational trophoblastic tumor, a rare cancer in women, is a disease in which cancer (malignant) cells grow in the tissues that are formed following conception (the joining of sperm and egg). Gestational trophoblastic tumors start inside the uterus, the hollow, muscular, pear-shaped organ where a baby grows. This type of cancer occurs in women during the years when they are able to have children. There are two types of gestational trophoblastic tumors: hydatidiform mole and choriocarcinoma.

If you have hydatidiform mole (also called molar pregnancy), the sperm and egg cells have joined, but there is no baby developing in the uterus. Instead, the tissue that is formed resembles grape-like cysts. Hydatidiform mole does not spread outside of the uterus to other parts of the body.

If you have choriocarcinoma, the tumor may have started from a hydatidiform mole or from tissue that remains in the uterus following an abortion or delivery of a baby. Choriocarcinoma can spread from the uterus to other parts of the body. A very rare type of gestational trophoblastic tumor starts in the uterus where the placenta was attached. This type of cancer is called placental-site trophoblastic disease.

NCI Cancerfax 208/01163.

Gestational trophoblastic tumor is not always easy to find. In its early stages, it may look like a normal pregnancy. You should see your doctor if you have bleeding from the vagina, if your uterus gets bigger after you have given birth or had an abortion, or if you are pregnant and you do not feel the baby move at the expected time.

If you have symptoms, your doctor may use several tests to see if you have gestational trophoblastic tumor, usually beginning by giving you an internal (pelvic) exam. Your doctor will feel for any lumps or strange feeling in the shape or size of the uterus. Your doctor may then do an ultrasound, a test that uses sound waves to find tumors. A blood test will also be done to look for high levels of a hormone called beta HCG (beta human chorionic gonadotropin). This hormone is present during normal pregnancy, but if you are not pregnant and the hormone is still found in your blood, it can be a sign of gestational trophoblastic tumor.

Your chance of recovery (prognosis) and choice of treatment depend on the type of gestational trophoblastic tumor you have, whether it has spread to other places, and your general state of health.

Stages of Gestational Trophoblastic Tumor

Once gestational trophoblastic tumor has been found, more tests will be done to find out if the cancer has spread from inside the uterus to other parts of the body (staging). Your doctor needs to know the stage of your disease to plan treatment. The following stages are used for gestational trophoblastic tumor:

- **Hydatidiform mole.** Cancer is found only in the space inside the uterus. If the cancer is found in the muscle of the uterus, it is called an invasive mole (choriocarcinoma destruens).

- **Placental-site gestational trophoblastic tumor.** Cancer is found in the place where the placenta was attached and in the muscle of the uterus.

- **Non-metastatic.** Cancer cells have grown inside the uterus from tissue remaining following treatment of a hydatidiform mole or following an abortion or delivery of a baby. Cancer has not spread outside the uterus.

Gestational Trophoblastic Tumor

- **Metastatic, good prognosis.** Cancer cells have grown inside the uterus from tissue remaining following treatment of a hydatidiform mole or following an abortion or delivery of a baby. The cancer has spread from the uterus to other parts of the body. Metastatic gestational trophoblastic tumors are considered good prognosis or poor prognosis.

  Metastatic gestational trophoblastic tumor is considered good prognosis if all of the following are true:

  1. Your last pregnancy was less than 4 months ago.
  2. The level of beta HCG in your blood is low.
  3. Cancer has not spread to your liver or brain.
  4. You have not received chemotherapy earlier.

- **Metastatic, poor prognosis.** Cancer cells have grown inside the uterus from tissue remaining following treatment of a hydatidiform mole or following an abortion or delivery of a baby. The cancer has spread from the uterus to other parts of the body.

  Metastatic gestational trophoblastic tumor is considered poor prognosis if any the following are true:

  1. Your last pregnancy was more than 4 months ago.
  2. The level of beta HCG in your blood is high.
  3. Cancer has spread to your liver or brain.
  4. You have received chemotherapy earlier and the cancer did not go away.
  5. The tumor began after you completed a normal pregnancy.

- **Recurrent.** Recurrent disease means that the cancer has come back (recurred) after it has been treated. It may come back in the uterus or in another part of the body.

Treatment Options Overview

How Gestational Trophoblastic Tumor Is Treated

There are treatments for all patients with gestational trophoblastic tumor. Two kinds of treatment are used: surgery (taking out the cancer) and chemotherapy (using drugs to kill cancer cells). Radiation therapy (using high-energy x-rays to kill cancer cells) may be used in certain cases to treat cancer that has spread to other parts of the body.

Your doctor may take out the cancer using one of the following operations:

- Dilation and curettage (D & C) with suction evacuation is stretching the opening of the uterus (the cervix) and removing the material inside the uterus with a small vacuum-like device. The walls of the uterus are then scraped gently to remove any material that may remain in the uterus. This is used only for molar pregnancies.

- Hysterectomy is an operation to take out the uterus. In the treatment of this disease, the ovaries usually are not removed.

- Chemotherapy uses drugs to kill cancer cells. It may be taken by pill or put into the body by a needle in a vein or muscle. It is called a systemic treatment because the drugs enter the bloodstream, travel through the body, and can kill cancer cells outside the uterus. Chemotherapy may be given before or after surgery or alone.

- Radiation therapy uses high-energy x-rays to kill cancer cells and shrink tumors. Radiation may come from a machine outside the body (external beam radiation therapy) or from putting materials that produce radiation (radioisotopes) through thin plastic tubes into the area where the cancer cells are found (internal radiation).

Gestational Trophoblastic Tumor

Treatment by Stage

Treatment of gestational trophoblastic tumor depends on the stage of your disease, your age, and your overall condition.

You may receive treatment that is considered standard based on its effectiveness in a number of patients in past studies, or you may choose to go into a clinical trial. Not all patients are cured with standard therapy and some standard treatments may have more side effects than are desired. For these reasons, clinical trials are designed to find better ways to treat cancer patients and are based on the most up-to-date information.

Hydatidiform Mole. Your treatment my be one of the following:

- Removal of the mole using dilation and curettage (D & C) and suction evacuation.

- Surgery to remove the uterus (hysterectomy).

- Following surgery, your doctor will follow you closely with regular blood tests to make sure the level of beta HCG in your blood falls to normal levels. If the blood level of beta HCG increases or does not go down to normal, you will have more tests to see whether the tumor has spread. Your treatment will then depend on whether you have non-metastatic disease or metastatic disease (see the treatment sections on metastatic or non-metastatic disease).

Placental-Site Gestational Trophoblastic Tumor. Your treatment will probably be surgery to remove the uterus (hysterectomy).

Non-Metastatic Gestational Trophoblastic Tumor. Your treatment may be one of the following:

- Chemotherapy.

- Surgery to remove the uterus (hysterectomy) if you no longer wish to have children.

Good Prognosis Metastatic Gestational Trophoblastic Tumor. Your treatment may be one of the following:

- Chemotherapy

- Surgery to remove the uterus (hysterectomy) followed by chemotherapy.

- Chemotherapy followed by hysterectomy if cancer remains following chemotherapy.

Poor Prognosis Metastatic Gestational Trophoblastic Tumor. Your treatment will probably be chemotherapy. Radiation therapy may also be given to places where the cancer has spread, such as the brain.

Reccurent Gestational Trophoblastic Tumor. Your treatment will probably be chemotherapy.

Chapter 11

Vaginal Cancer

What Is Cancer of the Vagina?

Cancer of the vagina, a rare kind of cancer in women is a disease in which cancer (malignant) cells are found in the tissues of the vagina. The vagina is the passageway through which fluid passes out of the body during menstrual periods and through which a woman has babies. It is also called the "birth canal." The vagina connects the cervix (the opening of the womb or uterus) and the vulva (the folds of skin around the opening to the vagina).

There are two types of cancer of the vagina: squamous cell cancer (squamous carcinoma) and adenocarcinoma. Squamous carcinoma is usually found in women between the ages of 60 and 80. Adenocarcinoma is more often found in women between the ages of 12 and 30.

The drug DES (diethylstilbestrol) was given to pregnant women between 1945 and 1970 to keep them from losing their babies (miscarriage). Young women whose mothers took DES are at risk for getting tumors in their vaginas. Some of them get a rare form of cancer called clear cell adenocarcinoma.

Like most cancers, cancer of the vagina is best treated when it is found (diagnosed) early. If you have any of these problems, you should see a doctor: bleeding or discharge not related to your periods (men-

---

NCI Cancerfax 208/01055.

struation), difficult or painful urination, pain during intercourse, and pain in the pelvic area.

Your doctor may use several tests to see if you have cancer. Your doctor will usually begin by giving you an internal (pelvic) exam. Your doctor will feel for lumps. Your doctor will then do a Pap smear, using a piece of cotton, a brush, or a small wooden stick to gently scrape the outside of the cervix and vagina in order to pick up cells. You may feel some pressure, but you usually do not feel pain.

If cells that are not normal are found, your doctor will need to cut a small sample of tissue (called a biopsy) out of the vagina and look at it under a microscope to see if there are any cancer cells. Your doctor should look not only at the vagina, but also at the other organs in the pelvis to see where the cancer started and where it may have spread. Your doctor may take an x-ray of your chest to make sure the cancer has not spread to your lungs.

Your chance of recovery (prognosis) and choice of treatment depend on the stage of your cancer (whether it is just in the vagina or has spread to other places) and your general state of health.

Stages of Cancer of the Vagina

Once cancer of the vagina has been found (diagnosed), more tests will be done to find out if the cancer has spread from the vagina to other parts of the body (staging). Your doctor needs to know the stage of your disease to plan treatment. The following stages are used for cancer of the vagina:

Stage 0 or carcinoma in situ. Stage 0 cancer of the vagina is a very early cancer. The cancer is found inside the vagina only and is in only a few layers of cells.

Stage I. Cancer is found in the vagina, but has not spread outside of it.

Stage II. Cancer has spread to the tissues just outside the vagina, but has not gone to the bones of the pelvis.

Stage III. Cancer has spread to the bones of the pelvis. Cancer cells may also have spread to other organs and the lymph nodes in the pelvis. (Lymph nodes are small bean-shaped structures that are found throughout the body. They produce and store cells that fight infection.)

Stage IVA. Cancer has spread into the bladder or rectum.
Stage IVB. Cancer has spread to other parts of the body, such as the lungs.

Recurrent. Recurrent disease means that the cancer has come back (recurred) after it has been treated. It may come back in the vagina or in another place.

Treatment Options Overview

How Cancer of the Vagina is Treated

Treatments are available for all patients with cancer of the vagina. There are three kinds of treatment: surgery (taking out the cancer in an operation) radiation therapy (using high-dose x-rays or other high-energy rays to kill cancer cells and shrink tumors) chemotherapy (using drugs to kill cancer cells).

Surgery is the most common treatment for all stages of cancer of the vagina. Your doctor may take out the cancer using one of the following:

- Laser surgery uses a narrow beam of light to kill cancer cells and is useful for stage 0 cancer.

- Wide local excision takes out the cancer and some of the tissue around it. You may need to have skin taken from another part of your body (grafted) to repair the vagina after the cancer has been taken out.

- An operation in which the vagina is removed (vaginectomy) is sometimes done. When the cancer has spread outside the vagina, vaginectomy may be combined with surgery to take out the uterus, ovaries, and fallopian tubes (radical hysterectomy). During these operations, lymph nodes in the pelvis may also be removed (lymph node dissection).

If the cancer has spread outside the vagina and the other female organs, your doctor may take out the lower colon, rectum, or bladder (depending on where the cancer has spread) along with the cervix, uterus, and vagina (exenteration).

You may need skin grafts and plastic surgery to make an artificial vagina after these operations.

Radiation therapy uses x-rays or other high-energy rays to kill cancer cells and shrink tumors. Radiation may come from a machine outside the body (external radiation) or from putting materials that produce radiation (radioisotopes) through thin plastic tubes into the area where the cancer cells are found (internal radiation). Radiation may be used alone or after surgery.

Chemotherapy uses drugs to kill cancer cells Chemotherapy may be taken by pill, or it may be put into the body by a needle in a vein. Chemotherapy is called a systemic treatment because the drugs enter the bloodstream, travel through the body, and can kill cancer cells outside the vagina. In treating vaginal cancer, chemotherapy may also be put directly into the vagina itself, which is called intravaginal chemotherapy.

Treatment by Stage

Treatment for cancer of the vagina depends on the stage of your disease, the type of disease, your age and your overall condition.

You may receive treatment that is considered standard based on its effectiveness in a number of patients in past studies, or you may choose to go into a clinical trial. Not all patients are cured with standard therapy and some standard treatments may have more side effects than are desired. For these reasons, clinical trials are designed to find better ways to treat cancer patients and are based on the most up-to-date information.

Stage 0 Vaginal Cancer. Your treatment may be one of the following:

- Surgery to remove all or part of the vagina (vaginectomy). This may be followed by skin grafting to repair damage done to the vagina.

- Internal radiation therapy.

Vaginal Cancer

- Laser surgery.

- Intravaginal chemotherapy.

Stage I Vaginal Cancer. Treatment for stage I cancer of the vagina depends on whether you have squamous cell cancer or adenocarcinoma.

If you have squamous cancer, your treatment may be one of the following:

- Internal radiation therapy with or without external beam radiation therapy.

- Wide local excision. This may be followed by skin grafting to repair damage done to the vagina.

- Surgery to remove the vagina with or without lymph nodes in the pelvic area (vaginectomy and lymph node dissection).

If you have adenocarcinoma, your treatment may be one of the following:

- Surgery to remove vagina (vaginectomy) and the uterus, ovaries, and fallopian tubes (hysterectomy). The lymph nodes in the pelvis are also removed (lymph node dissection).

- Internal radiation therapy with or without external beam radiation therapy.

- Wide local excision and removal of some of the lymph nodes in the pelvis followed by internal radiation (in selected patients).

Stage II Vaginal Cancer. Your treatment may be one of the following:

- Combined internal and external radiation therapy.

- Surgery followed by radiation therapy (in selected patients).

Stage III Vaginal Cancer. Your treatment say be one of the following:

- Combined internal and external radiation therapy.

- Surgery plus internal and external radiation therapy (in selected patients).

Stage IVA Vaginal Cancer. Treatment for stage IVA cancer of the vagina depends on whether you have squamous cell cancer or Adenocarcinoma. If you have stage IVA squamous carcinoma, your treatment usually is one of the following:

- Combined internal and external radiation therapy.

- Surgery plus internal and external radiation therapy (in selected patients).

If you have stage IVA adenocarcinoma, treatment is usually combined internal and external radiation therapy

Stage IVB Vaginal Cancer. If you have stage IVB cancer of the vagina, treatment may be radiation to relieve symptoms such as pain, nausea, vomiting, or abnormal bowel function. You may also choose to participate in a clinical trial.

Recurrent Vaginal Cancer. If the cancer has come back (recurred) and spread past the female organs, your doctor may take out the cervix, uterus, lower colon, rectum, or bladder (exenteration), depending on where the cancer has spread. Your doctor may give you radiation therapy or chemotherapy.

You may also choose to participate in a clinical trial of chemotherapy or radiation therapy.

Chapter 12

Vulvar Cancer

What Is Cancer of the Vulva?

Cancer of the vulva, a rare kind of cancer in women, is a disease in which cancer (malignant) cells are found in the vulva. The vulva is the outer part of a woman's vagina and looks much like a pair of lips. The vagina is the passage between the uterus (the hollow, pear-shaped organ where a baby grows) and the outside of the body. It is also called the birth canal.

Most women with cancer of the vulva are over age 50. However, it is becoming more common in women under age 40. Women who have constant itching and changes in the color and the way the vulva looks are at a high risk to get cancer of the vulva. You should see your doctor if you have bleeding or discharge not related to your periods (menstruation), severe burning/itching or pain in the vulva, or if the skin of the vulva looks white and feels rough.

Like most cancers, cancer of the vulva is best treated when it is found (diagnosed) early. If you have symptoms, your doctor may do certain tests to see if you have cancer, usually beginning by looking at the vulva and feeling for any lumps. Your doctor may then go on to cut out a small piece of tissue (called a biopsy) from the vulva and look at it under a microscope. You will be given some medicine to numb the area when the biopsy is done. You may feel some pressure, but you usually won't feel any pain. This test is often done in a doctor's office.

NCI Cancerfax 208/01038.

Your chance of recovery (prognosis) and choice of treatment depend on the stage of your cancer (whether it is just in the vulva or has spread to other places) and your general state of health.

Stages of Cancer of the Vulva

Once cancer of the vulva is diagnosed, more tests will be done to find out if the cancer has spread from the vulva to other parts of the body (staging). Your doctor needs to know the stage of your disease to plan treatment. The following stages are used for cancer of the vulva:

- **Stage 0 or carcinoma in situ.** Stage 0 cancer of the vulva is a very early cancer. The cancer is found in the vulva only and is only in the surface of the skin.

- **Stage I.** Cancer is found only in the vulva and/or the space between the opening of the rectum and the vagina (perineum). The tumor is 2 centimeters (about 1 inch) or less in size.

- **Stage II.** Cancer is found in the vulva and/or the space between the opening of the rectum and the vagina (perineum), and the tumor is larger than 2 centimeters (larger than 1 inch).

- **Stage III.** Cancer is found in the vulva and/or perineum and has spread to nearby tissues such as the lower part of the urethra (the tube through which urine passes), the vagina, the anus (the opening of the rectum), and/or has spread to nearby lymph nodes. (Lymph nodes are small bean-shaped structures that are found throughout the body. They produce and store infection-fighting cells.)

- **Stage IV.** Cancer has spread beyond the urethra, vagina, and anus into the lining of the bladder (the sac that holds urine) and the bowel (intestine); or, it may have spread to the lymph nodes in the pelvis or to other parts of the body.

Vulvar Cancer

- **Recurrent.** Recurrent disease means that the cancer has come back (recurred) after it has been treated. It may come back in the vulva or another place.

Treatment Option Overview

How Cancer of the Vulva is Treated

There are treatments for all patients with cancer of the vulva. Three kinds of treatment are used: surgery (taking out the cancer in an operation) radiation therapy (using high-dose x-rays or other high-energy rays to kill cancer cells) chemotherapy (using drugs to kill cancer cells).

Surgery is the most common treatment for cancer of the vulva. Your doctor may take out the cancer using one of the following operations:

- Wide local excision takes out the cancer and some of the normal tissue around the cancer. This is usually done in a doctor's office.

- Radical local excision takes out the cancer and a larger portion of normal tissue around the cancer. Lymph nodes may also be removed.

- Laser surgery uses a narrow beam of light to remove cancer cells.

- **Skinning vulvectomy** takes out only the skin of the vulva that contains the cancer.

- **Simple vulvectomy** takes out the entire vulva, but no lymph nodes. **Partial vulvectomy** takes out less than the entire vulva. **Radical vulvectomy** takes out the entire vulva and the lymph nodes around it.

- If the cancer has spread outside the vulva and the other female organs, your doctor may take out the lower colon, rectum, or bladder (depending on where the cancer has spread) along with the cervix, uterus, and vagina (pelvic exenteration).

You may need to have skin from another part of your body added (grafted) and plastic surgery to make an artificial vulva or vagina after these operations.

Radiation therapy uses x-rays or other high-energy rays to kill cancer cells and shrink tumors. Radiation may come from a machine outside the body (external radiation) or from putting materials that contain radiation through thin plastic tubes into the area where the cancer cells are found (internal radiation). Radiation may be used alone or before or after surgery.

Chemotherapy uses drugs to kill cancer cells. Drugs may be given by mouth, or they may be put into the body by a needle in the vein or muscle. Chemotherapy is called systemic treatment because the drug enters the bloodstream, travels through the body, and can kill cancer cells throughout the body.

Treatment by Stage

Treatment for cancer of the vulva depends on the stage of your disease, the type of disease, your age, and your overall condition.

You may receive treatment that is considered standard based on its effectiveness in a number of patients in past studies, or you may choose to go into a clinical trial. Not all patients are cured with standard therapy and some standard treatments may have more side effects than are desired. For these reasons, clinical trials are designed to find better ways to treat cancer patients and are based on the most up-to-date information.

Stage 0 Vulvar Cancer. Your treatment may be one of the following:

- Wide local excision or laser surgery or a combination of both.

- Skinning vulvectomy.

- Ointment containing a chemotherapy drug.

Vulvar Cancer

Stage I Vulvar Cancer. Your treatment may be one of the following:

- Wide local excision.

- Radical local excision while taking out all nearby lymph nodes in the groin on the same side as the cancer.

- Radical vulvectomy and removal of the lymph nodes in the groin and upper part of the thigh on both sides of the body.

- Radiation therapy alone (in selected patients).

Stage II Vulvar Cancer. Your treatment may be one of the following:

- Radical vulvectomy and removal of the lymph nodes in the groin and upper part of the thigh on both sides of the body. Radiation may be given to the pelvis following the operation if cancer cells are found in the lymph nodes.

- Radiation therapy alone (in selected patients).

Stage III Vulvar Cancer. Your treatment may be one of the following:

- Radical vulvectomy and removal of the lymph nodes in the groin and upper part of the thigh on both sides of the body. Radiation may be given to the pelvis and groin following the operation if cancer cells are found in the lymph nodes or only to the vulva if the tumor is large but has not spread.

- Radiation therapy and chemotherapy followed by radical vulvectomy and removal of lymph nodes on both sides of the body.

- Radiation therapy (in selected patients) with or without chemotherapy.

Stage IV Vulvar Cancer. Your treatment may be one of the following:

- Radical vulvectomy and removal of the lower colon, rectum, or bladder (depending on where the cancer has spread) along with the uterus, cervix, and vagina (pelvic exenteration).

- Radical vulvectomy followed by radiation therapy.

- Radiation therapy followed by radical vulvectomy.

- Radiation therapy (in selected patients) with or without chemotherapy.

Recurrent Vulvar Cancer. If the cancer has come back, your treatment may be one of the following:

- Wide local excision with or without radiation therapy.

- Radical vulvectomy and removal of the lower colon, rectum, or bladder (depending on where the cancer has spread) along with the uterus, cervix and vagina (pelvic exenteration).

- Radiation therapy plus chemotherapy with or without surgery.

- Radiation therapy for local recurrences or to reduce symptoms such as pain, nausea, or abnormal body functions.

- Clinical trials of new forms of therapy.

Part Two

The Road to Recovery: Treatments, Therapies and Coping

Chapter 13

Questions to Ask Your Doctor About Breast Cancer

The following lists of questions will help you ask your doctor about breast cancer. Each list covers a different topic: The first three focus on breast cancer diagnosis—for women who find a lump in their breast, those who are scheduling a routine mammogram, and those who are undergoing a breast biopsy. The last 6 lists provide questions about breast cancer surgery, after surgery considerations, radiation therapy, chemotherapy, hormone therapy, and breast reconstruction .

A List of Questions Can Help

Many people feel intimidated in the doctor's office. They're not sure what questions to ask, or forget their questions when they are ready to ask them. These lists will remind you of important questions to ask, so that you won't have to rely on your memory.

Feel free to add or delete questions depending on your own situation.

Photocopy the lists, take them to the doctor's office with you, and bring a pen. Writing down the answers to your questions means you can reread and think about them later when you are at home.

Ask a family member or friend to go with you to the doctor, to take notes, ask more questions, and help you recall what was said.

National Cancer Institute, November 1991.

"Questions To Ask Your Doctor" was produced by the National Cancer Institute with assistance from the Komen Foundation, Dallas, TX.

For more information, call the National Cancer Institute's Cancer Information Service at 1-800-4-CANCER. CIS information specialists provide callers with information and free publications on all aspects of cancer and local cancer-related services. Spanish-speaking CIS staff are also available.

IF YOU FIND A LUMP IN YOUR BREAST

1. Will you refer me to a mammography facility for a mammogram?

2. Does the mammography facility meet quality standards?

3. Can this lump be aspirated (fluid or cells removed with a needle)?

4. Will you refer me to a doctor who specializes in breast problems for further tests and/or treatment?

ASK THESE QUESTIONS TO BE SURE THAT YOU'RE GETTING YOUR MAMMOGRAM AT A QUALITY FACILITY

(Choose a facility that answers YES to these 5 questions.)

1. Do you use machines specifically designed for mammography? (Note: These are called "dedicated" mammography machines. Do not choose a facility that uses a machine that also takes x-rays of the bones and other parts of the body.)

2. Is the person who provides the mammogram a registered technologist?

3. Is the radiologist who reads the mammograms specially trained to do so?

Questions to Ask Your Doctor About Breast Cancer

4. Does the facility provide mammograms as part of its regular practice? (Note: The American College of Radiology suggests choosing a facility that performs at least 10 mammograms per week.)

5. Is the mammography machine calibrated at least once a year?

Answers to these questions will help you prepare for the procedure and steps that will follow.

6. Is there anything I should do to prepare for my mammogram?

7. What will the mammogram show?

8. Who gets the report of my mammogram? Can it also be sent to other doctors who treat me?

9. How long will it take to receive the mammography report?

10. What are the next steps if my mammogram finds a problem?

ABOUT BREAST BIOPSY

Answers to these questions will help you understand the procedures involved.

1. What type of biopsy will I have? Why? Will the entire lump be removed or just part of it?

2. Can the lump be aspirated (the fluid drained or a small number of cells removed) with a needle? How reliable is a needle biopsy?

3. How long will the biopsy or aspiration take?

4. Will I be awake during the biopsy or aspiration and can it be done on an outpatient basis?

Answers to these questions will help you prepare for the results of the biopsy.

1. If I do have cancer, what other tests should I have?

2. Will estrogen or progesterone receptor tests be done on the biopsied tissue you remove? What will these tests tell you? Will other special tests (flow cytometry and other markers for tumor aggressiveness) be done on the tissue?

3. Will you do a two-step procedure? (With a two-step procedure, the patient is informed of treatment options after the biopsy results are available. Any further surgery is done as a separate procedure.)

4. How visible will the biopsy scar be?

5. Are there any after effects of a biopsy? If so, what are they?

6. After the biopsy, how soon will I know if I have cancer or not?

7. After a biopsy, if cancer is found, how much time can I take to decide what type of treatment to have?

WHEN BREAST CANCER IS DIAGNOSED

Answers to these questions will help you understand your diagnosis.

1. What did my biopsy or needle aspiration show?

2. What kind of breast cancer do I have?

Questions to Ask Your Doctor About Breast Cancer

3. What were the results of my estrogen and progesterone tests? What were the results of the other tests (flow cytometry and other markers of tumor aggressiveness)?

4. What tests will I have before surgery to see if the cancer has spread to any other organs (liver, lungs, bones)?

Answers to these questions will help you determine the best treatment for you.

1. What are my treatment options? What procedure are you recommending for me and why?

2. What are the potential risks and benefits of these procedures?

3. (Ask this question if tests were not done during the biopsy.) Will estrogen and progesterone receptor tests be done on the tissue removed during surgery? What will these tests tell you? Will other special tests (flow cytometry and other markers of tumor aggressiveness) be done on the tissue?

4. What is your opinion about breast-conserving surgery (lumpectomy) followed by radiation therapy? Am I a candidate for this type of treatment?

5. Will I need additional treatment with radiation therapy, chemotherapy, and/or hormonal therapy following my surgery? If so, can you refer me to a medical oncologist?

6. Can breast reconstruction be done at the time of the surgery, as well as later? Would you recommend it for me?

7. What potential risks and benefits are involved?

8. If I choose not to have reconstruction, how good are currently available breast prostheses?

9. How long do I have to make a treatment decision?

10. What is a clinical trial? Is there a clinical trial that is enrolling patients with my type of breast cancer? If so, how can I learn more?

11. Could you recommend a breast cancer specialist for a second opinion?

Answers to these questions will help you prepare for the results of your surgery.

1. Where will the surgical scar(s) be?

2. What side effects should I expect after the operation?

3. How should I expect to feel after the operation?

AFTER BREAST SURGERY

Answers to these questions will help you play an active role in your recovery.

1. Are there special exercises I should be doing? What type do you recommend? How long should I continue them?

2. Are there any precautions I should take? (For example, if lymph nodes were removed, should I avoid getting shots in that arm or shaving under that arm?)

3. When will I be able to get back to my normal routine?

4. What can I do to ensure a safe recovery?

5. What problems, specifically, should I report to you?

Questions to Ask Your Doctor About Breast Cancer

Answers to these questions will help you prepare for follow-up visits to the doctor.

1. If additional therapy is being considered, can you refer me to a medical oncologist?

2. When the additional therapy is completed, who will be responsible for my follow-up care? How often should I return for an exam? For lab tests or x-rays?

3. What tests will be done at these times?

4. What will the tests tell us?

ABOUT RADIATION THERAPY

Answers to these questions will help you understand the reason for radiation therapy.

1. Why is radiation therapy being recommended?

2. Do you think that the size, location, and type of breast cancer I have will respond to radiation therapy?

Answers to these questions will help you prepare for the treatment.

1. How long will each treatment take? How long will the whole series last?

2. How soon should treatment begin?

3. Who will be responsible for my radiation treatments? Who will administer them?

4. Where will these treatments be done?

5. Can I come alone or should a friend or relative accompany me?

Answers to these questions will help you prepare for the treatment's effects on your lifestyle.

1. What side effects should I expect and how long might they last?

2. What are the risks of this treatment?

3. What are the precautions or prohibitions during treatment? After treatment (skin creams, lotion, underarm shaving, etc.)?

4. Can I continue normal activities (work, sex, sports, etc.) during treatment? After treatment?

5. Will the costs of the treatment be covered by my health insurance?

6. How often are checkups and tests required after treatment is completed?

7. Will other therapies be needed?

ABOUT BREAST CANCER CHEMOTHERAPY

Answers to these questions will help you understand the reason for chemotherapy.

1. Why is chemotherapy indicated in my case?

2. What is the significance of lymph node involvement?

3. How many of my lymph nodes are involved?

4. If my lymph nodes are not involved, should chemotherapy or hormone therapy still be considered?

Questions to Ask Your Doctor About Breast Cancer

Answers to these questions will help you understand the drugs involved and their effects.

1. What drugs will I be taking?

2. Why have you chosen these particular drugs for me?

3. What are the drugs supposed to do?

4. What are the short and long-term risks involved?

5. What are the possible side effects of this type of chemotherapy? Are they permanent?

6. Which side effects should I report to the doctor immediately?

Answers to these questions will help you prepare for your treatment and follow-up.

1. How soon should the chemotherapy be started?

2. How and where will the chemotherapy be given?

3. How long will each treatment take? How long will the whole series last?

4. Can I continue to work, exercise, etc. during these treatments?

5. Will I need to be admitted to the hospital during the course of my chemotherapy?

6. Can I come alone for treatments or should a friend or relative accompany me?

7. Are there other special precautions I should take while on chemotherapy or afterwards?

8. Will treatments be covered by my health insurance?

9. If I lose my hair, will the cost of a wig be covered by health insurance?

10. When the treatments are completed, how often will I need to be seen by the oncologist?

ABOUT HORMONE THERAPY

Answers to these questions will help you understand the hormone treatment.

1. Which hormones are you recommending for me and why?

2. What are the hormones supposed to do?

3. What are the short and long-term side effects of this hormone treatment?

Answers to these questions will help you prepare for the treatment itself.

1. How soon should the hormone therapy be started? How long will I be taking the hormones?

2. In what form and how often will the treatment be given?

3. Will I be given the hormone therapy along with other forms of treatment?

4. Are the costs of the hormone treatment covered by my health insurance?

ABOUT RECONSTRUCTIVE BREAST SURGERY

Answers to these questions will help you understand reconstructive surgery.

1. What are the types of reconstructive surgery?

Questions to Ask Your Doctor About Breast Cancer

2. What type is best for me and why?

3. What chance is there of rejection and/or infection of any implant?

4. Are there any other risks or side effects to consider?

5. What can be done if the operation is unsuccessful?

6. When is the best time for me to have reconstruction—at the same time as the mastectomy? Some time after surgery? After chemotherapy?

7. If I do not choose reconstruction, what prostheses, or breast forms, are available?

Answers to these questions will help you prepare for your reconstruction and follow-up.

1. How many operations are needed? How long a hospital stay is necessary for each? How much time is needed for recovery after each? Are there any medications to avoid before surgery?

2. Is there much pain after surgery? For how long?

3. Are special bras needed after surgery? Where do I purchase them?

4. How can I expect the reconstruction to look and feel? How will the reconstructed breast compare in appearance with my healthy breast? Will anything need to be done to the healthy breast?

5. Will I be able to detect a possible recurrence after reconstructive surgery?

6. Will my health insurance cover this type of surgery?

Chapter 14

Progress Against Breast Cancer

Nineteen years ago, at the age of 43, Joyce Fine of Bethesda, Md., had a radical mastectomy to treat breast cancer. She didn't discuss her disease much with anyone then, except her husband.

Twenty years ago and more, Fine remembers, cancer was not talked about. "Everything was secretive then. Obituaries of people with cancer read that they died of 'a lingering illness.'" Fine thinks that her father's mother may have had breast cancer, but she's not sure. The impression came from a single conversation she happened to overhear.

A New Attitude

There is today an unprecedented openness about breast cancer. Along with strides in diagnosis and treatment have come long overdue changes in attitudes and awareness about the disease. Happy Rockefeller, Betty Ford, Nancy Reagan, Jill Eikenberry, Shirley Temple Black, Gloria Steinem, and many other public figures have come forward in recent years to tell about their experiences, bringing breast cancer out of the closet and offering women hope and encouragement. But it's certainly not just because of the celebrities that breast cancer has captured the public's attention. For a disease that strikes 1 in about 10 American women (the American Cancer Society

---

FDA Consumer Reprint September 1991 DHHS Pub No. FDA 91-1176.

puts the figure at 1 in 9) it's almost become a rarity not to know someone who has had breast cancer.

Since the early 1970s, according to the National Cancer Institute, the incidence of breast cancer has increased about 1 percent a year. In 1970, there were about 69,000 newly diagnosed cases, compared with 150,000 in 1990. The number of deaths rose from 30,000 in 1970 to 44,000 in 1990.

Although researchers have identified several risk factors for breast cancer and are gathering data on possible others, one thing that's clear is that no woman can afford to be complacent. That fact came home to Ellen Weinberg of Chevy Chase, Md., when she was diagnosed last December.

"I had no risk factors at all," she says. "There was no family history. My son was born when I was 27. I did not start menstruating especially early. I grew up in a house where my dad was diabetic and a little overweight, so I've always had a low-fat diet. There was just nothing. The one mistake I made was that I didn't have a mammogram. I knew I should start having them at 40, but I was only 42, I was very healthy, I had no risk factors, and I felt no urgency. I just hadn't gotten around to it."

Risks: The Known

Some risk factors for breast cancer are clearly established, as are some factors known to reduce the chance of developing the disease. Although the average lifetime risk of breast cancer for a woman is 1 in 10, the actual risk of getting it in any given year is less than 1 in 100. A woman's risk rises continuously with age, but never exceeds 1 percent a year.

Breast cancer is more common in women from North America and Northern Europe and in women of high socioeconomic status. In the United States, women of European Jewish descent also have an increased risk. Certain types of benign (noncancerous) breast disease, radiation exposure, and family history of the disease are also established risk factors. Also, among post-menopausal women, obesity is associated with an increase in risk.

Women whose mothers or sisters have had breast cancer have two to three times the usual risk of developing the disease. The risk is greatest if the relative developed breast cancer before menopause or if both breasts were involved. Nevertheless, only 10 to 15 percent of women with breast cancer have a family history of the disease. As NCI researcher Susan Bates, M.D., says, the statement, "There's no breast cancer in my family" should provide a woman no security whatsoever.

In the Nov. 30, 1990, issue of *Science*, Stephen H. Friend, M.D., Ph.D., of the Massachusetts General Hospital Cancer Center, reported that certain alterations in a gene called p53 lead to increased susceptibility to breast and certain other cancers, all occurring at unusually young ages. About 100 families around the world have been identified with this rare syndrome, named Li-Fraumeni for the two scientists who first described it in 1969. Followup of the four families originally identified revealed 16 new cancer cases when only one would have been expected.

The p53 gene is one of a few tumor suppressor genes researchers have identified. These genes act to control normal cell processes, and cancer results when the gene is missing or damaged and other genetic changes occur. The p53 gene is transmitted through the father's side of the family as well as the mother's.

Another genetic trait associated with breast cancer is wet ear wax. The breasts and the glands that produce ear wax are both apocrine glands. According to NCI's *Breast Cancer Digest*, women with wet ear wax are twice as likely to develop breast cancer as those with dry wax. Wet ear wax is a dominant genetic trait in the United States—85 percent of whites and virtually all blacks in this country have wet ear wax. In Asia, where wet ear wax is rare, breast cancer is also much less prevalent.

A link between radiation and breast cancer has been established from studies of survivors of Hiroshima and Nagasaki and from women who have undergone radiation therapy or had repeated fluoroscopy, which was used many years ago to treat tuberculosis. The interval between exposure and disease development varies, but, according to Bates, the average is 20 years.

Women who begin menstruating before age 12, become menopausal after age 50, delay childbearing until after age 30, or who bear no children are also at higher risk. On the other hand, the risk is lower in women who have their first child before age 18 and in women who, because of surgical removal of the ovaries, become menopausal before age 35.

Risks: The Unknown

Reserpine (a drug for high blood pressure), chemicals in hair dyes, alcohol consumption, dietary fat, use of birth control pills, and estrogen therapy have all been suggested as risk factors, but results from various studies have been contradictory, and their role in disease development remains controversial.

Some research has indicated that birth control pills might increase the risk of breast cancer, particularly in pre-menopausal women between the ages of 45 and 55, in women with a family history of breast cancer, or among young women who use them before the first pregnancy. One long-term study, however, reported that neither short-term nor long-term (more than 11 years) use appeared to increase risk, even in these groups of women. For now, the Food and Drug Administration requires that birth control pills carry a label indicating that the association between oral contraceptives and breast cancer is not clear.

Women who receive estrogen replacement therapy (ERT) may also be at increased risk. ERT is recommended for some menopausal women to counteract hot flashes and sweating and to slow bone thinning (osteoporosis). ERT may also confer protection from cardiovascular disease. A recently published study of 118,000 female nurses followed for 10 years found a "modest" increase in risk in current users—more so with increasing age—but not in past users, even if therapy had lasted more than 10 years. The researchers, led by Graham Colditz, M.B., B.S. (British equivalent of M.D.), of Brigham and Women's Hospital in Boston, concluded that, "Though this increase in risk will be counterbalanced by the cardiovascular benefits, [there is a] need for caution in the use of estrogens."

Of increasing interest is the possible relation of a high-fat diet to breast cancer. The death rate from breast cancer is highest in countries, including the United States, in which the intake of fat and animal protein is high. For instance, Japanese women historically have a low risk for breast cancer, but that risk has been rising dramatically, concurrent with a "Westernization" of eating habits—that is, from a low-fat to high-fat diet. Within Japan, the risk is 8.5 times higher for wealthier women, who eat meat daily, than among poorer women.

When large populations move from a low-incidence area to a high-incidence area and adopt the local lifestyle, they tend to take on the cancer risk patterns of their new homeland. Among immigrants from Asia to the United States, the incidence of breast cancer typically rises somewhat in the first generation, then continues to rise in subsequent generations until it approaches that of the United States.

A study involving nearly 57,000 women, published in the March 6, 1991, *Journal of the National Cancer Institute*, found an association between breast cancer and fat intake that, the authors say, "appears unlikely to have arisen by chance," even though the link is not strong and two previous studies contradict their results. It could be that the issue is muddled because the difference in fat content between the lower fat and higher fat diets of the women studied may not be great enough to influence breast cancer development. Americans typically consume 40 percent of their calories in fat. A reduction to 30 percent may not be significant in reducing breast cancer risk.

To examine the question further, NCI has approved funding for a 15-year trial that includes 24,000 women aged 50 to 69 who typically eat 38 percent of their calories from fat. Forty percent of the women will be taught how to follow a diet with only 20 percent of calories from fat, and the rest will follow their usual diet. The study will compare the incidence of breast cancer, colorectal cancer, heart disease and overall mortality between the two groups.

Meanwhile, Bates advises that, "although there is not a definitive answer to the dietary fat hypothesis, the link seems to be plausible, and efforts to alter our diet would appear prudent."

The Estrogen Connection

These risk factors may appear unrelated, but a possible common thread may be estrogen. Estrogen causes breast cells to grow, and there may be times in a woman's life when the breast is more susceptible to cancer-causing substances in the environment.

"Most of the risk factors listed can in some way increase the exposure to estrogen," says Bates. "A longer menstrual history, the additional estrogens from birth control pills or from estrogen replacement at menopause, even a high-fat diet, alcohol, or just being overweight may increase the amount of estrogen in the bloodstream, or may increase the amount available to the woman's breast tissue."

An American Cancer Society study published in 1982 analyzed the contribution of 10 common risk factors by following more than 365,000 white women 30 to 84 years old for six years. One telling conclusion was that three-quarters of all breast cancer cannot yet be attributed to any known specific causes. "From the point of view of the clinician," the authors state, "all women should be treated as being at appreciable risk for breast cancer."

Nevertheless, it is important to remember that having one or more risk factors does not mean that a woman is certain, or even likely, to develop breast cancer. It means only that she may be at statistically greater risk than another woman.

Despite the continuing rise in the incidence of breast cancer, the death rate has remained fairly stable over the past 50 years. This can be attributed largely to earlier detection.

Anatomy of a Disease

The breast is a gland designed to produce milk. Milk ducts leading to the nipple originate from lobules inside 15 or 20 lobes arranged like spokes around a wheel. The spaces around and between the milk-producing lobes are filled with fat. Ninety percent of breast cancers arise from the milk ducts. When ductal carcinoma, as it is called, remains confined to the duct, it is called *in situ*, or intraductal, cancer. When the cells penetrate the walls of the duct and invade surrounding tissue, it is called invasive ductal cancer. About 5 percent of breast cancers are lobular carcinomas, which originate in the lobules.

Two atypical kinds of breast cancers are inflammatory breast carcinoma and Paget's disease. Whereas most breast cancers are slow growing and painless, inflammatory breast carcinoma progresses very rapidly and is painful, with symptoms resembling an infection. The breast is warm and reddened, and the skin may appear pitted like an orange peel. In Paget's disease, the nipple becomes crusted; cancer cells grow upward along the ducts from a malignancy deeper in the breast.

When an abnormality is detected in the breast by mammography, the doctor may recommend a biopsy. If a lump is found by palpation (feeling the mass), a biopsy is almost always necessary, regardless of the results of mammography. Exceptions may be certain lumps found in women who have histories of lumpy or cystic breasts.

The biopsy—surgical removal of all or part of the lump or suspicious area—allows a pathologist to examine the tissue and determine with certainty whether or not the lesion is cancerous. Eighty percent of palpable lumps are benign (not cancerous).

Biopsy does not always require hospitalization. It can be done as an outpatient procedure. Also, some biopsies are done by fine needle aspiration, using a local anesthetic. The doctor inserts a needle into the lump and tries to withdraw fluid. If it is a cyst, it will collapse when the fluid is removed. If it is solid, the doctor may remove some cells with the needle to send to the laboratory for analysis.

The common practice nowadays is to do a biopsy first and then schedule surgery, if necessary, within the next few weeks. Some women may still opt for the one-step procedure that was routine when Joyce Fine had her mastectomy. (Until the late 1970s, it was standard procedure for the patient having a biopsy to sign a consent form permitting the surgeon to remove the breast at the same time if the tumor was found to be cancerous.)

The interval with the two-step procedure, however, allows the woman time to find out about and choose among her treatment options, get a second opinion, and prepare for her hospital stay. The brief delay in treatment does not reduce the chances for a successful outcome. Some states have passed laws requiring that women be told a two-step procedure is their legal right and, in some cases, that they be given specific information about their options.

Progress in Therapy

In a recent talk on breast cancer, NCI's Bates remarked, "It has been said that a woman must know more about her disease in breast cancer than a physician. With the array of choices currently facing a woman diagnosed with breast cancer, this is more true now than ever before."

The choices that Bates refers to were not available to Joyce Fine when she had her mastectomy—a Halsted radical. This entailed removing the entire breast, underlying chest muscles, all the axillary (underarm) lymph nodes, and some additional fat and muscle. Fine's surgeon did not discuss with her possible treatment alternatives. The Halsted radical was the standard treatment for breast cancer in 1972.

"There was no discussion," Fine recalls. "He convinced me I had to have the tumor out as soon as possible and that I should sign a release that if they find at biopsy that it's cancerous, they should remove it right away."

The surgeon acknowledged that Fine could have a two-step procedure. "But he said that if I go that way, it would metastasize [spread] and I couldn't be put under anesthesia again soon," she says. "It would be a waiting period of a couple weeks, and I was so frightened I said I'd do it in one procedure. He made me feel as though if I didn't. I might be dead in two weeks."

And so, like so many women with breast cancer then, Fine went into surgery not knowing if she would leave the hospital physically the same as she entered, or minus one breast as the result of extensive, disfiguring surgery. "Beginning in the 1940s, studies were suggesting that so much surgery was not necessary," says Bates. "In Europe, by 1971, smaller operations were accepted, but in the United States, change was slow in coming. Surgeons were reluctant to abandon the Halsted radical mastectomy for fear of giving inadequate treatment."

Treating Early-Stage Disease

Both the surgery and the process Fine experienced now belong to medical history. Surgical treatment now emphasizes breast conservation-preserving the breast when possible. Lumpectomy (also called segmental mastectomy or tylectomy), in which only the tumor and a margin of surrounding tissue is removed, is light years away from the Halsted radical, both in its physical and psychological effects.

Radical mastectomy was based on the rationale that breast cancer started with a tumor in the breast and, over time, spread in an orderly fashion to the lymph glands under the arms and then, through the lymph and blood to other parts of the body—usually the lungs, liver, bone, or brain. Halsted's procedure was designed to remove the avenues of possible spread.

By the late 1970s, experts had determined that the Halsted radical mastectomy was not necessary. As Bates says, "It was a consensus that less is more."

This conclusion was based on research that changed the concept of how breast cancer progresses. It is now understood that very early in the disease (although exactly how early is not known), breast cancer cells travel through the blood and lymph to other parts of the body. In this process, called micrometastasis, the cancer is so small it can't even be detected with a microscope. Treatment now emphasizes removing the tumor while sparing the breast and controlling metastasis with the use of additional therapy that may include radiation, chemotherapy (drugs that kill cancer cells), hormone therapy, or a combination.

As new approaches to surgical and medical treatment have been tried, each method has had its supporters and dissenters. In 1957, NCI organized the National Surgical Adjuvant Breast Project (NSABP) to create a pool of data gathered from research on breast cancer treatments. In the late 1970s, scientists reviewed study results and determined that simple, or total, mastectomy, in which only the breast was removed, was as effective as the Halsted radical.

Then, in 1990, at a National Institutes of Health consensus development conference on treatment of early-stage breast cancer, a panel of experts agreed that still less-extensive surgery, lumpectomy, gave the same results if radiation followed surgery to kill any remaining cancer cells. The lymph nodes are also removed for examination during this procedure.

The panel concluded that breast conservation treatment is not only appropriate for most women with early-stage disease but also "is preferable because it provides survival equivalent to total mastectomy and also preserves the breast. Total mastectomy remains an appropriate primary therapy when breast conservation is not indicated or selected."

"Despite nearly 20 years of studies showing that survival with lumpectomy and radiation is equivalent to that of mastectomy, only one-fifth of women eligible for lumpectomy have the procedure. This may be due in part to the slowness of some surgeons to accept and offer, without subtle or explicit bias, the newer procedure," says Bates.

Wendy Schain, Ed.D., a participant at the NIH conference and psychosocial director of adult oncology at the Memorial Cancer Institute in Long Beach, Calif., says that of the 14 most recent studies examining the psychosocial consequences of breast surgery, all showed that patients with breast conservation therapy had significantly improved body images compared with patients who underwent mastectomy.

"For most of the kinds of psychological symptoms we measure, there are not vast differences in magnitude between the two treatment groups," she says. "But the issues underlying the different symptoms are very dissimilar. The depression in mastectomy patients is due primarily to feelings of disfigurement and concern about the impact on intimate relationships, whereas the underlying reasons for depression in breast conservation are fatigue and loss of vitality.

"Chemotherapy, whether following mastectomy or lumpectomy, is the single most psychologically undermining course of treatment," says Schain. "It pervades all areas of well-being, both physical and psychological, ranging from feelings of lowered self-esteem to energy drain and other physical distresses."

Schain says that some patients with lumpectomy seem to have some increased anxiety about recurrence, but that the studies on this are "pretty much split and should not be interpreted to mean that the cosmetic benefits gained from breast conservation would be offset by increased fear of recurrence."

Many factors govern the patient's reaction, she says, and much depends on the individual's psychological defenses and interpretation of treatment outcome. For example, for one woman, treatment with lumpectomy helps minimize her concern about the disease because she is reassured by the less-extensive surgery. The continued presence of her breast increases her comfort and reduces her fear. But another woman may react to the preserved breast with a concern over whether or not "they got it all."

Women who have multicentric breast cancer (cancers that develop at several locations within a single breast), or whose tumors are large relative to breast size and therefore would not have a good cosmetic result, are among those who may not be candidates for breast conservation.

No single procedure can be recommended as ideal for all patients. Women and their surgeons must base their decisions on the patient's medical status and her particular concerns. Her choice may be influenced by emotional considerations, finances, access to care, body image, and personal beliefs.

Adjuvant Therapy

Following either mastectomy or lumpectomy with radiation, additional (adjuvant) therapy is given to most women whose cancer has spread to the lymph nodes. This may be chemotherapy or hormone therapy, or both. A current controversy in treatment concerns whether or not to treat node-negative breast cancer patients (patients in whom the disease has not spread to the lymph nodes) with adjuvant therapy. Seven of ten node-negative women will never have a recurrence of disease. Of the remaining three, standard adjuvant therapy will prevent recurrence in one. Unfortunately, there is no way yet to predict which three will have a recurrence, nor which one of those will be helped by adjuvant treatment. The dilemma, says Bates, is, "Do we treat ten to help one, and potentially three, if our treatments can improve?"

The NIH consensus panel concluded that, "The decision to use adjuvant treatment [in node-negative patients] should follow a thorough discussion with the patient regarding the approximate risk of relapse without adjuvant therapy, toxicities of therapy, and its impact on quality of life." They further agreed that, except for patients in clinical trials, "it is reasonable not to employ adjuvant therapy in patients with tumors 1 centimeter or smaller because their chance of recurrence is less than 10 percent in 10 years." For patients with larger tumors, other predictors of recurrence should be considered.

Drug Therapy

Many drugs have been tried alone and in combination to find the best regimen to treat breast cancer. Cancer drugs can have serious side effects. They are designed to kill cancer cells, but they also affect other rapidly growing cells, such as blood-forming cells and those that line the digestive tract. As a result, they may lower resistance to infection, sap energy, and cause bruising or bleeding, nausea, vomiting, mouth sores, loss of appetite, hair loss, and other side effects. Premenopausal women may also experience hot flashes, vaginal dryness, painful intercourse, and irregular menstrual periods.

For Ellen Weinberg, the choice of treatment came with the chemotherapy, not surgery. (Because her cancer was multicentric, Weinberg had a total mastectomy.) She saw two oncologists about adjuvant therapy and got two different opinions.

"That's really where I was hoping there would be no discrepancy—that both would say the same thing. But of course they didn't," she says. One recommended CMF—a combination of cyclophosphamide (Cytoxan), methotrexate, and 5-fluorouracil. The second oncologist told her about CMF and another regimen, CAF, which uses doxorubicin hydrochloride (Adriamycin) instead of methotrexate. "He said that CMF would be fine for me and that CAF was a more aggressive treatment—that I would probably have more severe side effects with it—but he described adriamycin as having a very good track record."

Weinberg chose the CAF. "I knew I was buying myself a whole lot of trouble short-term, and I didn't know if the result was going to be any different long-term. And everyone said the prognosis was real good anyway. It was a sort of agony, but I came to that decision and I felt very comfortable with it."

Side effects of chemotherapy vary with each patient, according to the treatment given and the individual's reaction. Weinberg, who has had three of six treatments so far, says that for her, it is like being very sick with the flu. "You feel hot, cold, very lethargic, you get strange tingles and pains. Some people get achy. I feel toxic. I can't describe it any other way." She also had severe vomiting after the first treatment, but less so with the second, when she was given Marinol (oral marijuana derivative) to help reduce the vomiting. With the third treatment, Weinberg was given ondansetron hydrochloride (Zofran), which FDA had just approved (in March 1991) to combat nausea and vomiting associated with cancer chemotherapy. With Zofran, she didn't vomit at all, but the other side effects remained.

Hormone therapy, usually in the form of a drug called tamoxifen (Nolvadex), is most often given to women whose cancer cells are estrogen-receptor positive. Tamoxifen blocks estrogen from binding to the cell's receptors for that hormone, thus keeping the cells from getting the hormones they need to grow. Originally approved by FDA in 1977 for patients with advanced breast cancer and subsequently for patients with less severe disease, tamoxifen was approved for use in node-negative patients in June 1990. Hormone therapy can also produce a number of side effects, but they are usually not severe. They may include symptoms of menopause, such as hot flashes, missed periods, and vaginal dryness.

Tamoxifen is also being studied in England as a preventive agent for breast cancer, and a similar study is planned in the United States. NCI is funding an NSABP study, which will be designed to test the effectiveness of this drug in preventing a first occurrence of breast cancer. The study will eventually include about 16,000 women at high risk for the disease.

Treating Advanced Disease

Breast cancer that has advanced to Stage III or IV (see "Determining Therapy" below) requires chemotherapy or hormone therapy, or both, to treat its spread. Treatment may also include surgery or radiation therapy, or both, to control the breast tumor. Hormone therapy may be accomplished with drugs such as tamoxifen or, in premenopausal women, by removing the hormone-producing ovaries. Women whose cancer has spread beyond the breast to other parts of the body usually have less-extensive breast surgery, but receive hormonal therapy or more aggressive chemotherapy directed to treating both local and metastatic disease. If necessary, radiation may be used for local control.

Most tumors eventually develop drug resistance. New treatments under study for patients with advanced breast cancer involve removing some of the patient's bone marrow and administering high-dose chemotherapy to overcome drug resistance. This is followed by reinfusing the bone marrow to prevent life-threatening drug toxicity. This therapy is also being tried in patients at high risk of disease recurrence.

Other means of reversing drug resistance with various agents are under study. One such agent, verapamil (approved for treating high blood pressure), has been shown in laboratory studies to block a cell surface protein that pumps chemotherapy drugs out of a cell, thereby making it drug resistant.

Fortunately, most breast cancers are now detected at the earlier, more treatable stages. (See "Determining Therapy" below.) Seventy-five to 80 percent of women diagnosed with breast cancer in 1990 had small, localized tumors, and about two-thirds of those had no lymph node involvement. According to the American Cancer Society, the five-year survival rate for localized breast cancer has risen from 78 percent in the 1940s to 91 percent today.

Scientists are continually researching more effective treatments for both early and advanced breast cancer. It is important to remember that cancer risk and survival statistics are averages based on large numbers of people. The chance of developing breast cancer is unique to each individual, as is the chance of recovery of any given patient.

NCI's Bates sums up: "For the medical community, the direction is clear-research. For women, the direction is also clear-take charge. Eat right, avoid a diet and a lifestyle that might increase your risk of cancer. At the age of 40 begin to get mammograms and get them on schedule."

Determining Therapy

Treatment is based on the extent of the disease and the biology of the specific tumor. Evaluation of these factors guides the approach to surgery and, if needed, adjuvant therapy. In addition, a woman's age and menopausal status are significant. Breast cancer tends to be more aggressive in younger, pre-menopausal women.

First, based on tumor size and degree of metastasis, the disease is classified into one of the following stages:

- Carcinoma *in situ*: Very early breast cancer that has not invaded nearby tissues.

- Stage I: The tumor is localized and no larger than 2 centimeters (about 1 inch).

- Stage II: The tumor is no larger than 2 cm, but the cancer has spread to the underarm lymph nodes, or the cancer is between 2 and 5 cm (about 2 inches) and may or may not have spread to the lymph nodes, or the cancer is bigger than 5 cm, but has not spread to the lymph nodes.

- Stage III: The tumor is larger than 5 cm and has spread to underarm lymph nodes, or the tumor is smaller than 5 cm and the underarm lymph nodes have grown into other tissues, or the tumor has spread to tissues near the breast (such as the chest muscles and ribs) or to lymph nodes near the collarbone, or it is inflammatory breast cancer. (Inflammatory breast cancer is fast-progressing with infection-like symptoms in which the skin is warm and reddened and may appear pitted.)

- Stage IV: The cancer has spread to other organs of the body, usually the lungs, liver, bone, or brain.

Carcinoma *in situ* has a cure rate approaching 100 percent with surgery alone. Tumors of 1 cm or less also carry a particularly good prognosis—less than 10 percent recurrence in 10 years. In general, the risk of recurrence rises with increasing tumor size and lymph node involvement.

Breast tumor tissue can be examined for important "markers" that give clues to the aggressiveness of the disease and can, therefore, help guide therapy. Some of these markers are:

- Estrogen and progesterone receptors. Patients whose cancer cells have proteins (receptors) to which these hormones bind have a better prognosis because the cells can be treated with hormone therapy.

- Histologic type. Breast cancers vary in their cell type. For example, invasive ductal cancers can sometimes be categorized into further subtypes, such as mucinous, tubular and medullary. Lobular cancers are another cell type. The various types have different rates of growth and metastasis.

- DNA studies. The degree of disruption of DNA in the cell nucleus correlates with the disease aggressiveness. The more disarrayed the DNA, the greater the risk of relapse. Also, cells that divide more rapidly carry a poorer prognosis.

- HER-2 oncogene. This gene is sometimes found in tumors of patients whose cancer has spread. Detected early, it could predict metastasis and identify patients who would benefit from more aggressive treatment.

- Cathepsin D. High levels of this protein are associated with a poorer prognosis. Secreted by the cancer cells, cathepsin D may aid their spread to other parts of the body.

Reconstruction Options

Breast reconstruction after mastectomy used to be very complex, and the results were often disappointing. So, as recently as the 1960s, few women chose to have it done. Many were not aware it was a possibility. Since then, however, advances in plastic surgery have made breast reconstruction easier, more successful, and more popular.

Not every woman who has had a mastectomy chooses reconstruction. Some women decide against it because they don't want to have any more surgery or they feel the risks outweigh the benefits or for other reasons. Many women prefer to wear breast forms (prostheses).

For women who desire reconstruction, however, the option is now available with few limitations. Even women who have had radical surgery or whose skin has been grafted, damaged by radiation therapy, or is otherwise thin or tight can have successful reconstructive surgery.

Although some women have breast reconstruction during the same surgery as their mastectomy, many surgeons recommend waiting three to six months. This allows time to complete radiation or chemotherapy and for the mastectomy incision to heal.

There are three major types of breast reconstruction. "Simple" reconstruction uses a silicone gel breast implant. It is usually done in patients who have healthy chest muscles to support the reconstructed breast and enough good skin to cover the implant. "Latissimus dorsi" and "rectus abdominus" are used in patients with more extensive loss of muscle and skin. This situation is less common with the trend to less radical surgeries.

"Simple" Implant Placement

This operation takes one to two hours. It is usually done under general anesthesia, but local anesthesia is sometimes used and it can be done as outpatient surgery. A small incision is made along the lower portion of the breast near the mastectomy scar, and the implant is inserted in the pocket created under the chest muscle. A drain may be inserted temporarily to remove excess fluid. If the surgeon is able to make the reconstruction incision in the original mastectomy scar, there will be no additional scarring. In fact, the appearance of the mastectomy scar can be improved, but not eliminated, during this operation.

Silicone breast implants have been in use since the 1960s. As of 1989, about 2 million women have had them implanted—about one-fourth for reconstruction after mastectomy. (The rest have been for cosmetic surgery to augment or change the shape of the woman's natural breast.)

Many women have been highly satisfied with the appearance, size, and softness of their reconstructed breasts and have reported a number of psychological benefits. Some women, however, have had problems with the implants, prompting concern about their safety.

The most common problem associated with breast implants is capsular contracture. This occurs when scar tissue shrinks around the implant, making it feel hard and sometimes misshaping it. Other known health risks include false mammography results, infection, silicone leakage and migration to other parts of the body, and implant rupture. There have also been questions raised about the possibility of long-term risks that may include some immune reactions and carcinogenicity (ability to cause cancer). Experts are divided on these questions.

Silicone gel implants have been marketed under a "grandfather" clause in the Medical Device Amendments of 1976 which exempted them from standard pre-market approval. Because of the safety issues, FDA in June 1988 classified the implants into Class III—giving the agency authority to request safety and effectiveness data after 30 months. In April 1991 FDA published a final regulation requiring submission of the data.

The agency has received 1,200 comments about the benefits and risks of the devices and, although the comments varied, a significant number of women proposed that the implants remain available as long as consumers are fully informed of the potential risks.

Women who are considering breast reconstruction with silicone gel implants should discuss any concerns they may have with their plastic surgeons and possibly other health professionals, consumer groups, and women who have had the surgery. They can also ask the plastic surgeon for the printed information that comes in the implant package.

Latissimus Dorsi

"Latissimus dorsi" reconstruction gets its name from the broad flat back muscle that the surgeon moves to the chest to take the place of muscles that have been removed during the mastectomy. The surgeon also transfers skin and other tissue from the patient's back to the mastectomy site. An implant is then placed under the new muscle, and drains may be inserted temporarily. This operation takes longer and requires longer hospitalization than simple reconstruction. It leaves a scar on the back in addition to the mastectomy scar on the chest.

Rectus Abdominus

In this procedure, the surgeon transfers one of the two rectus abdominus muscles (the parallel vertical abdominal muscles) to the breast area, along with skin and fat from the abdomen. The surgeon shapes this flap of muscle, skin and fat into the contour of a breast. If there is enough abdominal tissue available, no implant is needed. One of the "side effects" of this procedure, which some might consider a benefit, is a tightening of the stomach, colloquially called a "tummy tuck." This procedure leaves a horizontal scar across the lower abdomen in addition to the mastectomy scar.

Nipple and Areola Construction

Breast reconstruction fashions the shape of the breast but does not always include a reconstructed nipple and areola (the dark skin around the nipple). Some women, who wish primarily to improve their appearance in clothing, choose not to have the additional one- to two-hour operation to reconstruct the nipple and areola. During this operation, the areola is most commonly fabricated from skin on the upper thigh or from behind the ear, and the nipple is created either from tissue from the newly created breast mound or from the other nipple. Skin from the vaginal lips can also be used to reconstruct the nipple and areola. If the reconstructed areola is not dark enough, ultraviolet light can be used to darken the skin.

Although breast reconstruction offers a more normal appearance both in and out of clothes, women should be aware that if there are scars from these operations they are permanent and that reconstruction does not restore lost sensation.

—by Marian Segal

Marian Segal is a member of FDA's public affairs staff.

Chapter 15

Breast Cancer: Understanding Treatment Options

As recently as a decade ago, most doctors considered removal of the breast the only treatment for breast cancer. The most common procedure was a radical mastectomy, the removal of the entire breast, the chest muscles under the breast, and the underarm lymph nodes. Breast cancer treatment almost always caused women serious physical and emotional trauma. Many women feared the treatment as much as the disease.

Today, radical mastectomies are rarely done. There has been much progress in the early identification and treatment of breast cancer. Beginning with the time a breast lump is found, women have a number of treatment options. As developments occur, doctors are continuing to learn about the advantages and disadvantages of these different treatments. Because of the different stages at which breast cancer is diagnosed, there is no one treatment that is best for all women.

If you discover a lump in your breast or if your doctor suspects you have breast cancer, now is the time to learn about the various treatments available, as well as their risks and benefits. This chapter will help you get started. The options available to you will depend on a number of factors, including the type of tumor, the extent of the disease at the time of diagnosis, your age, and your medical history. But your personal feelings about the treatment, your self-image, and your lifestyle will also be important considerations in your doctor's assess-

---

NIH 91-2675.

ment and recommendations. You and your doctor should discuss these treatment methods and how they apply to your situation.

Right now, you may be asking yourself, "Why me?" Cancer has suddenly intruded on your life and threatened your health and well-being. You don't have to lose control of your personal health, however. You can continue to take care of yourself by working in partnership with the health care professionals responsible for your treatment and safe recovery. By becoming informed, asking questions, and participating in treatment decisions, you can have a positive influence on your own well-being.

Biopsy: Learning If You Have Breast Cancer

If you have noticed a lump or other change in your breast, your doctor may recommend several tests to determine if you have cancer. After taking your medical history and performing a manual breast exam, your doctor may recommend a breast x-ray or mammogram. If the lump is suspected to be a cyst, your doctor may use a needle to drain fluid from the lump. Another test is a biopsy, in which tissue is removed and examined under a microscope by a pathologist. Part or all of the lump is removed under local or general anesthesia. Biopsy is the only certain way to diagnose breast cancer.

During the biopsy procedure, the surgeon removes the suspicious tissue and sends it to the pathology department to be analyzed. The pathologist will examine the tissue to see if it is benign or malignant. If it is malignant, the pathologist will try to identify the type of cancer cells present, how fast they reproduce, if the blood vessels or lymph system contains cancer cells, and if the cancer's growth is affected by hormones. All of this information allows your doctor to determine the best treatment for you.

There are two ways that a pathologist prepares the tissue for examination: a "frozen section," which is a quick procedure that takes about 30 minutes, and a "permanent section," which takes a day or two. The frozen section is a quick way of determining whether or not cancer is present. The permanent section is the most accurate method.

The Frozen Section

The frozen section is done while the patient is in the operating room; the surgeon does not continue the operation until the pathologist reports the results from the frozen section.

In the frozen section, the pathologist cuts thin slices of tissue and fast-freezes them to be able to look quickly at the tissue. The disadvantage of the frozen section is that the freezing process distorts the cells and the method is not always accurate.

The Permanent Section

The permanent section takes longer than a frozen section, usually a day or two. In this process, the tissue is treated by a series of chemical solutions that give a high-quality slide. The advantage of this process is that it is more accurate and allows the pathologist to make a more correct diagnosis. Permanent sections are always performed, even if a frozen section is done too.

If your lump is cancer, estrogen and progesterone receptor assay tests may be performed. These tests will determine if hormone treatment may benefit you.

Other diagnostic procedures may be performed including special blood tests, additional x-rays, radioisotope scans, and/or computerized body scans.

There are two basic options for having a biopsy: the one-step and the two-step procedures. In this procedure, biopsy, diagnosis of cancer, and breast removal are completed in a single operation.

The One-Step Procedure

With this procedure, you and your doctor must agree before surgery that your breast will be removed if the lump is cancerous. Your doctor will explain the full details of a mastectomy (surgical removal of the breast) before biopsy, even though the lump may not be cancerous. In the past, the one-step procedure was thought to be the best way to treat breast cancer. However, studies have shown that treatment can safely follow a biopsy by a week or two, even if the lump is cancerous.

The Two-Step Procedure

This method involves biopsy on one day; then, if the lump is cancerous, the treatment takes place within a couple of weeks. In many cases, the biopsy can be done on an outpatient basis, and it may be possible to perform the biopsy under local, rather than general, anesthesia. The short time between biopsy and treatment (which will not reduce the chances for success) allows time to examine the permanent section slides, to perform additional tests to determine the extent of the disease, to discuss treatment options, to gain another medical opinion, to make home and work arrangements, and to prepare emotionally for the treatment.

If you are going to have a biopsy, discuss these procedures with your doctor. The two of you can decide which option is best for you. Additional information about biopsy can be found in *Breast Biopsy: What You Should Know*, a National Cancer Institute booklet. *(This pamphlet is reproduced in this sourcebook. See the index or the table of contents for the page reference.)*

Breast Surgery

Mastectomy is the medical term for surgical removal of the breast. It refers to a number of different operations, ranging from those that remove the breast, chest muscles, and underarm lymph nodes, to those that remove only the breast. Other kinds of surgery remove only the breast lump.

The different types of breast surgery are described below. Based on the size and location of the lump, your doctor will recommend the type of surgery that offers you the best chance of successful treatment.

Most medical and surgical procedures carry some risk. The risk may be small or serious, frequent or rare. Because there is such a wide range of potential risks and benefits from the various treatments for the different stages and kinds of breast cancer, you should discuss with your doctor the particular benefits and risks of the treatment methods suitable for you.

Radical Mastectomy

This type of surgery removes the breast, the chest muscles, all of the underarm lymph nodes, and some additional fat and skin. It is also called a "Halsted radical" (after the surgeon who developed the procedure). A radical mastectomy was the standard treatment for breast cancer for more than 70 years and is still used today for some women.

Breast Cancer: Understanding Treatment Options

Advantages. Cancer can be completely removed if it has not spread beyond the breast or nearby tissue. Examination of the lymph nodes provides information that is important in planning future treatment.

Disadvantages. Removes the entire breast and chest muscles, and leaves a long scar and a hollow chest area. May cause lymphedema (swelling of the arm), some loss of muscle power in the arm, restricted shoulder motion, and some numbness and discomfort. Breast reconstruction is also more difficult.

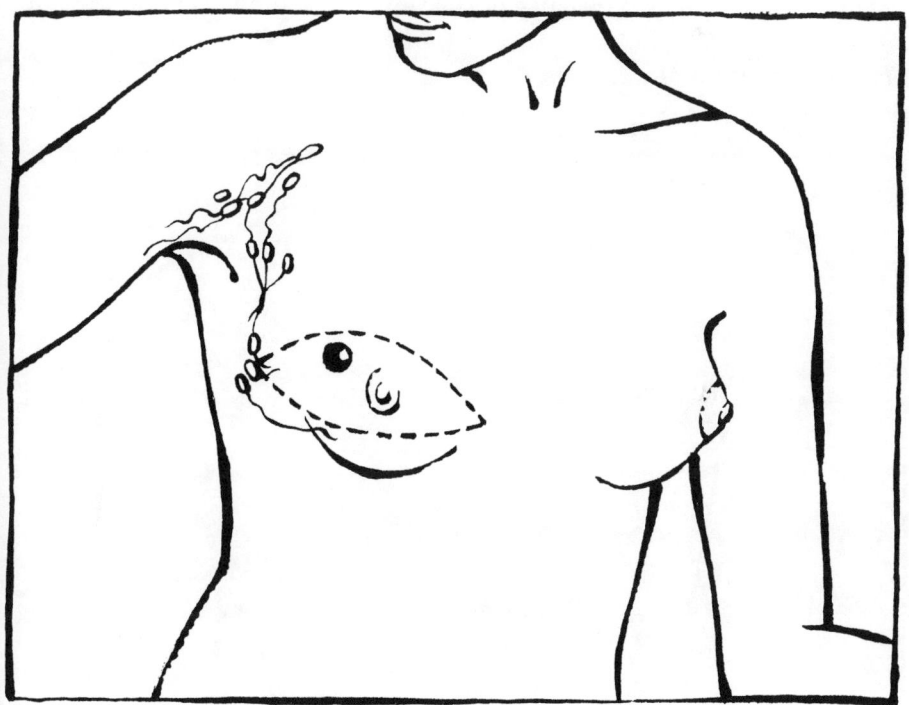

Figure 15.1. Radical Mastectomy

Modified Radical Mastectomy

This procedure removes the breast, the underarm lymph nodes, and the lining over the chest muscles. Sometimes the smaller of the two chest muscles is also removed. This procedure is also called "total mastectomy with axillary (or underarm) dissection" and today is the most common treatment of early stage breast cancer.

Advantages. Keeps the chest muscle and the muscle strength of the arm. Swelling is less likely, and when it occurs it is milder than the swelling that can occur after a radical mastectomy. Leaves a better appearance than the radical. Survival rates are the same as for the radical mastectomy when cancer is treated in its early stages. Breast reconstruction is easier and can be planned before surgery.

Disadvantages The breast is removed. In some cases, there may be swelling of the arm because of the removal of the lymph nodes.

Total or Simple Mastectomy

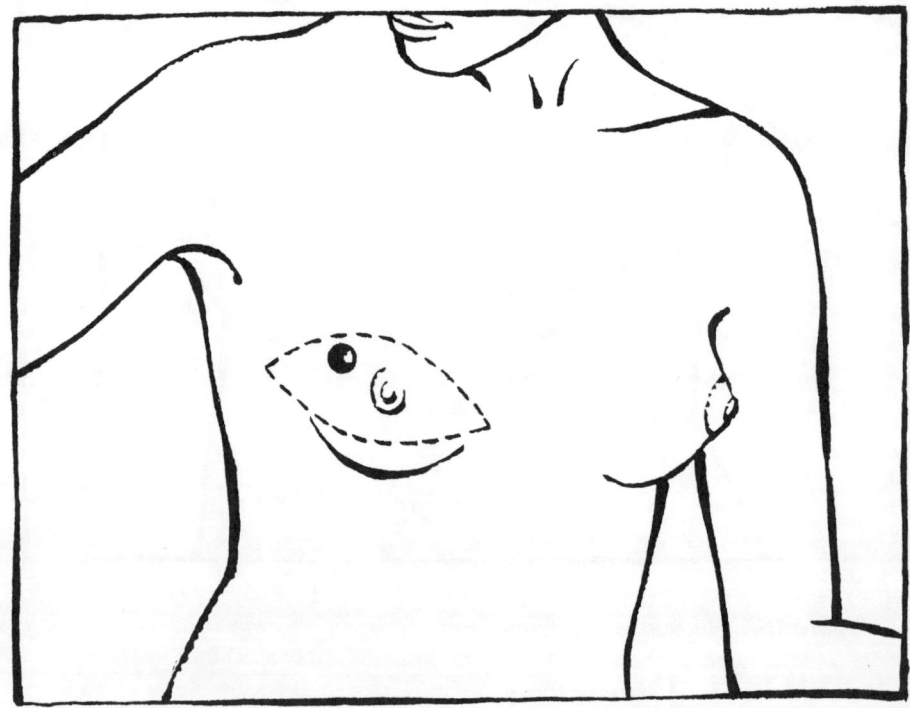

Figure 15.2. Total or Simple Mastectomy

This type of surgery removes only the breast. Sometimes a few of the underarm lymph nodes closest to the breast are removed to see if the cancer has spread beyond the breast. It may be followed by radiation therapy.

Advantages. Chest muscles are not removed and arm strength is not diminished. Most or all of the underarm lymph nodes remain, so the risk of swelling of the arm is greatly reduced. Breast reconstruction is easier.

Disadvantages. The breast is removed. If cancer has spread to the underarm lymph nodes, it may remain undiscovered.

Partial or Segmental Mastectomy

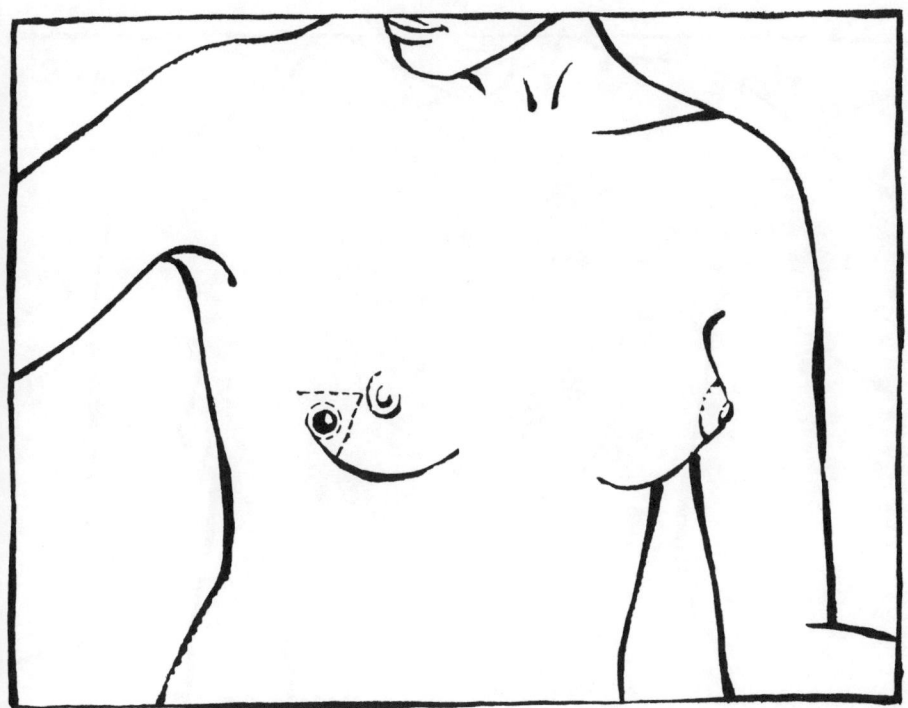

Figure 15.3. Partial or Segmented Mastectomy

This procedure removes the tumor plus a wedge of normal tissue surrounding it, including some skin and the lining of the chest muscle below the tumor. It is followed by radiation therapy. Many surgeons also remove some or all of the underarm lymph nodes to check for possible spread of cancer.

Advantages. If a woman is large-breasted, most of the breast is preserved. There is little possibility of loss of muscle strength or arm swelling.

Disadvantages. If a woman has small or medium sized breasts, this procedure will noticeably change the breast's shape. There is a possibility of arm swelling.

Lumpectomy

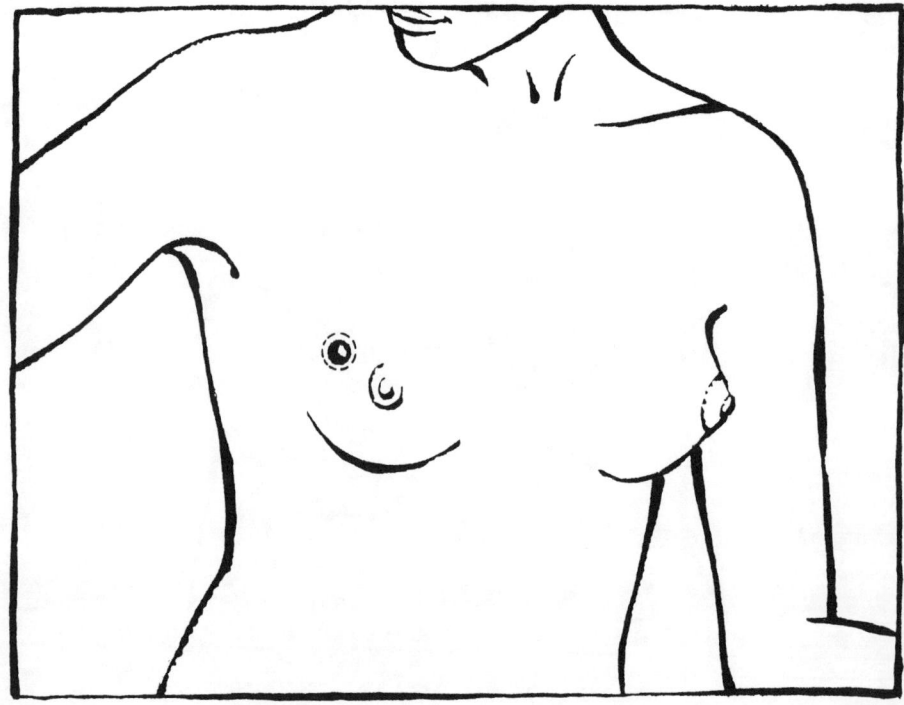

Figure 15.4. Lumpectomy

Breast Cancer: Understanding Treatment Options

Lumpectomy removes only the breast lump and is followed by radiation therapy. Many surgeons also remove and test some of the underarm lymph nodes for possible spread of cancer.

Advantages. The breast is not removed.

Disadvantages Small-breasted women with large lumps may have a significant change in breast shape. Scar tissue from the treatment may make it more difficult to examine the breast later. There is a possibility of arm swelling.

For more information, see the section "Mastectomy: A Treatment for Breast Cancer" in this sourcebook.

A Word About Breast Reconstruction

As you consider mastectomy as a treatment option, you should be aware of breast reconstruction, a way to recreate the breast's shape after a natural breast has been removed. This procedure is gaining in popularity, although many women are still unaware of it.

Today, almost any woman who has had a mastectomy can have her breast reconstructed. Successful reconstruction is no longer hampered by radiation-damaged, thin, or tight skin, or the absence of chest muscles.

Reconstruction is not for everyone, however. And it may not be right for you. After mastectomy, many women prefer to wear artificial breast forms inside their brassieres.

Both a general surgeon and a plastic surgeon may help you decide whether to have breast reconstruction. If possible, you should discuss breast reconstruction before your surgery because the position of the incision may affect the reconstruction procedure. However, many women consider the option of reconstruction only after surgery.

Radiation Therapy

Radiation therapy as primary treatment is a promising technique for women who have early stage breast cancer. This procedure allows a woman to keep her breast and involves lumpectomy followed by radiation (x-ray) treatment.

Once a biopsy has been done and breast cancer has been diagnosed, radiation treatment usually involves the following steps:

- Surgery to remove some or all of the underarm lymph nodes to see if the cancer has spread beyond the breast;

- External radiation therapy to the breast and surrounding area; and

- "Booster" radiation therapy to the biopsy site. For external radiation therapy, a machine beams x-rays to the breast and possibly the underarm lymph nodes. The usual schedule for radiation therapy is 5 days a week for about 5 weeks. In some instances, a "booster" or concentrated dose of radiation may be given to the area where the cancer was located. This can be done with an electron beam or internally with an implant of radioactive materials.

If you are having radiation therapy as primary treatment for early stage breast cancer, it should be done by a qualified, board-certified radiation therapist who is experienced in this form of treatment.

Advantages. The breast is not removed. Lumpectomy with radiation therapy as a primary treatment for breast cancer currently appears to be as effective as mastectomy for treating early stage breast cancer. Because this is a new treatment procedure, researchers are continuing to collect information on long-term results. Usually there is not much deformity of surrounding tissues. This skin usually regains a normal appearance after treatment is completed.

Disadvantages. A full course of treatment requires short daily visits to the hospital as an outpatient for about 5 weeks, as well as hospitalization for a few days if implant radiation therapy is used. Treatment may produce a skin reaction like a sunburn, and may cause tiredness. Itching or peeling of the skin may also occur. Radiation therapy can sometimes cause a temporary decrease in white blood cell count, which may increase the risk of infection.

Adjuvant Therapy

Recent studies have shown that women with early stage breast cancer may benefit from adjuvant (additional) therapy following primary treatment (mastectomy or lumpectomy with radiation therapy). These studies indicate that many breast cancer patients whose underarm lymph nodes show no sign of cancer (known as node negative) may benefit from chemotherapy or hormonal therapy after primary treatment. (These findings do not apply to women with preinvasive or *in situ* breast cancer.)

Until now, women whose underarm lymph nodes were free of cancer usually received no additional therapy because they have a relatively good chance of surviving the disease after primary treatment. But scientists know that cancer may return in about 30 percent of these women. Adjuvant therapy may prevent or delay the return of cancer.

Based on these findings, the National Cancer Institute has alerted doctors to consider using adjuvant therapy for their node negative breast cancer patients. Although there is strong evidence of the benefits of adjuvant therapy, there also are certain risks and expenses. Therefore, each woman should discuss her treatment options with her doctor.

The Breast Cancer Treatment Team

During your treatment you are likely to meet several health professionals who will perform the various tests and treatments your doctor recommends. It may be difficult at first to talk with them about your illness and your feelings about treatment. But each of them can offer information to help you feel more at ease. By talking with the professionals who care for you, you will come to understand more about cancer and its treatment and be better able to cope.

These are some of the specialists you may meet or hear about:

- **Anesthesiologist.** A doctor who administers drugs or gases to put you to sleep before surgery.

- **Clinical nurse specialist.** A nurse with special knowledge in a particular area, such as post-operative care or radiation therapy.

- **Medical oncologist.** A doctor who administers anticancer drugs or chemotherapy.

- **Pathologist.** A doctor who examines tissue removed by biopsy to see if the tissue is cancer.

- **Personal physician.** Your doctor, who will be responsible for coordinating your treatment and working with you to ensure that treatment is satisfactory. Your personal physician may be a surgeon, radiation oncologist, medical oncologist, or family physician.

- **Physical therapist.** A specialist who helps in rehabilitation after surgery by using exercise, heat, light, and massage.

- **Plastic surgeon.** A doctor who specializes in rehabilitative and cosmetic surgery. Plastic surgeons perform breast reconstruction.

- **Radiation oncologist.** A doctor who supervises radiation therapy.

- **Radiation therapy technologist.** A specially trained technician who helps the radiation oncologist give external radiation treatments.

- **Surgeon.** A doctor who performs surgery, such as biopsy and mastectomy.

Informed Consent: When Surgery is Recommended

When surgery is recommended, most health care facilities require patients to sign a form stating their willingness to permit diagnosis and medical treatment. This certifies that you understand what procedures will be done and that you have consented to have them performed.

Breast Cancer: Understanding Treatment Options

Before consenting to any course of treatment, ask your doctor for information on:

- The recommended procedure;
- Its purpose;
- Risks and side effects associated with it;
- Likely consequences with and without treatment;
- Other available alternatives; and
- Advantages and disadvantages of one treatment over another.

You are likely to discover that your anxiety over treatment decreases as your understanding of breast cancer and its treatment increases. Important decisions are always hard to make, particularly when they concern your health.

However, there are a number of things you can do to make decisions about breast cancer treatment easier. One is gathering information. You can:

- Talk with your doctor. There are a number of treatments that may be used for breast cancer. To make sure you will be comfortable with your decision to have a particular treatment, you may want to get another medical opinion.

- Gather additional information from published reports. Many articles and books have been written about breast cancer for patients and professionals. There is also much information available about cancer in general. Reading materials are available at local libraries and may be available through local offices of the American Cancer Society.

- Call the Cancer Information Service (CIS). This program, sponsored by the National Cancer Institute, is available to answer questions about cancer from the public, cancer patients and their families, and health professionals. Call this toll-free number and you will automatically be connected to the CIS office serving your area:

1-800-4-CANCER

Spanish-speaking CIS staff members are also available.

- Ask your doctor to consult PDQ. The National Cancer Institute has developed PDQ (Physician Data Query), a computerized database designed to give doctors quick and easy access to the latest treatment information for most types of cancer; descriptions of clinical trials that are open for patient entry; and names of organizations and physicians involved in cancer care. To access PDQ, a doctor may use an office computer with a telephone hookup and a PDQ access code or the services of a medical library with online searching capability. Cancer Information Service offices provide free PDQ searches and can tell doctors how to get regular access. Patients may ask their doctor to use PDQ or may call 1-800-4-CANCER themselves.

Some of the other things you might want to do before making a final decision about various treatments are:

- Discuss them with friends or relatives. Although you and your doctor are in the best position to evaluate treatment options, it sometimes helps to discuss your feelings with others whose judgment you respect. Often, close friends and relatives can provide insights that can help your own thinking.

- Talk with other women who have had breast cancer. Many women who have been treated for breast cancer are willing to share their experiences. Your local American Cancer Society (ACS) office may be able to direct you to such women through its Reach to Recovery program. This program, which works through volunteers who have had breast cancer, helps women meet the physical, emotional, and cosmetic needs of their disease and its treatment. Some ACS offices have volunteer visitors who have had a mastectomy, breast reconstruction, radiation, or chemotherapy. Sometimes they are able to meet with women before surgery. Contact your local ACS office for more information.

Remember that you have time to consider options. Except in rare cases, breast cancer patients do not need to be rushed to the hospital for treatment as soon as the disease is diagnosed. Most women have time to learn more about available options, make arrangements at

Breast Cancer: Understanding Treatment Options

medical facilities where treatments will be given, and organize home and work lives before beginning treatment. A long delay, however, is not advisable because it may interfere with the success of your treatment.

Chapter 16

Questions & Answers about Breast Lumps

It's natural to be concerned if you've found a lump in your breast. But . . . 80 percent of all breast lumps are benign, which means no cancer is present. After reading this chapter, you will know more about the normal changes that can occur in a woman's breasts. And you'll learn what to do if you find a lump or other change in your breasts. Most lumps are found by women themselves, either through regular breast self-exam or just by accident. Others are discovered during routine breast exams by a health professional and through mammograms, special x-rays of the breast.

About 20 percent of breast lumps are malignant (cancerous). However, if cancer is found at an early stage and treated promptly, the outlook is good. In fact, 85 to 95 percent of women with early breast cancer will be alive 5 years after diagnosis.

It is normal to be afraid when you find a lump in your breast. But don't let fear stop you from seeing a doctor right away if you think something is wrong. You will feel more confident about finding a breast lump early by:

- Having regular mammograms
- Having a regular breast exam by a health professional.
- Doing a monthly breast self-exam (BSE) as illustrated in this sourcebook.

NIH Pub No. 92-2401.

What is the difference between having a lump in the breast and simply having "lumpy" breasts?

The breasts are made up of ducts, lobes, and fat. Under the breasts are muscles and ribs. These normal features may make the breasts feel "lumpy" or uneven.

In addition, many women have changes in their breasts that are related to their monthly menstrual cycle. Swelling, tenderness, and pain in the breasts may occur before and sometimes during the menstrual period. At the same time, one or more lumps or a feeling of increased "lumpiness" may appear in the breasts. These symptoms are caused by extra fluid collecting in the breast tissue, which is normal. If the "lumpiness" or lumps do not go away after the end of your period, it is important to see a doctor.

If you are past menopause and you find any new lump or thickening in your breast, you should see your doctor.

What am I looking for when I do BSE?

You are looking for a lump that stands out as different from the rest of your breast tissue. Many women are confused about BSE because their breasts generally feel "lumpy." Becoming more familiar with your breasts by doing BSE each month will help you tell the difference between your normal "lumpiness" and what may be a change.

Ask your doctor or other health professional to do a breast exam with you and to explain what you are feeling in your breasts. They can make sure you are doing BSE correctly and thoroughly, which will make you feel more confident.

What should I do if I find a lump in my breast?

If you notice a lump in one breast, examine the other one. If both breasts feel the same, then what you feel is probably a normal part of your breast. You should, however, mention it to your doctor at your next visit.

If a lump of any size appears in either breast and does not go away after your menstrual period, see your doctor. The doctor may refer you to a specialist to discuss the need for further tests.

Questions and Answers about Breast Lumps

If you do not have a doctor of your own, your local medical society or the Cancer Information Service (CIS) may be able to help you find a doctor or breast clinic in your area. The toll-free telephone number of the CIS is 1-800-4-CANCER.

How is a breast lump evaluated?

Your doctor can evaluate a lump in a number of ways.

1. **Palpation** is a physical exam of the breast. The doctor examines each breast and underarm by feeling the tissue. Although a doctor can tell a lot by the way the lump feels, no one can be certain what a lump is just by palpation.

2. **Aspiration**, also called fine needle aspiration, can help the doctor discover whether the lump is a cyst (fluid-filled) or a solid mass of tissue. Aspiration is usually done in the doctor's office. First, the doctor uses a local anesthetic to numb the area. Then, the doctor inserts a needle into the lump and tries to withdraw fluid. If it is a cyst, removing the fluid will collapse it. The fluid may be sent to a laboratory for testing to be sure no cancer cells are present. When the lump is solid, the doctor sometimes removes a sample of cells with the needle. These cells are then sent to a laboratory for analysis.

3. A **mammogram** is a type of x-ray that creates an image of the breast on film or paper. It can help determine whether a lump is benign or cancerous. In fact, it often can detect cancer in the breast before a lump can be felt. The National Cancer Institute (NCI) suggests that beginning at age 40, all women should have a mammogram every 1 to 2 years. When a woman reaches 50, she should have a mammogram each year. A doctor may also recommend a mammogram if any sign or symptom of breast cancer is found, regardless of age.

Several other methods also are being studied. None is now reliable enough to be used alone, but they may be helpful when combined with other methods.

Ultrasound uses high-frequency sound waves to get an image of the breast and can help determine if a lump is a cyst or a solid mass. It is usually used along with palpation and mammography.

Diaphanography, or transillumination, shines a light through the breast to show its inner features.

Thermography measures the heat patterns in the breast to produce an image.

4. A **biopsy** is the only certain way to learn whether a breast lump or suspicious area seen on a mammogram is cancer. In a biopsy, the doctor surgically removes all or part of the lump and sends it to the laboratory for analysis. There are several biopsy methods that a doctor may use: needle biopsy, incisional biopsy, excisional biopsy, and mammographic localization with biopsy.

Occasionally the doctor will do a **needle biopsy** to remove a small amount of tissue from the lump. A needle biopsy can be performed in the doctor's office. This is most often done when cancer is suspected and the doctor hopes to confirm the diagnosis immediately. If cancer is not found, a more thorough biopsy will follow.

Once, it was thought that inserting a needle or cutting into a breast lump might cause cancer to spread. This is not true.

An **incisional biopsy** is the surgical removal of a portion of a lump. This procedure is often used when the growth is very large. Again, if no cancer is found, a more thorough biopsy may follow to make sure the entire lump is free of cancer.

In an **excisional biopsy** the doctor removes the entire lump. This is currently the "standard" biopsy procedure and the most thorough method of diagnosis. Incisional and excisional biopsies are usually done in the outpatient department of a hospital. Either a local or general anesthetic may be used.

Mammographic localization with biopsy (also known as needle localization) is used for suspicious areas such as microcalcifications (tiny specks of calcium) that cannot be felt but can be seen on a mammogram. During this procedure, the breast is x-rayed

Questions and Answers about Breast Lumps

and small needles are placed to outline the suspicious area for the surgeon, who then removes the tissue for biopsy. This can be done using a local anesthetic in the outpatient department of a hospital.

Your doctor may suggest one or more of these procedures to evaluate a lump or other change in your breast. The doctor may also suggest watching the suspicious area for a month or two. Because many lumps are caused by normal hormonal changes, this waiting period may provide additional information.

However, if you feel uncomfortable about waiting, speak with your doctor about your concerns. You also may want to get a second opinion, perhaps from a breast specialist or surgeon. Many cities have breast clinics where you can get a second opinion. The Cancer Information Service also may be able to help you locate doctors to consult.

What will the doctor be able to learn from a biopsy?

The biopsy can tell the doctor whether your lump is benign or malignant. If it is cancer, your doctor will talk with you about choices of treatments, and you may be advised to get a second opinion. (You can call the Cancer Information Service for NCI publications that deal with breast cancer treatment.)

If no cancer is found, you may be told that the lump or suspicious area is the result of a **fibrocystic condition, fibrocystic disease, benign breast disease**, or one of many other conditions. Remember, 80 percent of all breast lumps are not cancer.

What is a fibrocystic condition, fibrocystic disease, or benign breast disease?

Unfortunately, doctors do not agree on standard terms for benign breast changes. We prefer to use the term benign breast condition for those changes in a woman's breasts that are not cancerous. These include normal changes that occur during the menstrual cycle as well as benign lumps that can appear in the breast. If your doctor uses a different term, or one you do not understand, ask for an explanation.

How many women have a benign breast condition?

It is estimated that at least 50 percent of all women have irregular or "lumpy" breasts. In addition, many doctors believe that nearly all women have some benign breast changes beginning at age 30. A woman is more likely to have these breast changes if she has never had children, has had irregular menstrual cycles, has a family history of breast cancer, or is thin. Women who have had more than one child and women who are taking birth control pills have a reduced risk.

What are the symptoms of a benign breast condition?

Women may have increased "lumpiness" with tenderness, pain, and swelling just before their period begins. These symptoms lessen after the menstrual period, only to reappear the next month. Many women find that these symptoms disappear after menopause. Benign breast lumps may appear at any time. Some cause pain, others don't. They may be large or small, soft or rubbery, fluid-filled or solid, and movable. In addition, some benign breast conditions may produce a discharge from the nipple.

What kinds of benign breast conditions are there?

1. **Normal hormonal changes** may cause a feeling of fullness in the breast, which goes away after the menstrual period. This condition is most common in women 35 to 50 years of age.

2. **Cysts** are fluid-filled sacs that often enlarge and become tender and painful just before the menstrual period. Cysts are found most often in women 35 to 50 years of age. They usually are found in both breasts. There may be many cysts of different sizes. Some cysts are so small that they can't be felt; others may be several inches across.

3. **Fibroadenomas** are solid, round, rubbery, and freely movable breast lumps. Usually they are painless. They appear most often in young women between 15 and 30 years of age. Fibroadenomas occur twice as often in black women as in others. They are benign but should removed to be certain of the diagnosis. Fibroadenomas do not go away by themselves and may enlarge during pregnancy and breast-feeding.

Questions and Answers about Breast Lumps

4. **Lipomas** are single, painless lumps that are sometimes found in older women. They are made up of fatty tissue and are slow-growing, soft, and movable. They can vary in size from a dime to a quarter. Lipomas should be removed or biopsied to make sure that they are not cancerous.

5. **Intraductal papillomas** are small wart-like growths in the lining of a duct near the nipple. They usually affect women between 45 and 50 years old and can produce bleeding from the nipple.

6. **Mammary duct ectasia** is an inflammation of the ducts that causes a thick, sticky, gray-to-green discharge from the nipple. Without treatment, the condition can become painful.

7. **Mastitis (sometimes called "postpartum mastitis")** is most often seen in women who are breast-feeding. It is an inflammatory condition in which the breast appears red and feels warm, tender, and lumpy.

8. **Traumatic fat necrosis** occasionally appears in older women and in women with very large breasts. The condition can result from a bruise or blow to the breast, although the woman might not remember the specific injury. The trauma causes the fat in the breast to form lumps that are painless, round, and firm. Sometimes the skin around them looks red or bruised. Again, a doctor should examine the area.

A word of caution. If you find a change in your breast, do not use these descriptions to try to diagnose it yourself. There is no substitute for a doctor's evaluation.

What is the treatment for a benign breast condition?

Treatment varies, depending on the type of condition a woman has. If you have a single lump, it is usually removed in the biopsy. Most cysts are aspirated, and if they don't disappear, they are removed by surgery. Although there is no treatment for normal monthly breast changes, some studies have looked at various ways of treating the uncomfortable symptoms. The results of those studies do not all agree. You may wish to discuss the treatments described below with your doctor. For a long time doctors thought that eliminating beverages and foods that contain caffeine such as coffee, tea, cola, and chocolate (all of which also contain a substance called methylxanthine) would reduce monthly breast pain and tenderness. Recent studies have been unable to prove that such a change in diet affects symptoms. However, women continue to report to doctors that when they stop drinking coffee or eating chocolate, the pain and swelling in their breasts is less.

Vitamin E is another treatment that has been suggested. It is generally accepted that taking this vitamin may help reduce the symptoms of breast pain and tenderness. You should speak with your doctor before taking vitamin E.

Occasionally doctors will suggest an anti-hormone treatment (Danazol) when a woman has severe symptoms. Danazol may relieve pain and tenderness and decrease "lumpiness"; however, serious side effects are possible, and you should discuss all aspects of this treatment with your doctor if it is recommended.

Do doctors ever suggest more extensive surgery for benign breast disease?

In cases where a woman's breasts are extremely difficult to examine, when there have been many biopsies or there are biopsy-proven tissue changes that place that woman in a high-risk category and there is a family history of breast cancer, a doctor may suggest a prophylactic mastectomy. In this surgery, both breasts are removed. Some women then choose to have breast reconstruction.

If your doctor suggests this treatment, you should consider getting a second opinion, preferably from a breast specialist. Remember that there is no reason to hurry into this decision. You should be comfortable with your choice and learn everything about the procedure, its possible side effects, and your risks of future problems. Prophylactic mastectomy is a controversial treatment, and many doctors prefer instead to schedule frequent exams to check for any breast changes.

Will insurance pay for the diagnosis and treatment of a benign breast condition?

Talk with your doctor about your diagnosis and call your insurance company to ask about their coverage for benign breast conditions. Only a very small percentage of women with a benign breast condition are at greater risk of developing cancer. Despite this fact, some insurance companies have cancelled policies or raised premiums for women who have been diagnosed with "fibrocystic disease."

Can benign lumps turn into cancerous ones?

Benign lumps do not turn into cancer. However, cancerous lumps can develop near benign lumps and can be hidden on a mammogram. This is another reason why removal of a benign lump is usually recommended.

What are micro-calcifications?

They are tiny specks of calcium in the breast tissue that are sometimes detected by a mammogram. They can be related to a benign breast condition or breast cancer. In some cases, micro-calcifications are seen when there is no lump present. The pattern and location of micro-calcifications help the doctor determine if additional tests are needed.

What causes a discharge from the nipple and should I be concerned?

You should see your doctor whenever you notice a spontaneous discharge from the nipple (when something comes out without the breast being squeezed). The fluid may be clear, milky, bloody, or even green. If you have a discharge when you do BSE, you should also check with your doctor.

Many conditions can cause a discharge. The doctor will take a sample of the discharge and send it to a laboratory to be analyzed. Occasionally, the doctor may order special tests to help in diagnosing the cause of the discharge. Your doctor can then recommend treatment.

If you are pregnant, breast-feeding, or have recently had a baby, a milky fluid that comes out of both breasts is most likely related to your pregnancy. If you have questions or if the fluid is bloody, talk to your doctor.

What if I notice a lump in my breast during pregnancy?

During pregnancy, the milk producing glands become swollen and the breasts might feel lumpier than usual. It can be difficult to examine your breasts when you are pregnant, but you should continue to do so. Although not common, breast cancer has been diagnosed during pregnancy. So, if you have a question about the way your breasts feel, talk to your doctor.

Does every new lump need to be biopsied?

Not necessarily. If a new lump appears, you cannot be sure that it is benign, even if you have had a benign lump removed in the past. Your doctor should evaluate it and decide whether a biopsy is needed.

Is a biopsy going to change the shape of my breast?

Generally, a breast biopsy leaves only a minor scar, but this depends on the location and size of the lump and how deep it is in the breast. You should discuss the procedure with your doctor so you understand just what is going to be done and what the result is going to look like.

Does having a benign breast change mean I am at greater risk of developing breast cancer?

Generally, no. Most benign breast changes do not increase a woman's risk of getting breast cancer. Recent studies show that only certain, very specific breast changes, which are detected by biopsy, put a woman at higher risk of developing breast cancer. Most important, 70 percent of the women who have a breast biopsy for a benign condition are not at any increased risk of cancer. About 26 percent of breast biopsies show changes that slightly increase the risk of developing breast cancer, and only 4 percent show breast changes that moderately increase the woman's risk.

If your biopsy shows benign changes, discuss with your doctor what kind of changes were found and whether those changes increase your risk of developing breast cancer.

What other factors cause women to be at increased risk of getting breast cancer?

Age is a factor. The older you are, the greater your chance of getting breast cancer. About one in five women diagnosed with breast cancer has a family history of the disease. Other risk factors include having your first child after age 30, never being pregnant, getting your first period at an early age, or having a late menopause. Do not place too much faith in being "safe" if you have none of these risk factors what puts you at risk for getting breast cancer is that you are a woman. The majority of women who are diagnosed with breast cancer do not fall into any special "high-risk" category.

Questions to Ask Your Doctor

We hope that this chapter has answered many of your questions about non-cancerous breast lumps. However, no book can take the place of talking with your doctor. Feel free to ask the doctor any questions you have. If you do not understand the answer, ask your doctor to explain. It is helpful to write down questions as you think of them. The questions below are some of the most common that women have; you may have others. Jot your questions down and take this list with you when you see your doctor.

1. Do I need to have a mammogram? If yes, how often?

2. How often should I make an appointment to see you?

3. Will you teach me how to do breast self-examination (BSE) and check to see that I'm doing it properly?

4. What should I look for when I do BSE?

5. How can I distinguish lumps from the other normal parts of my breast?

6. What kind of lumps do I have?

7. Do you think I need to have a biopsy? If no, why not?

For Additional Information

For answers to questions you may have about breast lumps or breast cancer, call the following toll-free telephone number and you will be automatically connected to the Cancer Information Service office serving your area:

1-800-4-CANCER

Spanish speaking CIS staff members are available.

Chapter 17

Breast Biopsy: What You Should Know

You have a lump or other change in your breast. After you've had an examination, you're told that a biopsy must be performed to find out whether the lump is benign (non-cancerous) or malignant (cancerous).

A biopsy is a test that establishes the precise diagnosis of your breast problem. it is a simple procedure in which tissue is removed and examined under a microscope by a specially trained doctor called a pathologist. A biopsy can be performed either by inserting a needle to withdraw fluid or by taking tissue from the lump, or by surgically removing the entire lump or a portion of it. The tissue is then analyzed in a laboratory.

Before the Biopsy

When a surgical biopsy is necessary, you have a choice of two procedures that should be discussed and agreed upon by you and your doctor. You can have a biopsy on one day and schedule treatment, if necessary, for a later date. This is called a **two-step procedure.** The biopsy is usually done in a hospital, on either an inpatient or outpatient basis, with local or general anesthesia. The size and location of your lump will help the doctor decide which type of anesthesia is better for you.

NIH Pub No. 87-657.

Or you can choose to have a **one-step procedure**. Your biopsy will be done in the hospital under general anesthesia. While you are asleep, the suspicious tissue will be removed and analyzed. If cancer is found, your surgeon will immediately perform a mastectomy, the surgical removal of a breast.

This chapter will help you in making the decision between one-step and two-step procedures. It will also provide information on what to expect during the biopsy procedure. However, this chapter is only a starting point. You will want to discuss this information in more detail with your doctor, a nurse, your family, a close friend, or perhaps another woman who has had a biopsy. You may want to seek a second medical opinion.

You do not have to rush to make this decision. A short delay will not reduce your chances of successful treatment.

Before the biopsy, it is important to discuss with your doctor the estrogen and progesterone receptor assay tests. If your lump is cancer, these laboratory tests will determine if hormone treatment will benefit you now or in the future. If these tests are not performed at the time of the biopsy, this information may be very difficult to obtain later. Whether you choose a one-step or a two-step procedure, you should ask your doctor if arrangements have been made to perform these tests.

Any woman facing breast surgery who thinks she may be interested in breast reconstruction should discuss the options with her surgeon and a plastic surgeon before having the mastectomy. Breast reconstruction, a type of plastic surgery that rebuilds the breast, is growing in popularity, and the techniques of breast reconstruction have improved greatly over the past few years. Some women plan for reconstruction during the same surgery as their mastectomy; others decide on reconstruction several months or even years after mastectomy. For more information, contact the National Cancer Institute for a copy of *Breast Reconstruction: A Matter of Choice*. This booklet is reprinted in this sourcebook.

The One-Step Procedure

Although a biopsy is the only sure way to determine whether a lump is cancer, your doctor may be able to predict if a mastectomy will be likely. Under such circumstances, many women choose a one-step procedure. If you decide to have the one-step procedure, you will probably enter the hospital the evening before your biopsy. Some routine blood and urine tests will be performed and you will be asked to sign a consent form authorizing your doctor to remove all or part of your breast if the biopsy shows that the tissue is cancer. Shortly before your surgery you will be given some medication to help you relax, and then you will be taken to the operating room where the anesthesiologist will put you to sleep.

The surgeon will remove the suspicious tissue and send it to the pathology department where it will be analyzed. Thin slices of frozen tissue will be mounted on a slide for examination under a microscope. Analysis of this "frozen section" can be completed in just minutes. If the pathologist finds that the tissue contains cancer cells, your surgeon will perform a mastectomy. Surgery will take several hours and you will remain in the hospital for approximately a week to 10 days to recover from the breast surgery.

If the lump is not cancer, the surgeon will close the incision and bandage it; your surgery will be completed in about an hour. You may be discharged within a few hours or you may spend the night in the hospital. You should be able to resume your normal activities within a few days. However, for the next week or so, your breast may be sore and slightly bruised, and your incision may feel firm for 3 to 4 months.

If there is any question about whether the tissue is cancer, the surgeon will close the incision and wait for a "permanent section" to be done which takes several days.

The one-step procedure requires a doctor to explain the full details of a mastectomy to you before biopsy even though the lump may not be cancer. If the lump is benign, this may cause unnecessary concern. However, some women who choose the one-step procedure, and who turn out to have cancer, are relieved to know when they wake up from surgery that the cancer has already been removed.

The Two-Step Procedure

When the two-step procedure is chosen, you have a biopsy with local or general anesthesia, usually as an outpatient in a hospital, and then schedule treatment, if necessary, for a later date. You can use the time between the biopsy and treatment to have additional tests to find out the extent of the disease, to look into the kind of treatment you want to have, to seek another medical opinion, to prepare yourself emotionally, and to make home and work arrangements for the time you will be in the hospital.

The tissue removed during a two-step procedure is analyzed by both frozen section and a permanent section. Once the biopsy is complete, the incision is closed and bandaged. After the results of the biopsy are learned, treatment decisions are made. Treatment usually is scheduled within a few weeks. Studies have shown that a short delay between biopsy and treatment will not affect the spread of the disease or reduce the chances for successful treatment.

Outpatient Hospital Procedures for a Biopsy

If you are having a biopsy as an outpatient, you will be admitted to the hospital on the same day that you have your biopsy and go home later that day. Before you go to the hospital, your doctor or nurse will tell you when and where to check in and if there are any restrictions on what you should eat or drink before the biopsy. As a general rule, it is a good idea to leave your money and jewelry at home, but be sure to take your insurance card and Social Security number. Also, if you wear fingernail polish, remove it before going to the hospital. Your doctor will be checking your circulation during the recovery period by pinching the tip of the nail until it turns white and then watching how quickly the color returns to normal.

You will probably have some routine tests performed before your surgery such as urine and blood tests, a chest x-ray, and an EKG (electrocardiogram, which electrically record the activity of your heart). Sometimes the laboratory tests can be done several days before the surgery.

When it is time for your surgery, you will be taken to the operating room where you will be given local or general anesthesia. It usually takes about 30 minutes to an hour to remove the suspicious tissue.

After surgery you will be taken to the outpatient care area. Most women have very little discomfort following a biopsy, but if you had general anesthesia, you will probably be sleepy and want to rest. Your doctor may see you and tell you the results of the frozen section. If the tissue is also being analyzed by permanent section, it may be a few days before your doctor can let you know the diagnosis. Before you leave the hospital, you will be given instructions for taking care of the incision. If you have any questions, ask your doctor or nurse.

Depending on how you feel, you may be ready to go home 2 to 3 hours after the biopsy. Most doctors will suggest that a family member or friend meet you at the hospital and take you home. You've been under stress and you may feel weak or tired. Once you are at home, you will return to your usual activities within a day or two. Usually about a week after the biopsy your doctor will want to see you to remove the stitches and discuss further treatment, if needed.

Learn the Facts

Your doctor can answer your questions to help you decide between a one-step and a two-step procedure. The two-step procedure was recommended for most women at a meeting of breast cancer specialists held at the National Institute of Health in 1979. However, once you know the treatment options available to you, you may prefer the one-step procedure. Don't hesitate to ask questions and learn the facts. Then you will be sure that the decision you make is the right one for you.

Whichever biopsy procedure you select, you will probably want to learn more about the options for treatment, what's involved, what to expect, and how to prepare yourself in the event your breast lump is cancer.

Breast Cancer Treatment

Today's treatments for breast cancer are less disfiguring than ever before. Knowing the options for breast cancer treatment will help you play an active role in your health care.

Mastectomy

Mastectomy, the surgical removal of the breast, remains the most common treatment for breast cancer. There are several types of mastectomy, but total mastectomy with axillary dissection is the standard treatment for most breast cancers today. This operation removes the breast and lymph nodes under the arm, but leaves the chest muscles.

Radiation Therapy

Radiation therapy as a primary treatment for breast cancer is a promising technique for some women who have early stage breast cancer. This procedure allows a woman to keep her breast. Only the breast lump and some or all of the underarm lymph nodes are removed. The remaining breast tissue is then treated with radiation. In some cases, iridium implants are temporarily placed in the breast to supplement the external radiation therapy.

Research is currently underway comparing the effectiveness of radiation therapy with the traditional surgical approach, mastectomy. Preliminary study results are encouraging. Researchers are hoping that over time the survival rates for women who are treated with radiation therapy will remain comparable to those of women treated by mastectomy.

Chemotherapy and Hormone Therapy

Chemotherapy, the use of drugs to destroy cancer cells, is often used in addition to surgery or radiation therapy if the cancer has spread beyond the breast. Finally, depending on the results of estrogen and progesterone receptor assays, hormone therapy may also be used. Hormone therapy is a way of changing the balance of a woman's hormones to discourage the growth of certain tumors.

Awaiting the Diagnosis

Many women have said that bringing their suspicions of breast cancer to their physician was one of the most difficult and trying experiences of their lives. Waiting for the appointment to discuss your symptoms can heighten fear. When you visit the doctor there are tests, then additional waiting time for test results, and perhaps an appointment with another physician for a second opinion or referral. While waiting, you bear the stress of not knowing what you may have to cope with or how to plan for the future. These emotional concerns are common to women facing the possibility of breast cancer. You may not face all of the problems discussed below, and you may find other ways of dealing with the stressful situations you have to face. Throughout this waiting period, seek support from friends and loved ones, who usually want to help out in stressful times.

Breast Biopsy: What You Should Know

Uncertainty

An unpredictable situation frequently causes a great deal of stress. This is especially true for a woman about to undergo a breast biopsy. You may feel better if you:

- Talk over your fears and concerns with someone close to you. It is very important for you to be open about your feelings with those people who are important to you. Also, expressing healthy anger can give you some vitality and the energy to cope with the unknown. Openness can set the tone for continued sharing. This is a good time to find ways of talking frankly. Don't hide your hurt or pain; share it. You are under a great deal of stress. Don't hesitate to seek professional help to deal with your anxiety or anger.

- Think through how you would deal with a diagnosis of cancer and what sorts of plans you'd make. Spend time learning about treatment options and considering what your needs are: someone to care for your children, who can fill in for you at work, etc. Look into the best medical facility and kind of care that are available to you. Find out what others in your situation have done and learn from their experiences.

Fear of Cancer

Cancer is frightening, however, it can be treated successfully, and it is not necessarily fatal. More than 5 million Americans who have been treated for cancer are considered cured. If you need to have treatment, you may have to adjust your daily activities temporarily, but most cancer patients return to their usual lifestyle. Many women who have been treated for breast cancer say that they discovered new sources of strength within themselves to cope with the emotional demands they faced.

Fear of Loss

If you think you may have breast cancer, you are naturally concerned about the possibility of losing a breast. The emotions and concerns about sex and intimacy related to that loss are another difficult aspect of the disease. If a mastectomy is necessary, you (and your partner) may experience depression and grief similar to those associated with other losses. Coping with loss is different for each woman, but recognizing and talking about your feelings—which may include anger, frustration, sadness, and fear—can help. These feelings lessen with time, and you may even find that your relationships with loved ones are stronger than before.

Chapter 18

Mastectomy:
A Treatment for Breast Cancer

You've been diagnosed as having breast cancer and your doctor has recommended a mastectomy. If you're like most women, you probably have many concerns about this treatment for breast cancer.

Surgery of any kind is a frightening experience, but surgery for breast cancer raises special concerns. You may be wondering if the surgery will cure your cancer, how you'll feel after surgery—and how you're going to look.

It's not unusual to think about these things. More than 100,000 women in the United States will have mastectomies this year. Each of them will have personal concerns about the impact of the surgery on her life.

This chapter is designed to ease some of your fears by letting you know what to expect from the time you enter the hospital to your recovery at home. It may also help the special people in your life who are concerned about your well-being.

Over the years, mastectomy has proven to be an effective treatment for breast cancer. Today, doctors may choose from a range of procedures depending on the extent of the disease at the time of diagnosis, the patient's medical history, her age, the type of tumor, and other factors. You can feel confident that your doctor is taking steps to see that you can continue to lead an active and full life.

Though breast surgery and recovery will cause you to take time out from your normal routine, it need not cause a permanent change

NIH Pub No. 91-658.

in your lifestyle. Like hundreds of other women who have had mastectomies, you can plan to continue doing the things you enjoy—whether it's working, raising a family, maintaining your home and personal relationships, or pursuing other interests.

When surgery is recommended, most health care facilities now require patients to sign a form stating their willingness to permit diagnosis and medical treatment. This is to certify that you understand what procedures will be done and have consented to have them performed.

Consent to surgical or other treatment is only meaningful if given by a patient who has had an opportunity to learn about recommended alternatives and to evaluate them. Before consenting to any course of treatment, be sure your doctor lets you know:

- The recommended procedure;
- Its purpose;
- Risks and side effects associated with it;
- Likely consequences with and without treatment;
- Other available alternatives; and
- Advantages and disadvantages of one treatment over another.

Even if you want your doctor to assume full responsibility for all decision making, you are likely to discover that your concerns about treatment decrease as your understanding of breast cancer and its treatment increases.

Types of Surgery

Mastectomy is the most common treatment for breast cancer today. As recently as 15 years ago, many doctors considered radical mastectomy the only procedure. It removed the entire breast, the chest muscles under the breast, and all underarm lymph nodes, leaving a hollow chest area. Many women feared the treatment as much as the disease.

Thanks to medical advances, there is now a wide range of effective procedures that may be used, depending on the individual case. In addition to the radical mastectomy, also called a "Halsted radical," surgical options include:

- **Modified radical mastectomy.** Removes the breast and the underarm lymph nodes and the lining over the chest muscles. Sometimes the smaller of the two chest muscles is also removed. This procedure is also called a "total mastectomy with axillary (or underarm) dissection" and today is the most common treatment of early stage breast cancer.

- **Total or simple mastectomy.** Removes only the breast. Sometimes a few of the underarm lymph nodes closest to the breast are removed to see if the cancer has spread beyond the breast. May be followed by radiation therapy.

- **Partial or segmental mastectomy.** Removes the tumor plus a wedge of normal tissue surrounding it, including some skin and the lining of the chest muscle below the tumor. It is followed by radiation therapy. Many surgeons also remove some or all of the underarm lymph nodes to check for possible spread of cancer.

- **Lumpectomy.** Removes the breast lump and is followed by radiation therapy. Many surgeons also remove and test some of the underarm lymph nodes.

Breast Reconstruction

Since you are about to have breast surgery, you should be aware of breast reconstruction, a way to recreate a breast shape after a natural breast has been removed. Though this procedure is gaining in popularity, many women are still unaware of it.

Some women have reconstruction at the same time as their mastectomies; others have it done several months or even years later. Almost any woman who has had a mastectomy can have her breast reconstructed. Successful reconstruction is not hampered by radiation-damaged, thin, or tight skin, or the absence of chest muscles.

Reconstruction isn't for everyone, however. And it may not be right for you. After mastectomy, many women prefer to wear an artificial breast form, called a prosthesis, inside their brassieres.

Both a general surgeon and a plastic surgeon can help you decide whether to have breast reconstruction. If possible, this should be discussed before your surgery because the position of the incision may affect the reconstruction procedure. However, many women consider breast reconstruction only after surgery. For more information on breast reconstruction, see the section Breast Reconstruction: A Matter of Choice.

Questions to Ask Your Doctor

Before Surgery

- What kind of procedure are you recommending?
- What are the potential risks and benefits?
- Am I a candidate for any other type of procedure?
- What are the risks and benefits of those alternatives?
- How should I expect to look after the operation?
- How should I expect to feel?

After Surgery

- When will I be able to get back into my normal routine?
- What can I do to ensure a safe recovery?
- What problems, if any, should I report to you?
- What type of exercises should I do?
- How frequently should I see you for a checkup?

In The Hospital

Hospital procedures and policies vary, but there are a number of things you probably can expect to have happen when you check in for surgery.

You will probably be admitted the afternoon before your operation so that some routine tests, such as blood and urine tests and a chest x-ray, can be performed. Shortly before the operation, the surgical area (breast and underarm) will be shaved, and you may be given some medicine to help you relax.

When it is time for surgery, you will be taken to the operating room and an anesthesiologist will put you to sleep. Electrocardiogram sensors will be attached to your arms and legs with adhesive pads to check your heart rate during surgery. The surgical area will be cleaned and sterile sheets will be draped over your body, except for the area

Mastectomy: A Treatment for Breast Cancer

around the operation. Depending on the procedure, surgery will take between 2 and 4 hours. When you awaken from surgery, you will be in the recovery room. Your breast area will be bandaged and a tube will be in place at the surgical site to drain away any fluid that may accumulate. Your throat may be sore from the tube that was placed in it to carry air to your lungs during surgery. You may also feel a little nauseated and have a dry mouth—common side effects of anesthesia.

You will spend an hour or so in the recovery room. Oxygen will be available in case you need it to ease your breathing. Wires may be taped to your chest to measure your heartbeat. An intravenous (IV) tube will be inserted into a vein in your arm to give fluid, nourishment, or medication after surgery. The IV will probably be removed after you begin to drink and eat.

It's common to feel drowsy for several hours after surgery. You may also feel some discomfort in your breast area. Some women experience numbness, tingling, or pain in the chest, shoulder area, upper arm, or armpit. Others feel pain in the breast that was removed. Doctors are not sure why this "phantom pain" occurs, but it does exist; it's not imaginary. If you are in pain, ask for medication to relieve it.

After you return to your room, a nurse will frequently check your temperature, pulse, blood pressure, and bandage. The nurse will ask you to turn, cough, and breathe deeply to keep your lungs clear after the anesthesia. You may also be encouraged to move your feet and legs to improve your blood circulation. Although each woman reacts to surgery differently, you will probably discover that by the next day you will be able to drink some juice or broth and, with help, to sit up in bed and walk from your bed to a chair in your room. Your doctor will probably encourage you to walk around and eat solid food as soon as possible.

You will be taking sponge baths for a few days after surgery until your incision starts to heal. Before you leave the hospital, ask the doctor or nurse for instructions on taking care of your incision. When you have permission to bathe or shower, do so gently and pat, don't rub, the area of your incision.

The average stay in the hospital is 7 to 10 days. Before you leave, the tube that drains fluid from your incision will be removed. Some of your stitches may also be removed before you leave the hospital. The remaining stitches will be taken out within 1 to 3 weeks at the doctor's office or clinic.

With your doctor's permission, a Reach to Recovery volunteer may visit you in the hospital. Reach to Recovery is an American Cancer Society program that brings volunteers who have had mastectomies together with breast cancer patients. A volunteer will be able to discuss with you any concerns you may have about coping with your mastectomy. She may also give you a lightweight, fiber-filled or cotton breast form to fasten inside your bra, robe, or nightgown while you are recuperating.

Exercising After Mastectomy

Exercising will help you ease the tension in your arm and shoulder and will hasten your recovery. You will probably be able to begin exercising within a few days of your operation. Your doctor, nurse, or physical therapist can show you what exercises to do. The key is to exercise only to the point of pulling or pain. Don't push yourself.

Ask your doctor if you might begin with these few simple movements:

- Lie in bed with your arm at your side. Raise your arm straight up and back trying to touch the headboard.

- Raise your shoulders. Rotate them forward, down, and back in a circular motion to loosen your chest, shoulders, and upper back muscles.

- Lying in bed, clasp your hands behind your head and push your elbows into the mattress.

- With your elbow bent and your arm at a 90 degree angle to your body, rotate your shoulder forward until the forearm is down and then backward until it is up.

- With your arm raised, clench and unclench your fist.

- Breathe deeply.

- Rotate your chin to the left and right. Cock your head sideways.

Mastectomy: A Treatment for Breast Cancer

In addition to exercises such as these, many communities offer swimming, exercise, and dance classes specifically for breast cancer patients.

Precautions

A problem that may arise after treatment is swelling of the arm on the side of the mastectomy. Called lymphedema, this condition is caused by the loss of underarm lymph nodes and their connecting vessels.

Because the lymph nodes have been removed, circulation of lymph fluid is slowed, making it harder for your body to fight infection. You should take special care of your arm to prevent infection. (If you have had breasts removed, ask your doctor about any special precautions.)

Follow these simple rules:

- Avoid burns while cooking or smoking;
- Avoid sunburns;
- Have all injections, vaccinations, blood samples, and blood pressure tests done on the other arm when ever possible;
- Use an electric razor with a narrow head for underarm shaving to reduce the risk of nicks or scratches;
- Carry heavy packages or handbags on the other arm;
- Wash cuts promptly, treat them with antibacterial medication, and cover them with a sterile dressing;
- Check often for redness, soreness, or other signs of infection;
- Never cut cuticles; use hand cream or lotion instead;
- Wear watches or jewelry loosely, if at all, on the operated arm;
- Wear protective gloves when gardening and when using strong detergents, etc.;
- Use a thimble when sewing;
- Avoid harsh chemicals and abrasive compounds;
- Use insect repellent to avoid bites and stings; and
- Avoid elastic cuffs on blouses and nightgowns.

Call your doctor at once if your arm becomes red, swollen, or feels hot. In the meantime, try to keep your arm over your head and periodically pump your fist.

Though you should be cautious, it's also important to use your arm normally. Don't favor it or keep it dependent.

Recovering At Home

After breast surgery, there are a number of steps you can take to ensure a safe physical recovery. Your physical health will not be your only concern, however. A mastectomy often has a dramatic emotional impact as well.

Taking Care of Yourself

Once you are home, you should continue to exercise until you have regained the full use of your arm. As you increase your exercise and daily activities, be careful not to overdo. Take clues from your body; rest before you become overly tired.

To keep your skin soft and to promote healing, you may want to massage your incision gently with cocoa butter or vitamin E cream. As time goes by and the incision begins to heal, the redness, bruising, and swelling will disappear. As you are healing, be sure to watch for any signs of infection such as swelling, inflammation, tenderness, or drainage. If you see any of these signs or develop a fever, call your doctor.

Although each woman recovers from a mastectomy at her own rate, you will probably discover that within 2 to 3 weeks after surgery you will be doing most of the things you have always done. Within about 6 weeks you will be able to resume your normal activities. Over time the numbness under your arm will decrease, but total feeling may not return for a long time. After you've had a mastectomy, you'll have a lot of things on your mind. You may think about the fact that you've just been treated for a serious disease. You've had an operation that has changed your appearance, perhaps your self-image. You might wonder how the mastectomy will affect your lifestyle and your personal relationships. You might even be unsure how to act toward your family and friends.

Adjusting Emotionally

Though every woman reacts to mastectomy differently, these types of concerns are common. Just as you will be taking action to help yourself physically recover from treatment, you can take steps to ease your emotional adjustment as well.

Expressing your feelings to your doctor and the people you love can be important emotional medicine. If you try to handle your problems alone, everyone will lose. You will lose chances to express yourself, your family and friends will lose opportunities to share your difficulties and help you work through them, and your doctor may not understand what you need to fully recover.

Remember, your family and close friends can be your strongest supporters. But chances are, they aren't quite sure how they can show their support. You can help them by being open and honest about the way you feel.

Others Are Willing To Help

In addition to talking with your doctor, your nurse, and the people closest to you, you may also want to talk with other women who have had similar experiences.

As described earlier, Reach to Recovery is an American Cancer Society program designed to help patients meet the physical, emotional, and cosmetic needs related to breast cancer and its treatment. Women who have had mastectomies volunteer to participate in the program by sharing their experiences with others. All volunteers are carefully selected and trained. If your doctor authorizes a visit from a Reach to Recovery volunteer, she will contact you about an appointment while you are in the hospital or shortly after you go home. When you get together, she'll bring a kit containing a temporary breast form and information for husbands, children, other loved ones, and friends. She'll be prepared to discuss all aspects of mastectomy, including your personal concerns. Programs vary from city to city, so contact your local American Cancer Society chapter for more information.

ENCORE is a national YWCA discussion and exercise program for women who have had breast cancer. This once-a-week 90-minute program consists of floor and swimming pool exercise sessions and group discussions. Contact your local YWCA for more information about ENCORE.

If informal approaches to dealing with your feelings don't work, consider professional help. Psychiatrists, psychologists, social workers, nurses, and religious counselors can help you adjust.

Intimacy

Whether you are single or married, you are likely to wonder how your mastectomy will affect your intimate relationships. Your partner will also have concerns. You can help each other by expressing them.

Intimate relationships are built on mutual love, trust, attraction, shared interests, common experiences, and a host of other feelings. A mastectomy will not necessarily change these feelings. What it may change is some of the physical aspects of lovemaking—what's pleasurable to you and what's not. It may also temporarily affect your partner's and your attitude toward intimacy.

After mastectomy you will still be the person your partner has come to love and enjoy. You can bring new closeness to your relationship by talking about the changes in your body, accepting them, and reaffirming your joy of being alive and being together.

At first, there may be some awkward moments. It may be helpful to let your partner see your body soon after surgery to decrease the anxiety both of you feel. Sometimes a partner is afraid that touching a mastectomy incision will hurt you. Let your partner know what's comfortable to you and what's not.

Sometimes a partner assumes that you will not be ready for sex for some time after surgery. Women often interpret this waiting as rejection. You may prevent this potential problem by letting your partner know when you feel ready for sex, that you still need your partner, and that it is important for you to know that your partner still finds you attractive and desirable.

Helping Children Cope

Children react to illness in a variety of ways. Some feel angry at their mothers for becoming ill. Others are frightened. Still others worry that they might have caused the illness.

Although you may be tempted to protect your children by not telling them about your operation or the disease that caused it, it's usually better to be honest. Even young children sense when something is wrong. Preschool children often feel deserted when their mother goes to the hospital. And if she returns feeling weak or depressed, they may become frightened. Adolescents sometimes suddenly change their behavior because they fear their mother's illness will keep them from maintaining the independence they have begun to enjoy. If you can avoid imposing too much responsibility on your teenage children, and if you share some of your feelings with them, you may be able to keep their problems to a minimum.

It is a good idea to tell your children the truth as simply and positively as possible. Be careful not to burden them with any more information than is necessary. Encourage their questions, and answer those questions honestly. You will probably find that talking helps your children to accept your illness and the temporary disruption it causes.

Common Questions About Breast Surgery

Q. Is breast surgery dangerous?

A. Doctors have been performing mastectomies for many years and are continuing to improve their techniques. There are risks associated with any kind of surgery, however. Risk depends on a lot of things, including your age, your medical history, your response to anesthesia, and your general health. After considering these factors, your doctor will recommend the type of surgery that will offer you the most benefit with the least amount of risk.

Q. How frequently should I plan to see a doctor after a mastectomy?

A. Your surgeon will tell you when to schedule your first postoperative exam. The two of you will then decide whether you should continue to make regular visits to the surgeon, or to a medical oncologist, an internist, a gynecologist, or a family practitioner. Most doctors believe that women treated for breast cancer should have professional exams every 3 to 6 months for the first 3 years after surgery. More information on follow-up exams, possible signs of recurrence, and taking care of yourself can be found in *After Breast Cancer: A Guide to Followup Care*, available from the National Cancer Institute.

Q. What is chemotherapy and when is it used?

A. Chemotherapy is the use of drugs to treat cancer. (Remember, a mastectomy treats only the cancer in the breast.) Anticancer drugs are used to reach areas of the body where cancer cells may be hiding, and to destroy them before they multiply and hurt the normal cells and organs.

Breast Self-Examination

After a mastectomy, breast self-examination (BSE) should be part of your routine. You will want to examine your natural breast and the surgical site once a month to note any changes in the way they look or feel. Though you may have been doing self-exams before your surgery, you will have to relearn what's considered "normal" for you now. About half the women who have mastectomies report that their remaining breast becomes larger. If you menstruate, the best time to do BSE is 2 or 3 days after your period ends, when your breast is least likely to be tender or swollen. If you no longer menstruate, pick a day, such as the first day of the month, to do BSE. Here is how to do BSE:

1. Stand before a mirror. Inspect your breast for anything unusual, such as any discharge from the nipple, or puckering, dimpling, or scaling of the skin. Inspect the scar for new swelling, lumps, redness, or color change. Although redness can be a result of irritation from your bra or prosthesis, report it to your physician. The next two steps are designed to emphasize any change in the shape or contour of your breast. As you do them, you should be able to feel your chest muscles tighten.

2. Watching closely in the mirror, clasp your hands behind your head and press your hands forward.

3. Next, press your hands firmly on your hips and bow slightly toward your mirror as you pull your shoulders and elbows forward.

The next part of the exam is done while standing. Some women do it in the shower because fingers glide over soapy skin, making it easy to concentrate on the texture underneath.

4. Raise your arm on the unoperated side. Using three or four fingers of your other hand, explore your breast firmly, carefully, and thoroughly. Beginning at the outer edge, press the

Mastectomy: A Treatment for Breast Cancer

flat part of your fingers in small circles, moving the circles slowly around the breast. Gradually work toward the nipple. Be sure to cover the entire breast. Pay special attention to the area between the breast and the underarm, including the underarm itself. Feel for any unusual lump or mass under the skin.

5. Gently squeeze the nipple and look for a discharge. Raise your arm on the operated side. Use three or four fingers of your opposite hand and begin at the top of the scar. Press gently, using small circular motions, and feel the entire length of the scar. Look for thickenings, lumps, and hard places. As with your breast, familiarity with your scar makes it easier to notice any changes. Lumps, thickening, and inflammation are among changes you should bring to the attention of your doctor.

6. Steps 4 and 5 should be repeated lying down. Lie flat on your back, raise your arm on the unoperated side over your head, and place a pillow or folded towel under your shoulder. This position flattens the breast and makes it easier to examine. Use the same circular motion described earlier.

Shopping for a Permanent Prosthesis

Ask your doctor when it's appropriate for you to shop for a permanent breast form. You can probably begin shopping as soon as you're feeling strong and the swelling and tenderness are gone from the incision. If you are planning to have breast reconstruction, you may want a prosthesis before it's time for your surgery.

Breast forms are available in many shapes and sizes Some prostheses feel like plastic bags, some are rubbery, some feel very much like skin. They may be covered with a soft fabric, polyurethane, or a silicone envelope, and they may be filled with foam rubber, water, air, chemical gel, polyethylene materials, polyurethane foam, silicone gel, or ceramic particles. Like natural breasts, prostheses vary in weight, and their consistency varies from very soft and pliable to relatively firm. Some brands have models specifically for the right or left side;

some are made with a modified nipple and can be worn with or without a bra. Custom-made forms, which adhere to the chest wall and closely match the remaining breast, are also available.

Small prostheses, sometimes called equalizers, are available for women who have had lumpectomies or segmental mastectomies. Women whose reconstructive surgery does not replace the nipple or whose breast form does not have a nipple may choose a nipple prosthesis. Extremely lightweight forms are available to wear in a nightgown or with leisure clothes.

When selecting your prosthesis you'll also need to find a properly fitting bra that will hold the breast form in place. You may be able to wear the same bra you have always worn if it fits well and does not have underwires. Special postmastectomy bras are available. They are built up to cover a larger area of the chest and have wider straps and pockets inside the cup to hold the prosthesis. You can sew a pocket into your swimsuit and your standard bras to keep the breast form in place. Breast prostheses are sold in surgical supply stores, in lingerie and corset shops, and in the underwear departments of large department stores. Many stores that sell breast forms also carry lingerie and sportswear specially designed for women who have had mastectomies. Look in the Yellow Pages under "Brassieres" or "Surgical Appliances." Reach to Recovery volunteers can often provide information on types of permanent prostheses and a list of where they are available locally.

Before you go out to try various breast forms, you should call ahead and see if the supplier has a professional fitter to meet with you. More than a dozen different breast forms are on the market, and the only way to find the best one for you is to try them on. Your breast form should feel comfortable, have a natural contour and consistency, and remain in place when you move. It may feel heavy at first, but you will get used to the extra weight. Ask the fitter if the form absorbs perspiration or other chemicals from the skin and how to clean and care for your prosthesis. Most prostheses are guaranteed for 1 to 5 years.

Prices for breast forms range from $7 to $265. Custom-made forms are more expensive. The expense is covered, at least partly, by most medical insurance policies. A written prescription from your doctor will help ensure payment. If your insurance does not cover a prosthesis, you may be able to deduct the cost as a medical expense on your income tax.

Mastectomy: A Treatment for Breast Cancer

If you want some emotional support when you shop, ask your partner or a good friend to go with you. Wear a form-fitting blouse or sweater so you can see how the form will make you look.

The most important thing to do is shop around. It's worth your time to find a prosthesis that feels comfortable and keeps you looking your best.

Chapter 19

Breast Reconstruction: A Matter of Choice

Thanks to recent advances in plastic surgery techniques, a mastectomy need not have the same physical and emotional consequences it did in the past. Women of all ages who have had all or part of a breast removed are finding that breast reconstruction can be a step toward restoring their bodies and their former lifestyles.

Whether you are about to have a mastectomy or have already had your surgery, the information given in this chapter may answer some of your questions about breast reconstruction and ease your concerns.

Although the procedure is gaining in popularity, many women still are unaware that a breast can be reconstructed after surgery. The fact is that today virtually any woman who has had a mastectomy for breast cancer can have her breast reconstructed. Radiation-damaged skin, grafted, thin, or tight skin, and the absence of chest muscles are no longer obstacles to successful reconstruction.

Its Your Choice

Reconstruction isn't for everyone, however. And it may not be right for you. Many women prefer to wear breast forms rather than having additional surgery. The important thing is that most breast cancer patients have a choice. This chapter is designed to help you decide whether breast reconstruction is for you.

NIH Pub No. 91-2151.

The decision to have plastic surgery is a personal one. It depends on a lot of things, including your self-image, but the issue goes beyond simple vanity. Breast reconstruction can help promote a sense of wellness. It can also help your family or others close to you to resolve their feelings about your having had cancer.

You may be thinking about breast reconstruction because you believe it will help you feel "whole" again. Or it may make it easier for you to get back to a normal routine after a period of illness.

Here's what some women have to say about breast reconstruction:

"I decided to have reconstruction because...

- ... I wanted to be able to wear all my favorite clothes including bathing suits and low-cut dresses."
- ... I felt it would help me regain my sense of femininity; make me feel more attractive."
- ... I tried wearing a breast form and found it uncomfortable and inconvenient."

"Reconstruction was not the best choice for me because...

- ... I was perfectly comfortable with a breast form."
- ... the idea of having additional surgery was too frightening. I wasn't willing to take the risk."
- ... I wasn't satisfied with the results my doctor told me I could expect."

You may agree with any of these women, or have your own ideas about whether or not to have breast reconstruction. The first step in deciding is to get additional information about all aspects of the surgery.

Reconstructive Surgery

Plastic surgeons have been developing methods of breast reconstruction since the late 19th century. Until the late 1960's, however, the standard surgical procedure was very complex and the results were often disappointing. Few women chose to have the operation.

Breast Reconstruction: A Matter of Choice

Two medical advances have made reconstruction more popular in recent years:

- Creation of **silicone gel implants** and
- Development of ways to transfer skin and muscle to the chest area from other areas of the body.

These advances have helped make breast reconstruction an option for many women who have had surgery for breast cancer, including those who have had **radical mastectomies**.

Reconstruction of the entire breast, including the nipple and areola (the dark-colored skin around the nipple), is a procedure that may require two or more operations over 6 to 12 months' time. A hospital stay of several days to a week is usual for each operation in the process.

Several types of breast implants are used in reconstruction. Generally, they are soft, fluid-filled sacs, available in various sizes. The surgeon chooses the size and shape that will best match the patient's opposite breast.

The simplest type of implant is a sac made of tough, elastic silicone rubber and filled with silicone gel or other fluids. Silicone implants are an improvement over liquid silicone injections, which were once used for breast enlargements but have now been banned by the Food and Drug Administration. There is no evidence that silicone gel implants cause cancer.

Common Procedures

Like any other type of plastic surgery, breast reconstruction is a personalized procedure. There are three major types: simple implant placement, tissue expansion, and tissue transfer. Your doctor will recommend the best one for you after considering the type of mastectomy performed, your postsurgery treatment, your skin and muscle conditions, your breast size, and other factors.

"Simple" Implant Placement

This procedure, which may be done as outpatient surgery, is used when the patient has a healthy chest muscle and enough good-quality skin to cover the implant. In this procedure, the surgeon makes a small incision, usually through the mastectomy scar, and inserts the implant in a pocket created under the chest muscle. A drain may be inserted to remove fluid that may accumulate during the next few days, and the incision is then closed. The operation takes 1 or 2 hours. It is usually done while the patient is under general anesthesia, but local anesthesia is sometimes used. The appearance of the mastectomy scar can be improved during the reconstruction, but the scar cannot be eliminated. If the surgeon makes the incision in the original mastectomy scar, there will be no additional scarring.

Tissue Expansion

A temporary tissue expander may be used when there is good-quality skin and muscle but the quantity is not enough to cover an implant that matches the size of the opposite breast. In this procedure, the remaining tissue is gradually stretched so that an implant that matches the opposite breast can be inserted. While the woman is under local or general anesthesia, the surgeon makes an incision in the mastectomy scar and inserts the deflated tissue expander under the skin and muscle. (In some instances, the expander may be inserted at the time of the mastectomy.) After the tissue expander is in place, it is filled with a small amount of sterile fluid. The operation takes 1 to 1 1/2 hours. During the next 8 to 12 weeks, the patient visits her doctor's office on the average of once a week where the doctor injects additional fluid, gradually enlarging the expander and stretching the tissue over it. While this expansion is taking place, the patient can keep up her normal activities, with little or no discomfort. Then, when the tissue has stretched enough to hold an implant of the desired size, the surgeon removes the tissue expander and inserts the permanent implant. This last step can be done on an outpatient basis, usually with local anesthesia.

Tissue Transfer

There are three kinds of breast reconstruction that involve the moving, or transfer, of tissue from one part of the body to another.

"Latissimus dorsi" reconstruction. This procedure may be used when more radical surgery has removed more of the chest

Figure 19.1.
"Simple" Implant Placement

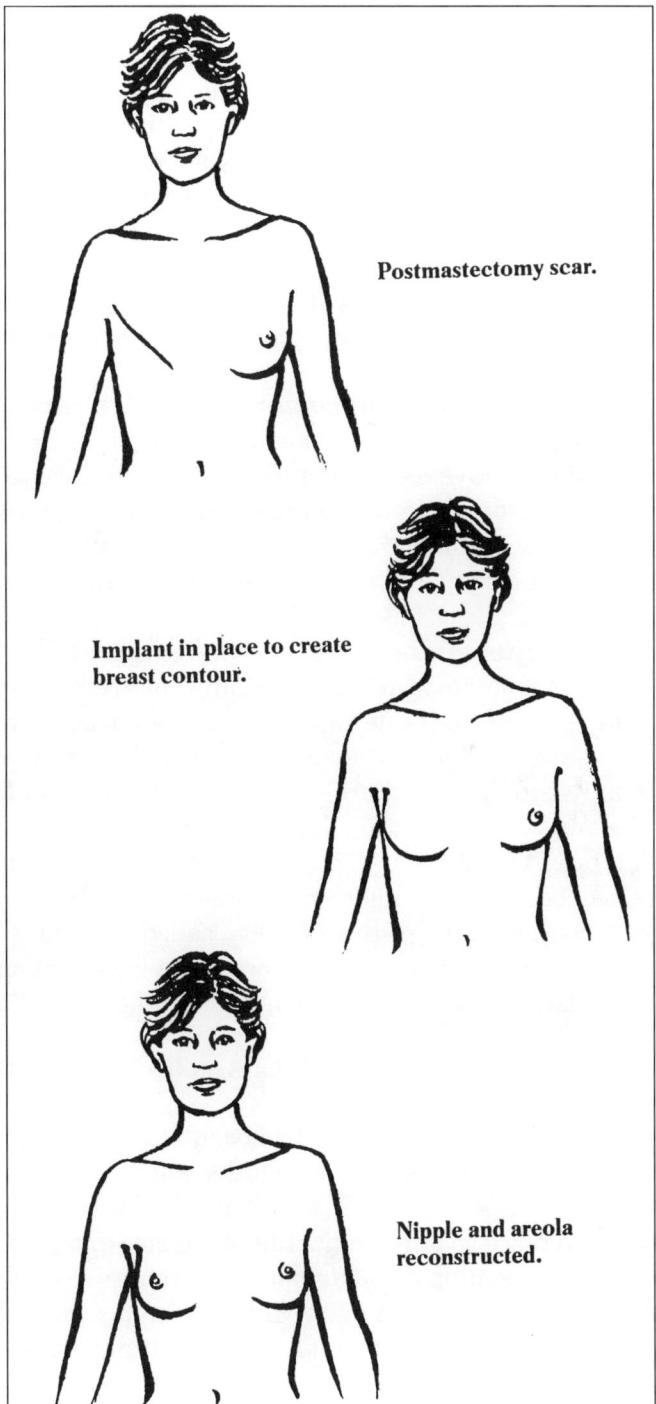

muscles and a large amount of skin, leaving too little soft tissue to hold and cover an implant. During this operation, the surgeon transfers skin and muscle from the patient's back to the mastectomy site. To create a new muscle on the front of the chest, the surgeon uses the latissimus dorsi, a broad, flat muscle on the back below the shoulder blade. An implant is then placed under the new chest muscle. Drains may be inserted and kept in place for several days after surgery to remove fluid. The operation takes several hours and patients stay in the hospital for about a week. This procedure leaves a scar on the back in addition to the mastectomy scar on the chest. (See Figure 19.2)

Abdominal advancement reconstruction. This procedure is often used for women who are large breasted. During this operation, the surgeon advances skin and fat from the chest and abdomen below the mastectomy site to the breast area. The advantages of this procedure are good match of skin color and texture, less scarring to other areas of the body, and relative ease of performance.

"Rectus abdominus" reconstruction. This procedure is also used for women whose mastectomy has removed a lot of skin and muscle. To move tissue to the chest, the surgeon transfers one of the two parallel vertical abdominal muscles (the rectus abdominus muscles) to the breast area along with skin and fat from the abdomen. The surgeon shapes this flap of muscle, skin, and fat into the contour of a breast. If there is enough abdominal tissue available, no implant is needed. Transferring tissue from the abdomen to the chest also results in tightening of the stomach, called a "tummy tuck." This procedure leaves a horizontal scar across the lower abdomen in addition to the mastectomy scar on the chest. (See Figure 19.3)

Recreating the Nipple and the Areola

After the breast shape has been reconstructed, most doctors prefer to wait several weeks or months before doing surgery to construct the nipple and areola. This is done to allow the new breast tissue to settle in place so minor adjustments in size and position can be carried out when the nipple and areola are reconstructed. Women who are primarily concerned with improving their appearance in clothing may be satisfied with reconstruction of the contour alone and choose not to have the nipple and areola reconstructed.

Breast Reconstruction: A Matter of Choice

Figure 19.2.
"Latissimus Dorsi" Reconstruction

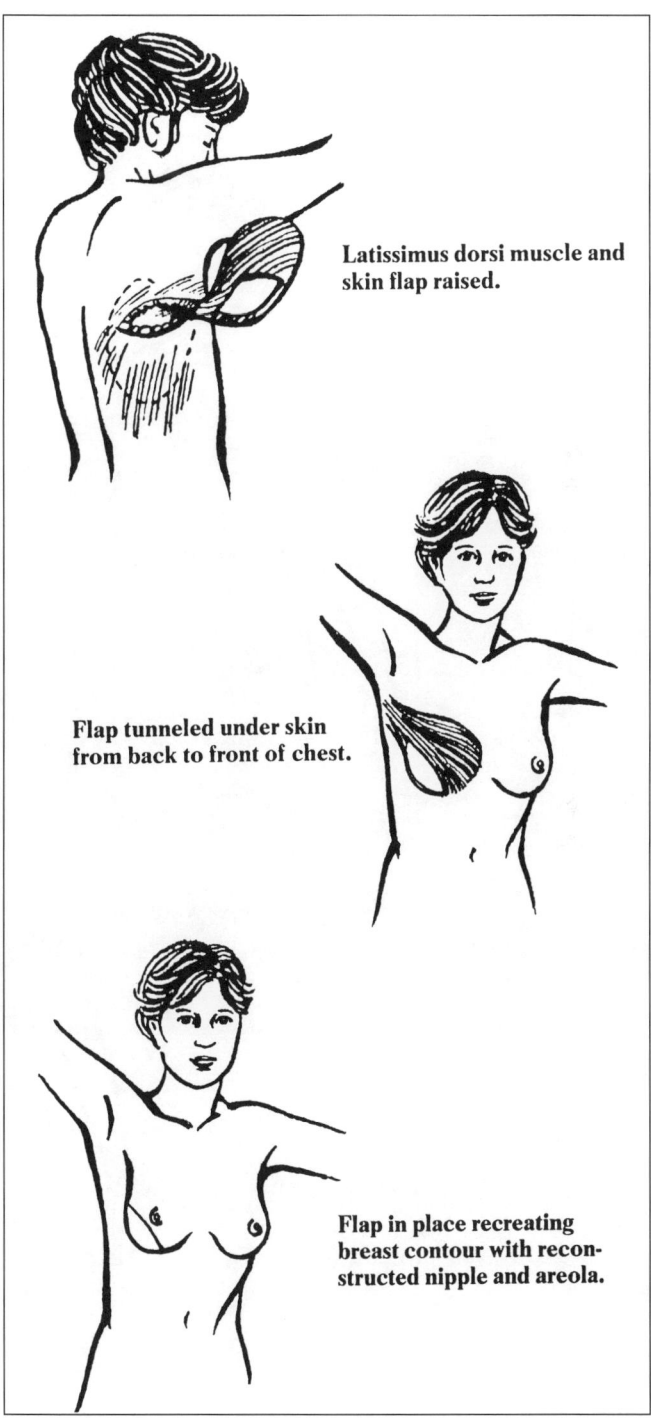

Latissimus dorsi muscle and skin flap raised.

Flap tunneled under skin from back to front of chest.

Flap in place recreating breast contour with reconstructed nipple and areola.

Cancer Sourcebook for Women

Figure 19.3. "Rectus Abdominus" Reconstruction

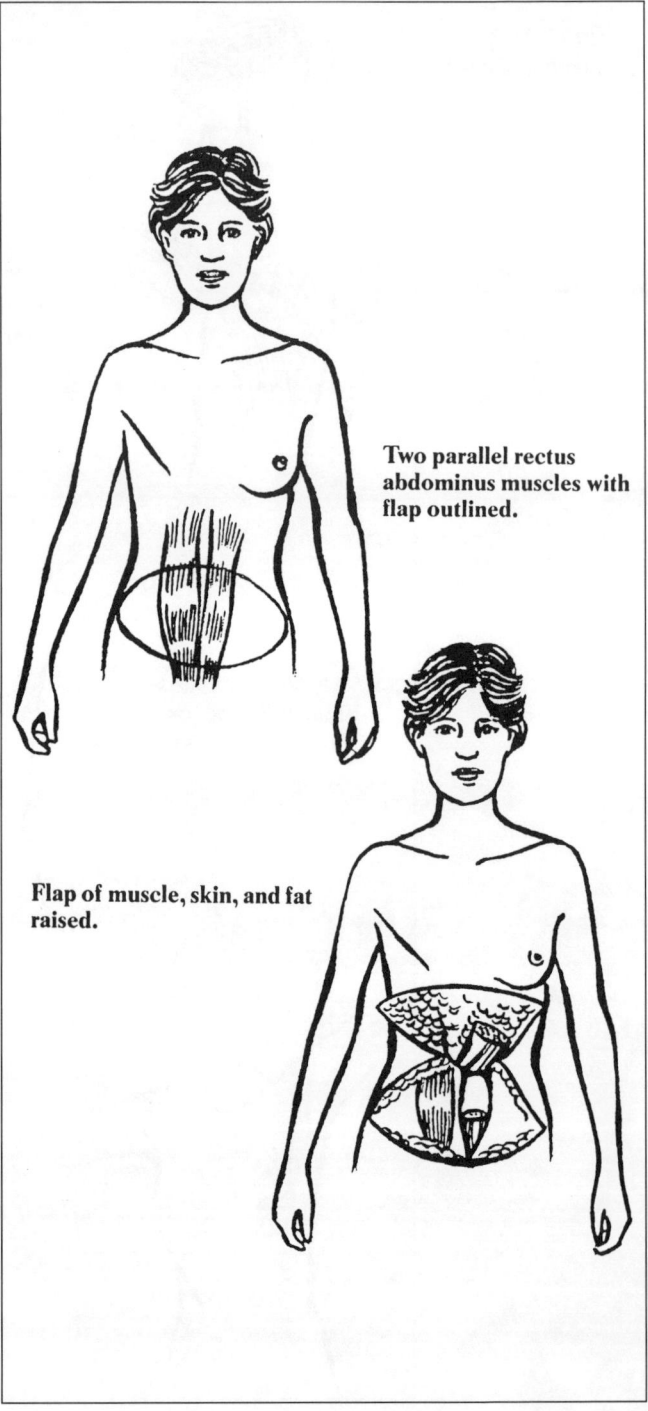

Two parallel rectus abdominus muscles with flap outlined.

Flap of muscle, skin, and fat raised.

Reconstruction of the nipple and areola can be accomplished in a variety of ways. The operation usually takes between 1 and 2 hours.

The most common technique for reconstructing the areola is to use the skin from the upper inner thigh or skin from behind the ear. The nipple is usually reconstructed by using tissue from the newly created breast mound or by grafting a piece from the opposite nipple. In another technique, skin from the vaginal lips can be used to reconstruct the nipple and areola. If the reconstructed areola is not dark enough, ultraviolet light may be used to improve the color match.

Possible Complications

As with all surgical procedures, there are certain risks associated with breast reconstruction. You should discuss possible complications and side effects with your doctor before having any operation. In breast reconstruction, complications may arise if a woman's body reacts unfavorably to a foreign substance, the implant. In about 20 percent of patients, the body's response causes a problem known as "capsular contracture" where the body creates a firm, fibrous capsule around the implant to protect itself. The capsule may become very thick, creating a spherical "baseball" appearance and possibly causing discomfort. Sometimes a contracture softens, as it is absorbed by the body, and improves. Frequently, the surgeon can manipulate it by hand to split the capsule, and the implant then assumes its normal size and shape. Contractures may need to be released surgically.

There are a number of other possible complications. If an infection occurs at the breast site, the implant may have to be removed until the infection heals; it can usually then be replaced. The implant may also have to be temporarily removed if large areas of skin die. Sometimes all or part of a transferred muscle may fail to survive. If the abdominal tissue is used, there is a small chance of an abdominal hernia developing.

Women who are considering reconstructive breast surgery should be aware that mastectomy and reconstruction scars are permanent, although the degree of scarring varies among individuals. As with any other type of plastic surgery, it is difficult to predict the overall result. Also, you should not expect that the reconstruction will restore the sensation lost through mastectomy. Any surgery on the breast can damage the sensitive nerves in that area.

Common Questions About Breast Reconstruction

What does a reconstructed breast look like?

The breast created by inserting an implant under the chest wall muscle does not look like a natural breast, but small differences won't be noticeable in clothing. The new breast will probably look more flattened than tapered. It may have a more youthful appearance than the natural breast, in that it may not droop as much. Plastic surgeons may be able to show you photographs of reconstructed breasts, but you should not expect your reconstructed breast to look like any other woman's.

Does a reconstructed breast feel different?

Breast implants are designed to be much like a natural breast in weight and density, so you should feel a balance between the reconstructed breast and its partner. The fluid-filled sacs are soft and pliable, like natural breast tissue. In place, the implant can move about to some extent, so the reconstructed breast may have some "bounce" to it. The skin over the breast will, of course, feel natural to the touch because it's your own skin; but sensations in the surgical area will probably be diminished. If abdominal tissue is used, the texture will be more like that of a normal breast.

Can a plastic surgeon match my natural breast?

While plastic surgeons make every attempt to match the opposite breast, a reconstructed breast is rarely an exact duplicate of its partner in size, shape, or contour. This is true of a reconstructed nipple and areola as well. Often, surgeons will suggest modifying the natural breast to give a more balanced appearance. Operations on the natural breast may be done at the time of the reconstruction or in a second operation. The most common types of modifications to the natural breast are reduction, enlargement, or lifting. If a woman is at high risk of developing cancer in the remaining breast, a surgeon may recommend a prophylactic mastectomy. With one technique that is sometimes used, the procedure removes most underlying tissue from the natural breast but leaves the skin and nipple. The operation could be followed by immediate reconstruction.

Breast Reconstruction: A Matter of Choice

What if I'm not pleased with the results?

Your level of satisfaction with the reconstruction will depend in large part on your expectations before the operation. Be sure to discuss them with your doctor before you decide to proceed. If an implant is used, after the operation you will be instructed to massage and exercise the muscles surrounding your implant. If you are dissatisfied with the results, after waiting a few months or the skin and muscle to stretch and for the reconstructed breast to take on a more natural appearance, discuss your concerns with your plastic surgeon. Often, the position or the size of the breast mound can be adjusted under local anesthesia.

How long must I wait after surgery before having my breast reconstructed?

Surgeons have different opinions about the most desirable waiting period. Most believe that the mastectomy incision should be well healed and the skin easily movable and elastic before reconstruction. This generally takes from 3 to 6 months. Some surgeons feel that no delay is necessary; they may create a new breast at the same time the natural breast is removed. Most recommend that reconstruction be delayed until chemotherapy and/or radiation therapy are completed. Your feelings also play an important role in the timing of reconstructive surgery. You should be comfortable with your decision before giving the signal to proceed. In most cases, reconstruction can be successfully performed even years after a mastectomy.

How much will breast reconstruction cost?

Plastic surgeon's fees vary with the complexity of the procedure. For example, simple insertion of an implant costs less than other procedures; creation of a nipple increases the cost. Fees also vary considerably in different parts of the United States. Hospital costs are extra. Most health insurance plans now cover part of the cost of breast reconstruction, because it is considered corrective surgery for postmastectomy rehabilitation, not cosmetic surgery. Some insurance companies, however, do not cover rehabilitation of any kind. Ask your insurance company representative if reconstruction is covered under your policy.

How long is the recovery period?

Depending on the extent of the operation, most women are able to resume normal activities in 2 to 3 weeks. It may be several more weeks before they can do strenuous exercise, however.

Do I continue breast self-examination after reconstruction?

By all means. Breast reconstruction does not cause cancer to come back, nor does it prevent recurrence. After reconstruction, you will continue to have periodic physical and laboratory exams. In addition, you should examine both of your breasts monthly, following your doctor's instructions.

Could a breast implant hide a new cancer?

Plastic surgeons and radiologists believe there is little or no difficulty in promptly detecting a recurrence of cancer, either beneath or around an implant, using examination by hand or mammography (x-rays of the breast). If cancer were to recur in the reconstructed breast, it would most likely be located just under the skin and be easy to find.

Making Decisions About Reconstruction

After a mastectomy, you may decide to have your breast reconstructed, to use an artificial breast form, or to make no attempt to alter your appearance. It's a choice that can have a significant impact on your lifestyle. And it is a choice that you need not make immediately or without help. In considering reconstruction, you should:

- Talk with your doctor about the benefits and risks;

- Consult one or more plastic surgeons about the best procedure for your particular situation;

- Talk with women who have had reconstructive surgery and those who have chosen not to have it; and

- Discuss your concerns with family members and friends.

Choosing a Plastic Surgeon

Both a general surgeon and a plastic surgeon may help you decide whether to have reconstructive surgery. If possible, you should discuss reconstruction with the doctor before you have surgery for breast cancer because the position of the mastectomy incision may affect the reconstruction procedure. However, many women consider the option of reconstruction only after surgery. A time lag, even if it's years, between mastectomy and reconstructive surgery need not be an obstacle to the success of the procedure.

In choosing a plastic surgeon, you will want some one who is technically competent and well-experienced in this procedure. Your surgeon should also be someone who is sensitive to the emotional issues associated with breast reconstruction. You may want to talk with a number of doctors. Discussing your feelings openly will help you decide if you are comfortable with a particular doctor.

Most mastectomies performed today are the modified radical type in which the breast and the underarm lymph nodes are removed but the chest muscles remain. After a modified radical mastectomy, the reconstruction procedures are relatively straightforward and can be performed successfully by nearly all plastic surgeons. Women who have had radical mastectomies might seek a surgeon with exceptional expertise in breast reconstruction.

Your doctor may be able to recommend a plastic surgeon. In addition. You can contact the following organizations:

- **American Society of Plastic and Reconstructive Surgeons.** This professional society may give you names of board-certified members in your area. Write to the ASPRS (444 East Algonquin, Arlington Heights, IL 66005) or call its patient referral service (800-635-0635).

- **The American Cancer Society (ACS).** Call your state or local unit (listed under American Cancer Society in the telephone book) to see if it has names of surgeons who perform reconstruction.

- **Medical societies.** Your local medical society also may recommend qualified surgeons who perform breast reconstruction.

Sharing Experiences With Other Women

Your surgeon and plastic surgeon may be able to refer you to other breast cancer patients they have treated. Other women who have made a decision about having reconstruction can provide insight that may help you decide what's best for you. Many women who have had reconstructive surgery are happy to meet with others considering the procedure. The American Cancer Society's Reach to Recovery Program is one means to meet such volunteers. Another is the YWCA's ENCORE program for postoperative breast cancer patients. For more information, contact your local units of ACS and YWCA.

Other Resources

The Cancer Information Service (CIS) is a nation-wide toll-free telephone program sponsored by the National Cancer Institute. Trained information specialists are available to answer questions about mastectomy and breast reconstruction as well as to provide information about other aspects of cancer. Write to the Office of Cancer Communications, National Cancer Institute, Bethesda, MD 20892, or call the toll-free CIS telephone number at:

1-800-4-CANCER

Spanish-speaking CIS staff members are also available.

The American Cancer Society offers a slide presentation on breast reconstruction through its Reach to Recovery Program and a bibliography listing articles, books, and pamphlets on the subject. Contact your state or local ACS unit or write to ACS national head-quarters at 1599 Clifton Rd., NE, Atlanta, GA 30329.

The National Cancer Institute has developed PDQ (Physician Data Query), a computerized database designed to give doctors quick and easy access to:

- The latest treatment information for most types of cancer;
- Descriptions of clinical trials (treatment studies); and
- Names of organizations and physicians involved in cancer care.

Breast Reconstruction: A Matter of Choice

To get access to PDQ, a doctor may use an office computer with a telephone hookup and a PDQ access code or the services of a medical library with online searching capability. Cancer Information Service offices (1-800-4-CANCER) provide PDQ searches and can tell doctors how to get regular access to the database. Patients may ask their doctor to use PDQ or may call 1-800-4-CANCER themselves. Information specialists at this toll-free number use a variety of sources, including PDQ to answer questions about cancer prevention, diagnosis, and treatment. The list of questions below can help you in getting the information you need to consider before you decide to have breast reconstruction. You may have other questions that are not listed here. If so, write them in at the end of a photocopy of the list; then take them with you when you consult a plastic surgeon.

- What type of surgery would you recommend for me? Why?
- What are the risks and benefits associated with it?
- What is your experience with operations of this type?
- May I see photographs of other patients who have had breast reconstruction?
- May I talk with other patients about the operation?
- What can I expect my reconstructed breast to look and feel like? Right after the surgery? In 6 months? In a year?
- How long will I be in the hospital?
- How long is the recovery period after surgery?
- What will I have to do to ensure a safe recovery?
- How much will it cost?
- When can I have the operation?
- What else should I consider in determining whether to have reconstructive surgery?
- Others?

When you visit the plastic surgeon, be prepared for a candid discussion of your expectations for breast reconstruction and your understanding of the impact it will have on you and those close to you. Your motivation for considering breast reconstruction is another area that the surgeon will want to know about.

Breast Self-Examination

After reconstruction, breast self-examination (BSE) should be part of your routine. You will want to examine your natural breast and the reconstructed breast once a month to note any changes in the way they look or feel. Although you may have been doing self-exams before your surgery, you will have to relearn what's considered "normal" for you now. About half the women who have mastectomies report that their remaining breast becomes larger.

If you menstruate, the best time to do BSE is 2 or 3 days after your period ends, when your breast is least likely to be tender or swollen. If you no longer menstruate, pick a day, such as the first day of the month, to do BSE.

Here is how to do BSE:

1. Stand before a mirror. Inspect your breast for anything unusual, such as any discharge from the nipple, or puckering, dimpling, or scaling of the skin. Inspect the scar for new swelling, lumps, redness, or color change. Although redness can be a result of irritation from your bra or prosthesis, report it to your physician.

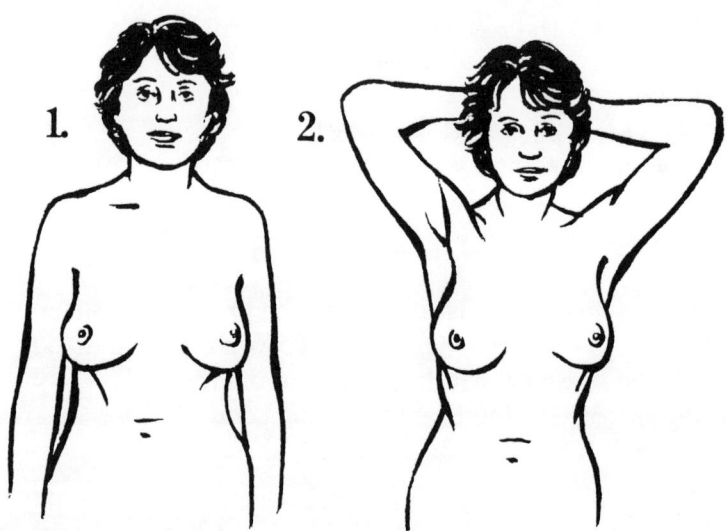

Figure 19.4.

Breast Reconstruction: A Matter of Choice

The next two steps are designed to emphasize any change in the shape or contour of your breast. As you do them, you should be able to feel your chest muscles tighten.

2. Watching closely in the mirror, clasp your hands behind your head and press your hands forward.

3. Next, press your hands firmly on your hips and bow slightly toward your mirror as you pull your shoulders and elbows forward.

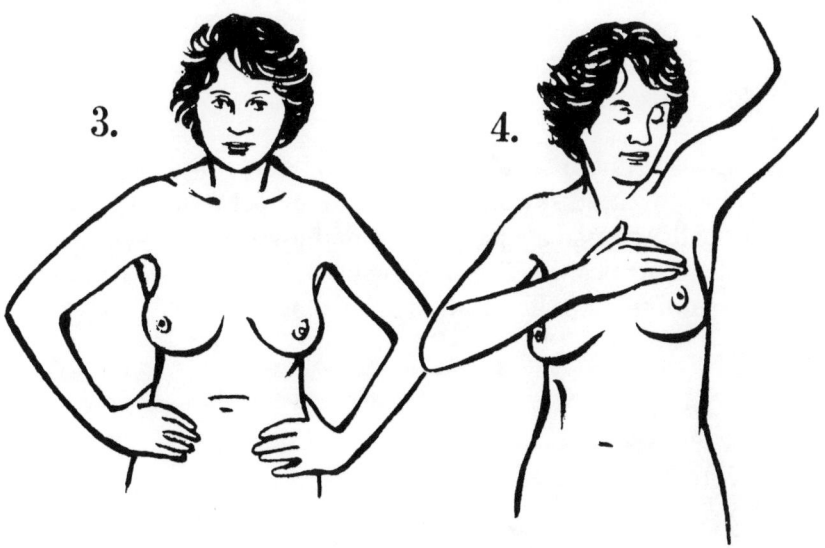

Figure 19.5.

The next part of the exam is done while standing. Some women do it in the shower because fingers glide over soapy skin, making it easy to concentrate on the texture underneath.

4. Raise your arm on the unoperated side. Using three or four fingers of your other hand, explore your breast firmly, carefully, and thoroughly. Beginning at the outer edge, press the flat part of your fingers in small circles, moving the circles

slowly around the breast. Gradually work toward the nipple. Be sure to cover the entire breast. Pay special attention to the area between the breast and the underarm, including the underarm itself. Feel for any unusual lump or mass under the skin.

5. Gently squeeze the nipple and look for a discharge. Raise your arm on the operated side. Use three or four fingers of your opposite hand and begin at the top of the scar. Press gently, using small circular motions, and feel the entire length of the scar. Look for thickenings, lumps, and hard places. As with your breast, familiarity with your scar makes it easier to notice any changes. Lumps, thickening, and inflammation are among changes you should bring to the attention of your doctor.

6. Steps 4 and 5 should be repeated lying down. Lie flat on your back, raise your arm on the unoperated side over your head, and place a pillow or folded towel under your shoulder. This position flattens the breast and makes it easier to examine. Use the same circular motion described earlier.

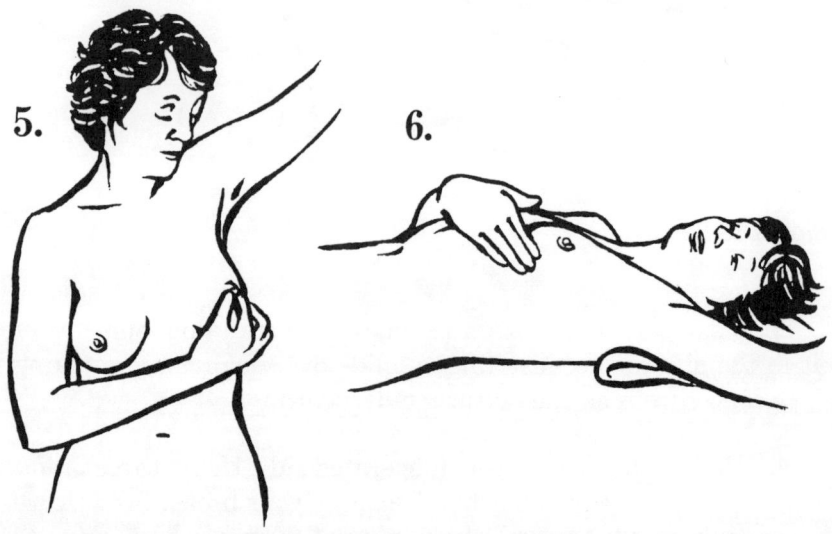

Figure 19.6.

Chapter 20

Survival Following Breast-Sparing Surgery vs Mastectomy

The 1990 NIH Consensus Development Conference on the Treatment of Early Stage Breast Cancer concluded that "breast conservation treatment is an appropriate method of primary therapy for the majority of women with stage I and II breast cancer and is preferable because it provides survival equivalent to total mastectomy and axillary dissection while preserving the breast".

The extensive review of the existing data that led the panelists to this conclusion in 1990 depended heavily on the NSABP B-06 trial, the largest randomized test of mastectomy versus breast sparing procedures. The submission of fraudulent data by one investigator in the B-06 trial created a need to validate the Consensus Conference conclusions. Fortunately however, these conclusions did not depend entirely on the results of the B-06 trial alone. There have been five other randomized trials reported in the scientific literature that also support this conclusion. In order to further evaluate these different therapeutic options, the authors performed a literature review of these trials and used this information to conduct a meta-analysis.

The five published studies, excluding B-06, include trials from: (1) The Danish Breast Cancer Group (J Natl Cancer Inst Monogr 11:19-25, 1992); (2) The EORTC (J Natl Cancer Inst Monogr 11:1518, 1992); (3) The Gustave-Roussy (Radiother Oncol 14:177-184, 1989); (4) The NCI-Bethesda (J Natl Cancer Inst Monogr 11:27-32, 1992); and (5) The NCI-Milan (Eur J Cancer 6:668-670, 1990). These five trials have

---

NCI Cancerfax 208/400020.

a total of 1,407 patients randomized to conservative surgery and breast irradiation versus 1,407 patients randomized to mastectomy. The results of this meta-analysis demonstrate that, without the B-06 trial, both types of treatment yield equivalent results in terms of overall survival.

The odds ratio of comparing the likelihood of death for patients who received mastectomy compared to patients who received breast sparing surgery is 0.964, which approaches equivalent results, with a 95 percent confidence interval of 0.804 to 1.157. Thus, even without the B-06 trial, there is substantial evidence that breast sparing procedures and mastectomy are comparable.

If the conservative surgery and breast irradiation arm (minus patients treated at St. Luc Hospital) and the mastectomy arm (minus patients treated at St. Luc Hospital) from the NSABP B-06 trial are included in the analysis, then there are a total of 1,962 patients treated with conservative surgery and breast irradiation versus 1,899 patients treated with mastectomy. The addition of the B-06 patients does not change the overall results, although the statistical power of the conclusions are strengthened. The odds ratio of death comparing mastectomy to breast sparing surgery is 1.035, which is still nearly equivalent, with a 95 percent confidence interval of 0.892 to 1.200.

Whenever a trial is designed to prove equivalence between two treatment options, the sample size should be large enough to ensure the critical difference is outside the 95 percent confidence interval. However, the use of meta-analysis to combine results from similar trials does increase the sample size and allows us to infer that, even in the worst case scenario, survival after mastectomy cannot be more than 11 percent better than that seen with breast conservation. This tight confidence interval makes it unlikely that meaningful differences exist between breast sparing procedures and mastectomy.

—by Jeffrey Abrams, M.D.,
Timothy Chen, Ph.D.,
and Ruthann Guisti.

Chapter 21

Breast Implants

Regulatory History of Breast Implants

FDA was given the responsibility for regulating medical devices such as breast implants by the Safe Medical Devices Amendment of 1976. Under this law, FDA requires manufacturers of new devices that might pose a risk to submit scientific evidence showing that they are safe, effective and properly labeled before the agency allows them on the market.

The many devices already in use when the 1976 Amendment was passed were allowed to remain in commerce with the understanding that the agency would eventually require scientific evidence of their safety and effectiveness, just as if they were new. Both silicone gel-filled and saline-filled silicone breast implants were among the products covered by this provision, called the "grandfather clause" of the Amendment.

Silicone Gel-Filled Breast Implants

Several years ago, when FDA asked the manufacturers of silicone gel-filled breast implants to submit the required evidence of safety and effectiveness, it became apparent that much of the information was not available. This did not necessarily mean that the implants were unsafe, but it did mean that FDA could not—as the law requires—vouch for their safety.

FDA Information Update June 1994 with revisions.

FDA therefore decided in April, 1991 to remove the gel-filled implants from the market and allow them to be used only in controlled clinical studies.

A year later, FDA announced that the studies would be conducted in three phases identified as Urgent Need, Open Availability or Adjunct, and Core studies. The Urgent Need phase began in the summer of 1992, and the Open Availability or Adjunct phase in the fall of 1992.

As of June, 1994 it is not known exactly when the third phase will begin because the Core studies will take more time to set up. Once it starts, each study will run 3-5 years. To enroll in a study, contact your surgeon who can find out from the manufacturer of the implants which hospitals or doctors offices are taking part in trials in your geographical area.

Saline-Filled Breast Implants

The manufacturers of saline-filled breast implants were notified by FDA in January 1993 that the agency requires proof of their products' safety and effectiveness. Pending the submission of the data, saline-filled breast implants, which contain salt water—part of the body's fluids—rather than silicone gel, remain on the market.

Deciding About Breast Implant Surgery

Before exploring the possibility of a breast implant surgery, it is advisable to consider other alternatives for breast reconstruction and augmentation. Such options include wearing an external artificial breast form (prosthesis) or undergoing a surgical procedure called the "flap" technique.

This technique involves moving skin, muscle and fat to the breast area from the abdomen, back, or buttock to rebuild the breast, leaving a scar where the skin was lifted. This is a major operation and, for medical reasons, it is not suitable for everyone.

Another matter to be considered early in the decision-making process is why some women choose reconstruction or augmentation with implants and why others do not. There are no studies that provide definite answers regarding either the effectiveness or the safety of breast implants, but some of the frequently cited factors are listed below.

Breast Implants

A few reasons why some women decide for implants:

- to replace an external breast prosthesis
- to avoid being constantly reminded of their cancer diagnosis
- to allow for a more comfortable active life-style
- to avoid embarrassment in public dressing areas
- to help create a look that makes them feel more comfortable with or without clothes
- to improve their self-image

A few reasons why some women decide against implants:

- they want to avoid more surgery following the implantation
- they feel the risks of the surgery, anesthesia and implants outweigh the benefits
- they are satisfied with their external prosthesis
- they are concerned over the unknown potential risks for them and their children with respect to breast implants

In considering these and other factors it is important to gather information from your doctor, from women who have undergone mastectomies, and from members of support groups.

Your Expectations

Your consideration of breast implants should be based on realistic expectations of the outcome.

To help you get an idea of what results may be possible, look at "before" and "after" pictures of patients who have had this surgery. Your doctor may have some to show you. Keep in mind, however, that there is no guarantee that your results will match those of other women.

Your results will depend on many individual factors, such as your overall health; chest structure and body shape; healing capabilities (which are hindered by radiation and cytotoxic chemotherapy, smoking, alcohol and various medications); bleeding tendencies; prior breast surgery(ies); infection; surgical skill and experience; and the type of surgical procedure. Also keep in mind that usually it takes more than one operation to get the results you want, especially if you want your nipple rebuilt.

Scarring is a natural outcome of surgery, and your doctor will try to keep scars as subtle as possible. She or he can explain the location, size, and appearance of the scars you can expect to have. For most women, they will fade over time to thin lines, although the darker your skin, the more prominent the scars are likely to be. If you have had a mastectomy, your doctor may be able to insert your implant through your mastectomy scar.

Remember also that an implant is artificial and the body reacts to it. Like anything else, implants age over time and may need to be replaced. Therefore, you should not expect your implant to last indefinitely, even though it may be serviceable for many years.

In balancing the pros and cons of a breast implant, you should consider the surgical procedures of implantation as well as the adverse effects of breast implants as reported to FDA by users.

The Surgery

General Description: Although some procedures can be performed on an outpatient (not hospitalized) basis or under local anesthesia, most surgical implant procedures require general anesthesia.

Depending on the technique used and whether or not surgery is performed on one or both breasts, breast implant surgery can last anywhere from one to several hours. Prior to surgery, your doctor should discuss with you the extent of surgery, the estimated time it will take, and the choice of drugs for anesthesia and for pain and nausea.

The length of the hospital stay will vary according to the type of surgery, the development of any postoperative complications, as well as your general health.

Implant Surgery: Inserting an implant under existing skin and tissue is possible if there is enough skin. If a mastectomy and implant surgery are done at the same time, the surgeon usually can use the mastectomy incision for inserting the implant into a pocket created under the skin.

The pocket may be located either behind (submuscular) or in front of (submammary) the chest muscle. Ask about the pros or cons of each technique. Your doctor will explain which is the best placement for you and why.

Implants may be inserted at the time of surgery, or a temporary "tissue expander" may be used. The surgeon should discuss which approach will be undertaken. If a temporary expander is used, the surgeon removes it in a later operation after the skin has stretched sufficiently. It is then replaced with an implant.

Recreation of the Nipple and Areola: After your breast has healed from the original implant surgery, you may want your nipple and areola (darker skin around the nipple) rebuilt. This procedure can usually be performed on an out-patient basis. Ask your surgeon to explain the various ways this can be done.

Postoperative Recovery: The health care provider should describe to you the usual postoperative recovery process, the possible complications that can arise, and the length of time to complete recovery from the effects of the surgery. Following the operation, as with any surgery, some pain, swelling, bruising, and tenderness can be expected to occur, but they should disappear with time. Medications for pain and nausea can be prescribed. Some women may experience fever, infection or bleeding. Patients should be instructed on appropriate wound care, and what to expect on wound healing.

The length of your stay in the hospital will vary, depending on the type of surgery you have had and your general health.

When implants are used as part of your surgery, your surgeon may advise you to massage your breast to reduce pain or the incidence of capsular contracture. If so advised, you should be taught the proper technique, as well as how often and how long to massage. This technique, however, is controversial. Some health care providers believe it can increase gel bleed and rupture of the implant(s).

Follow-Up: Ask your surgeon about follow-up care including future, routinely scheduled examinations; any limits to your activities; any particular precautions you should take; do's and don'ts; and when you can return to your normal routine.

The Risks of Implant Surgery

There are always potential adverse reactions and complications that the surgeon should discuss with the patient well in advance of surgery both with regard to the proposed surgical procedure and the implant itself. A week of more before the surgery, ask your surgeon and anesthesiologist or anesthetist for full risk information including the patient package insert and a copy of the hospital informed consent form.

Anesthesia Risks: General anesthesia involves risk. For a full understanding of each risk and the statistical chances of being exposed to it, explore the subject with your anesthesiologist or anesthetist before the surgery.

The following risks and complications can occur:

- Nausea/vomiting after operation
- Problems with intubation (e.g., chipped teeth, sore throat)
- High fever (uncommon)
- Seizures, stroke, heart attack, coma (rare)
- Death (rare)

There are no studies of anesthesia and breast implants. However, in a study of 45,090 outpatient, rather than in-patient (in the hospital) surgical procedures (similar in complexity to cosmetic breast surgery) involving some form of anesthesia care, there were no deaths and only one major complication clearly related only to anesthesia.

Thus, the risk of anesthesia in healthy patients is very low, and there appear to be no special problems associated with breast implants and anesthesia. However, chemotherapy or radiation therapy may cause cardiac damage or increase cardiac risk, and thus increase the risk for anesthesia. Other concurrent medical problems may increase the risk as well.

Surgical Risks: Breast reconstruction and augmentation entails potential risks or adverse reactions directly connected with the surgery. Discuss these risks or adverse events or reactions with your anesthesiologist and surgeon in detail before your surgery. The following complications may result from the placement of any foreign object in the body, including a breast implant:

- **Hematoma** is a collection of blood or a blood clot from a leak in a blood vessel that forms, within hours after surgery, in the surgical pocket where the implant has been placed. If this happens, swelling, pain, and bruising may result.

- **Infection or sepsis** is not a frequent problem but may be troublesome or even serious if it occurs. If you notice signs of infection such as pain, redness, swelling, tenderness and fever, report them to your doctor immediately.

  If infection does not subside promptly with the appropriate treatment removal of the implant may be indicated. After the infection has completely cleared, the implant can usually be replaced.

- **Hemorrhage** (abnormal bleeding) may be a result of abnormal bleeding tendencies, chemotherapy or other medications, or the surgery itself.

- **Thrombosis** (abnormal clotting)

- **Skin necrosis** occurs when there is not enough blood supply to the skin. This may happen because the circulation to the remaining tissue has been changed by the mastectomy or other trauma to the breast area.

The chance of skin necrosis may be increased as a result of radiation treatments, cortisone-like drugs used to reduce capsular contracture, an implant that is too large for the available space, or from smoking.

In some cases of necrosis, the surgeon may have to remove the implant to prevent infection. If necrosis is severe enough, the implant may force its way through the skin.

Risks of Silicone Gel-filled and Saline-filled Breast Implants

FDA's Device Experience Network tracks adverse events reports involving all breast implants.

Between January 1, 1985 and June, 1994, the agency received 77,318 adverse reaction reports—including 68 deaths—associated with the silicone gel-filled breast implants.

During the same time, the Device Experience Network received 12,426 reports, including 3 deaths, involving the saline-filled breast implants.

The reported adverse effects included both known risks, which are experienced by some women and are clearly associated with these devices, and possible risks, which might exist but have not been proven at this time.

Known Risks

In addition to the risks of surgery, the most common of the known risks or adverse reactions or events for silicone gel-filled and saline-filled breast implants are:

- **Capsular contracture** is a tightening of the scar tissue that normally forms around the implant. This can sometimes cause pain, hardening of the breast, or changes in its appearance.

- **Calcium deposits** can form in surrounding tissue, and can cause pain and hardening.

- **Implant rupture** may occur slowly as with silicone implants or suddenly, as happens more often with saline implants. Rupture or leakage allows the filling inside the implant envelope to be released into surrounding tissue. Rupture may be sudden and recognized or unrecognized by the woman. If the problems are severe, the implants may have to be removed permanently.

- **Changes in nipple or breast sensation** may result from the surgery.

Possible Risks

Interference with Mammogram Readings: The presence of breast implants requires a special mammography technique and increases the technical difficulty of taking and reading mammograms. This interference may delay or hinder the early detection of breast cancer by "hiding" suspicious lesions in the breast on a mammogram.

Also, it may be difficult to distinguish any calcium deposits formed in the scar tissue around the implant from a tumor when interpreting the mammogram. Remember to check with your doctor, radiologist, and mammography technologist to make certain that you are receiving the proper mammography techniques.

Several factors affect the success of special mammography techniques in imaging the breast tissue in women with breast implants. The procedure involves pushing the implant back and gently pulling the breast tissue into view. Therefore such factors as location of the implant, the degree of capsular contraction, relative size of the breast tissue to implant size and other factors may affect how well the breast tissue can be imaged.

Other imaging methods, e.g., magnetic resonance imaging (MRI) and ultrasound, may be helpful in assessing the integrity of an implant and in evaluating other breast problems. For example, ultrasound can be useful in differentiating between cystic and solid masses. These methods have not, however, been proven useful in detecting early breast cancer in asymptomatic women, whether or not they have implants. Additionally, the imaging procedures used to detect early signs of breast cancer are different from those used to evaluate the integrity of the implant. The techniques used in mammography to evaluate the implant may differ from those techniques used to evaluate the breast tissue.

Silicone: The envelope of both silicone gel-filled and saline-filled breast implants contains silicone. Silicone is thought to cause an array of reported signs and symptoms, many of which are not limited to women who have implants filled with silicone-gel. As yet, however, there is no scientific proof that confirms or disproves such association.

Silicone gel-filled implants may rupture or "bleed" silicone through the implant envelope, causing silicone to reach distant parts of the body. The manufacturers of the implants have been unable to supply FDA with the actual percentage of women who experience such bleed or rupture over time. The manufacturers also do not have data on how many women with or without implants have the various problems reported as possibly associated with silicone breast implants.

Clinical trials should help to answer these question. See the index for information on the status of the studies.

Autoimmune-like Disorders: These are disorders of the body's defense, or "immune" system. Signs include: pain and swelling of joints; tightness, redness or swelling of the skin; swollen glands or lymph nodes; unusual and unexplained fatigue; swelling of the hands and feet; and unusual hair loss.

These signs are not specific to autoimmune disorders, and many women with or without breast implants have one or more of these symptoms from time to time. However, those who have immune-related disorders (which are relatively rare in the general population) usually experience a combination of these and other signs that do not disappear.

Some recent research conducted in animals has shown that silicone gel of the type used in breast implants can increase antibody production in these animals. Antibodies are substances produced in the blood which can produce a specific immunity to a specific germ or virus. However, clinical studies as yet are inconclusive in demonstrating any link between silicone and effects on the human immune system. Autoimmune-like disorders have been found in women with breast implants, some of whom have reported a reduction in symptoms after their implants were removed. It has been suggested that even the very small amounts of silicone that "sweat" through the implant could cause such autoimmune-like disorders as lupus, scleroderma and rheumatoid arthritis in some women.

One study has shown that some women with breast implants produced antibodies against their own collagen (a connective tissue protein), but it is not known whether this might increase their risk of actually developing an autoimmune-like disorder.

A recent study which followed women with breast implants for 7-10 years, found that they did not have a higher rate of immune-related disorders than women without the implants. The study was too small to rule out the possibility of a very small increase in these diseases in breast implant patients, and it did not rule out the possibility that the effects could occur after the tested period. The study did show, however, that most women are unlikely to experience these kinds of effects within the first decade after implantation.

Fibrositis/Fibromyalgia-like Disorders: Some physicians have reported that a few of their patients have developed these disorders after receiving breast implants. However, there is no conclusive evidence at present that women with breast implants have an increased risk of developing these disorders.

Cancer: Thus far, only one lab study in mice, described below, shows any evidence that silicone in breast implants could increase the risk of cancer. Long-term clinical studies presently underway should provide better answers to this question within the next few years.

A study published in the July 20, 1994 *Journal of the National Cancer Institute* shows that silicone gel can induce a rare form of cancer, plasmacytoma, in laboratory mice. Plasmacytomas are similar to a rare human blood cell cancer call B-cell multiple myeloma.

The relevance of this study to women with silicone gel-filled breast implants is not yet known. In the study silicone gel was injected into the abdomens of the mice, and the two strains of mice in the study are bred to be susceptible to plasmacytomas. FDA is aware of a few cases of women with breast implants who have developed multiple myeloma. However, there is no evidence at this point that women with breast implants are more susceptible to this disease than other women. Since multiple myeloma occurs throughout the population, some cases are expected to develop in women both with and without implants. Based on a rate of four new cases in 100,000 persons in the United States, and considering the differing rates of various segments of the population, epidemiologist expect that over the last six years, about 155 cases of multiple myeloma would have occurred in women with breast implants, whether or not they had the implants.

FDA and researchers are asking physicians to report cases of multiple myeloma in their breast implant patients. Signs and symptoms of the disease include weakness and fatigue, bone pain, kidney failure, recurrent bacterial infections and anemia. For some patients, weakness and fatigue may be the primary symptoms.

This reinforces FDA's advice to women who have breast implants. The agency has said in the past that these women should stay on the alert for signs of problems and see their doctors if these occur, but that women who are not experiencing problems need not have their implants removed.

Pregnancy: At this time the effects of a mother's breast implants on a growing fetus are unknown.

Breast Feeding: It is not known whether the small amounts of silicone that "bleed" from gel-filled silicone breast implants or from the silicone envelope encasing the saline-filled silicone implants can find their way into breast milk; and, if this were to occur, whether it could affect the child. One published report suggests a few children of women with breast implants have abdominal pain and swallowing problems, but it is not known whether these problems are related to breast implants. Further study is needed to answer this question.

Breast augmentation surgery generally does not interfere with a woman's ability to nurse her baby. As mentioned above, however, some surgical procedures may affect the shape and function of the nipple as well as the sensation of the nipple and that of surrounding breast tissue.

Reconstructive surgery may affect breast feeding to a greater degree, depending on the surgery. Such questions should be posed to the surgeon prior to implant surgery.

Saline-filled Implants: Leakage or rupture from saline-filled implants results in release of salt water, which is not foreign to and does not remain in the body. But because saline-filled implants use a silicone envelope, whose long-term safety has not been demonstrated, the saline-filled implants may not be without risk. Moreover, if a saline-filled implant leaks or ruptures, it deflates and usually must be removed or replaced, which requires new surgery.

Possible Risks of Silicone Gel-filled Breast Implants Coated with Polyurethane Foam

These implants were removed from the U.S. market in January 1990, and the company is no longer making them. About 10 percent of women with implants have this type. The coating was intended to reduce the risk of capsular contracture. In addition to the risks listed above, there are special questions about silicone gel-filled breast implants that are coated with polyurethane foam:

Cancer: On July 31, 1991, an FDA advisory committee found that over a long period of time the polyurethane coating can chemically break down under laboratory conditions to release very small amounts of a substance called 2-toluene-diamine (TDA), which can cause cancer in animals. No such association with cancer has been made in humans, and there is insufficient evidence to justify having polyurethane-coated breast implants removed because of concerns about cancer.

Breast Feeding: Concerns have also been raised about whether the TDA from the polyurethane-coated implants could find its way into breast milk and whether this might pose a risk to a nursing infant. To help answer this and other questions about polyurethane-coated implants, FDA is requiring the manufacturer to conduct studies on these implants, analyzing breast milk, blood, and urine for TDA. This will take some time, as reliable test methods must be developed before these studies can be done. Women who use these implants and are concerned about nursing their infants should consult with their doctors.

Special Medical and Physical Considerations

In addition to the risks outlined above, breast implants may have implications for your individual risks and benefits. To gain understanding of these potential short- and long-term effects, it is important to discuss with your health providers the following risk factors:

Changes in the physical properties of the implanted breast(s): What are the chances that you will experience any of the following: movement or discomfort of the implant on lying down or raising the arm; altered sensation to heat, cold, touch; changes in the sensation of the breast during sexual excitement; feel the edges of the implant under the skin?

Changes in the appearance of the breasts: What is the possibility that your breasts may not match for such reasons as capsular contracture; shifting; side effects resulting from the use of cortisone around the implant(s); the use of different-sized implants; differences in the healing processes between the two breasts; the thickness of your chest skin after mastectomy; tissue changes resulting from radiation treatments, or other medical reasons?

Other considerations: What are the effects of medications, smoking and alcohol use on the ability to do the implantation surgery and achieve good cosmetic results?

- How is the implantation surgery affected by past or future radiation (x-ray) therapy treatments for breast cancer?

- Are there any medical contraindications to either the surgery under general anesthesia, or to the implants themselves?
- Does a history of prior problems with breast implants predispose a woman to problems, if so, which ones?
- What effect do anticancer medications, in particular, cytotoxic chemotherapy, have on the ability to conduct the surgery and have positive results?

After you have considered the pros and cons of breast implants and discussed the matter with your doctor, you may need to decide on which type of implant to choose. While this matter should be also explored with your doctor, the next two sections answer some of the most frequently asked questions about the current options.

Availability of Silicone Gel-Filled Implants

Under what circumstances are silicone gel-filled implants available?

Because of scientific concerns about the possible short- and long-term effects of silicone gel-filled breast implants, these devices are only available to women who are enrolled in a clinical study sponsored by the implant manufacturer and approved by FDA. At this time, one manufacturer, Mentor Corporation, has been approved by FDA to conduct such a study. More than 7,000 patients have enrolled so far, with about 11,000 implants to be studied. This study will look at short-term risks, such as capsular contracture and rupture of silicone gel-filled implants. It will be about three years before the researchers will be able to come to any conclusions about these short-term risks.

Any woman who needs the implants for breast reconstruction can enroll in the study. This includes those who have had breast cancer surgery or a severe injury to the breast, or who have a medical condition causing a severe breast abnormality. Those who must have an existing implant replaced for medical reasons, such as rupture of the implant, are also eligible. Women who want the implants for breast augmentation (enlargement) cannot be enrolled in these studies.

More completely controlled studies are planned to investigate the safety of the implants in greater detail. Those studies will enroll a limited number of women who want the implants for breast augmentation, as well as those having them for reconstruction.

Will the studies address all of the safety issues related to silicone gel-filled breast implants?

No. The research studies are prospective clinical investigations. This means that they are designed to follow new patients after they receive the implants and look for specific benefits or problems. Other types of safety questions will be answered in other studies.

For example, questions about possible long-term effects, such as immune-related disorders or cancer, will be addressed by studies of those who already have the implants. Two of these studies, sponsored by implant manufacturers, are underway at New York University and the University of Michigan. The results of these trials are coming in, and more are expected over the next few years. A third study on long term effects will begin this year under the sponsorship of the National Cancer Institute, part of the National Institutes of Health (NIH).

Other kinds of safety questions will be answered by laboratory studies conducted by the manufacturers under an FDA-imposed timetable. These include the chemical makeup and effects of silicone material that "bleeds" out of the implant shell, the strength of the implant shell and its resistance to rupture, and the physical and chemical changes that implants may undergo in the body.

Will silicone gel-filled breast implants continue to be available in the future?

This is uncertain at the moment. Mentor Corporation (the sole active manufacturer of gel-filled implants at this time) has announced that it will stop manufacturing silicone gel-filled breast implants within the next couple of years. McGhan Medical Corporation intends to resume manufacturing silicone gel-filled implants, but it is uncertain when that will happen.

How can a woman enroll in a study on silicone gel-filled implants?

To enroll in a study, a woman who is interested in silicone gel-filled implants for breast reconstruction should first contact the doctor she chooses to perform the implant surgery. The doctor will then make the necessary arrangements with the implant manufacturer.

Before the woman can be enrolled, her doctor must certify that she qualifies medically for the implant. She will have to sign a special Informed Consent Form, certifying that she has been told about the risks of the implants, and that she will be enrolled in a registry so that she can be notified in the future, if necessary, about new information on the implants.

Can a woman who wants silicone gel-filled implants for breast augmentation still get them?

Silicone gel-filled implants are no longer available for breast augmentation. However, at this time women can still have their breasts enlarged with saline-filled silicone implants.

Availability of Saline-Filled Silicone Implants

What's the status of saline-filled silicone breast implants?

The saline-filled silicone implants are still on the market for both reconstruction and augmentation. However, FDA has notified the manufacturers of these implants that they will be required to submit safety and effectiveness information in conjunction with their Premarket Approval (PMA) applications, just as the manufacturers of the gel-filled implants were required to do.

FDA held a public hearing on June 2, 1994 to solicit public comment on the timing of its call for data from manufacturers of saline-filled implants. Implant manufacturers, consumers, and health professionals and representatives of other organizations made presentations. Issues that were discussed included: the perceived safety or hazards of these implants; the status of manufacturers' studies to develop data required by FDA; the availability of these implants for both augmentation and reconstruction patients; and the use of saline-filled implants as controls in studies of silicone gel-filled implants.

After FDA calls for manufacturers of saline filled implants to provide the information, the saline-filled implants will be allowed to remain on the market only if FDA decides that the information submitted by the manufacturers shows that the implants are safe and effective.

Information to Obtain For Your Records

If you are going to be fitted with a breast implant, there are several important items of information you should get from your doctor before the surgery. They are:

Manufacturer's Sticker: A copy of the "sticker" identifies the brand of the implant you will receive, its size and the manufacturer's lot number. This data should be part of your record. It will be useful if you should you have problems following surgery or seek care by another health provider.

Package Insert: You should also receive a copy of the manufacturer's package insert for the particular breast implant you will use. Each package insert contains important information about the precautions to be taken and the risks associated with the specific brand of implant. You should use this insert as a basis for discussion about the surgery with your doctor, and keep the paper for future reference.

Other Frequently Asked Questions

What about Insurance Coverage?

Most insurance companies cover the costs of breast reconstruction after mastectomy, but do not cover augmentation. Before surgery, be sure to get in writing answers from your insurance company to these questions:

- Does my policy cover the costs of the implant surgery, the implant, the anesthesia, and other related hospital costs?
- To what extent?
- Does it cover treatments for medical problems that may be caused by either the implant or the reconstruction?
- Does it cover explanation?

Alternative Implants

Are there other types of breast implants available besides silicone gel-filled and saline-filled implants?

No other breast implants are currently available, although researchers are developing other types of devices. FDA has given conditional approval for a pilot study of 50 patients to evaluate certain characteristics of a new breast implant, the Trilucent Adjustable Breast Implant, made by LipoMatrix Inc. of Neuchatol, Switzerland. This new implant is filled with triglyceride, a purified form of soybean oil. Triglycerides are used as nutrients for intravenous feeding in adults and infants. The shell is made of a silicone elastomer like the shells used with saline-filled and silicone gel-filled breast implants. Each implant will have a unique identifier accessible by non-invasive means. In addition to this study in the U.S., the Trilucent implant is undergoing limited clinical trials in Europe.

The U.S. pilot study is designed to evaluate certain characteristics, such as capsular scarring tendencies, implant identification methods, and whether mammograms can better detect breast masses with the Trilucent implant than other breast implants. Long-term clinical trials would be required if the manufacturer decides to market the Trilucent implant.

FDA has drafted guidance for the testing of alternative breast implants, outlining the requirements and types of preclinical and clinical data that would be necessary for a complete pre-market approval application (PMA).

Alternatives to Silicone Breast Implants Workshop

The draft guidance on testing alternatives was presented and discussed at an FDA scientific workshop on Alternatives to Silicone Breast Implants on Friday, October 21, 1994 in Washington, D.C. This scientific workshop focused on the elements of the testing requirements for alternative breast prostheses: chemical characterization of materials, mechanical testing, preclinical biological testing, clinical testing including study design, quality of life considerations, requirements for Investigational Device Exemptions (IDEs) and Pre-market Approval Applications (PMAs), and post-market surveillance. The workshop included discussion and information exchange by invited scientific authorities. Public participation included written questions facilitated by an invited moderator. FDA accepted additional written comments until December 2, 1994. Transcripts of the workshop may be purchased by written request only from either Freilicher & Associates, 11923 Parklawn Drive, Suite 203, Rockville, Maryland 20852 (301-881-8132) or Freedom of Information Public Records and Documents Center, 5600 Fishers Lane, HFI-35, Rockville, Maryland 20857.

Advice for Women With Implants

Below are answers to some of the questions frequently asked by women with implants:

What is the proper way of examining my breasts?

Like all women, those with breast implants should perform regular breast self-examinations and have regular examinations by their personal physicians, their surgeons or other health professionals trained in breast examination. For women with breast implants, these examinations take on added importance because they can help to detect complications that might be due to the implants.

Women with implants should examine their breasts each month so they can detect changes. For women who menstruate, the best time to examine the breasts is two or three days after the menstrual period ends, when the breasts are least likely to be tender or swollen. Women who no longer menstruate should examine their breasts at the same time each month.

To examine your breasts, first stand in front of a mirror and look for anything unusual, such as changes in the shape or appearance of your breasts or nipples. Then lie down on your back to allow for a better examination of tissue which flattens and spreads out for deeper palpitation.

With your right arm raised above your head, use the flat surface of your fingertips of your left hand to feel your breast. Move your fingers in one of three ways: in a circular motion in a clockwise fashion; in strips (like mowing the lawn); or in a radiant pattern. Feel around the breast to feel for any unusual lump, swelling, or mass under the skin of your right breast.

You should also feel for any swelling of glands or lumps in your armpit. Follow the same procedure for the other breast. Repeat the exam while standing if you have time.

Pay particular attention to changes in the firmness, size, or shape of your breasts. Be attentive to pain, tenderness, or color changes in the breast area, or any discharge or unusual sensation around the nipple. Any of these changes should be reported promptly to a physician, as should any other concerns about your breasts.

Do I need to get regular mammograms?

Women with breast implants who are in an age group where routine mammograms are recommended should be sure to have these examinations at the recommended intervals. (Those who have had breast cancer surgery on both breasts should ask their doctors whether mammograms are still necessary.)

It is important to make sure that personnel at the mammography facility are trained and experienced in the special techniques needed to perform mammography on patients with breast implants. If these techniques are not used, there is a greater chance that breast cancer or ruptured implant will go undetected. At this time, facilities that are certified to FDA standards may—but are not required to—have personnel appropriately trained in these techniques. So, it is important to ask.

Under a new law, the Mammography Quality Standards Act of 1992, all mammography facilities must be certified by FDA to lawfully continue their services after October 1, 1994. All facilities in operation will be required to display a certificate. The law requires that mammography facilities pass federal inspections, and meet standards covering:

- mammography equipment

- personnel involved in mammography, including the interpreting physician, the radiologic technologist and the medical physicist

- quality assurance and quality control, and

- record-keeping and reporting.

The new law is aimed at ensuring that all facilities provide high quality mammography.

Women with implants should always inform the radiologist and mammography technologists about the implants before mammography is performed. That way they can be sure that special techniques for detecting breast abnormalities are used, and can take extra care when compressing the breasts to avoid rupturing the implant.

What are the symptoms of implant rupture?

Some of the signs and symptoms of rupture may include: pain, tingling, numbness, burning, changes in breast size or shape, and changes in sensation.

Implants may rupture without causing symptoms, but women should not have routine mammograms (breast x-rays) just to detect these "silent" ruptures. Mammograms do not necessarily detect ruptures.

As mentioned earlier, the imaging procedures used to detect early signs of breast cancer are different from those used to evaluate the integrity of the implant. The mammography techniques used to evaluate the implant may also differ. Other methods of detecting implant rupture, such as ultrasound, computed axial tomography (CAT) scans, and magnetic resonance imaging (MRI), are still being studied and are not recommended for detecting breast cancer or for routine screening for rupture.

What factors increase the chance that an implant will rupture?

The chance of rupture may increase the longer the implant has been in the body. Injury to the breast also increases the chance of rupture, as may closed capsulotomy, a technique used to correct capsular contracture by squeezing the breast to soften the scar tissue. Closed capsulotomy was commonly practiced in the past, but is not currently recommended.

Should a woman with breast implants nurse her infant?

No one knows whether the small amounts of silicone that "bleed" from silicone gel-filled breast implants or if any silicone from the silicone shell encasing the saline-filled silicone implants can find its way into breast milk; and, if this were to occur, whether it could affect the child. So, FDA does not know if it is safe for a woman with breast implants to nurse. As a result, women must make this challenging benefit-risk decision with the help of their health care providers.

Are there concerns about the children of women with implants?

No one knows if the children of women with breast implants are more likely to have health problems. Only very limited research has been conducted on issues related to breast-feeding with breast implants or risks to the fetus while in utero. Some women are concerned that their children's health problems might be linked to exposure to silicone during pregnancy or while nursing, but at this time there is no scientific evidence to either support or refute their views and concerns. FDA will follow any research in this area and will provide this information to women as it becomes available. Meanwhile, women with breast implants who have questions about risks while pregnant or breast feeding should consult their doctor and carefully weigh the risks and benefits. If their children develop health problems that may be associated with breast implants, these adverse events should be reported to FDA's MedWatch program.

One preliminary study, based on 11 children, suggested that breast-fed children of women with silicone breast implants may be at risk of developing abnormal esophageal motility—a reduction in the normal wave-like motion of their esophagus which moves food toward the stomach. The authors have stated that this is an inconclusive, preliminary report and in FDA's view, deficiencies in the study design make it difficult to draw any conclusions from the data presented. Further study may yield more definitive results.

Is there a test to detect silicone in the body, or to determine whether an individual is sensitive to silicone?

There is no widely available, standardized test to detect silicone in the body. Some large, sophisticated research laboratories can detect the presence of silicone or silicon (an indirect measure of silicone) in blood, tissue, and urine, but the meaning of these test results is unknown.

Some researchers are attempting to develop a test that can detect antibodies to silicone in blood. However, even if such antibodies were detected, the significance would be unclear. Antibodies to silicone would not necessarily indicate that silicone is harmful, or that a person would necessarily have an adverse reaction to it. FDA has not approved any tests for general marketing to determine the level of silicone in the body.

Even if simple techniques to detect silicone were available, they might not be useful in detecting a rupture, because small amounts of silicone ordinarily "bleed" even from intact implants. Further, since silicone is found in food and many other products, including commonly used medicines and cosmetics, the tests would not easily determine whether the silicone came from the implant or another source.

Determining that silicon or silicone is present in body fluids does not indicate whether a person is sensitive to these substances or at risk for any specific disease. There is presently no test available for the general public to determine if a person reacts to silicone or silicon.

How can a woman find out what kind of implant she has?

This information should be in her medical records. She can contact the hospital or other facility where she had the surgery, or ask her surgeon. Women who want this information should seek it as soon as possible, since physicians and hospitals do not necessarily keep medical records indefinitely.

Should a woman have her breast implants removed?

FDA is not recommending that a woman have her implants removed if she is experiencing any problems. But if she is experiencing symptoms that may be related to her implants, she should contact her physician or surgeon in order to discuss the next course of action.

In addition to direct breast symptoms such as hardening, some women have reported problems that could be associated with their implants. The reported symptoms include:

- Swelling and/or joint pain or arthritis-like pain
- Hardening of the breast tissue
- Swelling of the hands or feet
- Numbness
- Unusual hair loss
- Loss of energy
- Unexplained and unusual fatigue
- Increased vulnerability to colds, viruses and flues
- Connective-tissue disorders, such as lupus, scleroderma, or rheumatoid arthritis
- Tightness, redness or swelling of the skin
- Swollen glands or lymph nodes

If you have these symptoms and they do not subside, you should see your doctor to determine 1) whether the symptoms are related to the implants, or 2) if these complaints stem from another health problem. Depending on the situation, your physician may refer you to a rheumatologist or other specialist for further evaluation. You should tell your doctor of the presence of an implant, and he or she should discuss your complaints in terms of their possible relationship to an implant. The physician or the patient should report any serious adverse reactions to FDA's Medwatch Program.

What is the status of the class action legal settlement?

FDA is not involved in any aspect of the class action legal settlement, and has no connection with the Multi-District Litigation. The following announcements are included merely as a service to consumers:

The original deadline for registration was December 1, 1994; a grace period was given extending the date until March 1, 1995. Although the March 1, 1995 deadline for registration has passed, citizens of the U.S., legal resident aliens, and individuals who had their breast implant surgery performed within the U.S. may still register by contacting the 24-hour Settlement Line (1-800-887-6828). For specific information, a Claims Assistance Hotline number is 513-651-9770. Over 365,000 people have registered with the settlement.

U.S. Federal Court Judge Sam S. Pointer has created a Claims Advisory committee to assist him in eliminating fraud and abuse by attorneys who are representing women in the Multi-District Litigation. **Women do not require an attorney to file a claim in the Multi-District Litigation, nor are they required to pay any attorneys' fees.** The settlement is structured so that attorneys' fees and expenses will be paid from a separate fund. If any woman feels her attorney may be guilty of fraudulent or abusive practices, she may contact Ernest H. Hornsby, chairman of the Claims Advisory Committee. Telephone: 205-793-2424. FAX: 205-793-6624.

MEDWATCH: Reporting Problems with Implants to FDA

Women or their health care providers can report problems or adverse events with breast implants through MEDWATCH. An adverse event is any undesirable experience associated with the use of a drug or medical product in a patient. The event is serious and should be reported when the patient outcome is:

Death: Report if the patient's death is suspected as being a direct outcome of the adverse event.

Life-threatening injury or illness: Report if the patient was at substantial risk of dying at the time of the adverse event or it is suspected that the use or continued use of the product would result in the patient's death.

Hospitalization initial or prolonged: Report if admission to the hospital or prolongation of a hospital stay results because of the adverse event.

Disability: Report if the adverse event resulted in a significant, persistent, or permanent change, impairment, damage or disruption in the patient's body function/structure, physical activities or quality of life.

Congenital anomaly: Report if there are suspicions that exposure to a medical product prior to conception or during pregnancy resulted in an adverse outcome in the child.

Medical or surgical intervention required to prevent permanent impairment or damage: Report, if you suspect that the use of a medical product may result in a condition which required medical or surgical intervention to preclude permanent impairment or damage to a patient.

To report, use MEDWATCH form 3500. If you are a consumer call 1-301-443-3170 for a form. If you are a health professional to receive a form or to report by phone call 1-800-332-1088. The form may be mailed, faxed to 1-800-332-1088, or sent by modem to 1-800-332-7737.

Keep a copy of the completed MEDWATCH form for your records.

Breast Implant Resource Groups

The following list provides sources of information and organizations involved in the breast implant issue. The list is provided for information purposes only and does not constitute an endorsement by the Food and Drug Administration or Omnigraphics of the information or recommendations they may provide.

Breast Implant Product Information

Manufacturer: Gel-filled Implants

Baxter Healthcare Corp.
1 Baxter Parkway
Deerfield, Illinois 60015
1-800-323-4533

Bioplasty, Inc.
1385 Centennial Drive
St. Paul, Minnesota 55113
1-800-328-9105

Breast Implants

Dow Corning Corporation
PO Box 994
Midland, Michigan 48686-0994
1-800-442-5442

McGhan Medical Inc.
700 Ward Drive
Santa Barbara, California 93111
1-800-624-4261

Mentor Corp.
S425 Hollister Avenue
Santa Barbara, California 93111
1-800-235-5731

Porex Technologies
500 Bohannon Road
Fairburn, Georgia 30213
1-800-241-0195

Surgitek
3037 Mt. Pleasant Street
Racine, Wisconsin 53404
1-800-634-4397

Manufacturers: Saline-filled Silicone Implants

Bioplasty, Inc.
1385 Centennial Drive
St. Paul, Minnesota 55113
1-800-328-9105

CUI Corporation
1035 Cindy Lane
Carpinteria, Californla 93013
1-800-872-4749

Dow Corning Corporation
PO Box 99 4
Midland, Michigan 48686-0994
1-800-442-5442

McGhan Medical Inc.
700 Ward Drive
Santa Barbara, California 93111
1-800-525-9151

Mentor Corp.
5425 Hollister Avenue
Santa Barbara, California 93111
1-800-235-5731

Medical Management and Surgical Information

Physician and Nursing Groups

American Academy of Cosmetic Surgery
Howard A. Tobin, M.D.
President
401 No. Michigan Ave.
Chicago, IL 60611-4267
Phone: (312) 527-6713
Fax: (312) 644-1815

American Cancer Society
Robert A. Smith, Ph.D.
Senior Director, Detection Programs
1599 Clifton Rd., N.E.
Atlanta, GA 30329
Phone: (404) 329-7610
Fax: (404) 636-5567

Breast Implants

American College of Surgeons
David Winchester, M.D.
Medical Director, Cancer Dept.
55 E. Erie St.
Chicago, IL 60611
Phone: (312) 664-4050
Fax: (312) 440-7014

American Medical Association
M. Roy Schwarz, M.D.
Senior Vice President
515 North State St.
Chicago, IL 60610
Phone: (312) 464-4370
Fax: (312) 464-5896

American Nurses Assn.
Karen S. O'Connor, M.A., R.N.
Director, Practice, Economics, and Policy
600 Maryland Ave., S.W., Suite 100W
Washington, DC 20024-2571
Phone: (202) 554-4444 x270
Fax: (202) 554-2262

American Society for Aesthetic Plastic Surgery
444 E. Algonquin Road, Suite 110
Arlington Heights, IL 60005
Plastic Surgery Information Service
1-800-635-0635
(Will provide a list of board-certified plastic surgeons who primarily perform cosmetic procedures.)

American Society of Plastic and Reconstructive Surgeons
444 E. Algonquin Road
Arlington Heights, Illinois 60005
1-800-635-0635
(Will assist in finding a plastic surgeon for consultation.)

Arthritis Foundation
Public Education
PO Box 19000
Atlanta, GA 30326
Phone: (404) 872-7100, Ext. 6350
1-800-283-7800
(Will provide information on arthritis and lists of specialists in arthritis)

National Medical Association
Rosemary Davis
Executive Vice President for Administrative Affairs
1012 10th St., N.W.
Washington, DC 20001
Phone: (202) 347-1895
Fax: (202) 892-3293

Consumer and Patient Information

AS IS (American Silicone Implant Survivors)
1288 Cork Elm Drive
Kirkwood, Missouri 5-122
Phone: (314) 821-0115
Fax: (314) 821-0199
For on-line computer access:
On Prodigy the call number is JanetVanWinkle (KQHP64A);
On America On-Line the call number is Janetas is.
(Quarterly newsletter for $25.00 a year donation.)

Boston Women's Health Book Collective
PO Box 192
West Somerville, Massachusetts 02144
Phone: (617) 625-0271
(Information package for a $10.00 donation.)

Breast Implant Information Foundation
P.O. Box 2907
Laguna Hills, CA 92654-2907
Phone: (714) 448-9928

Breast Implants

Children Afflicted by Toxic Substances (CATS)
60 Oser Avenue, Suite 1
Hauppauge, New York 11788

East Coast Connection
New York/New Jersey
Breast Implant Support Group
7002 Boulevard East 15c
Guttenberg, NJ 07093
For monthly support group meeting information call:
(212) 802-5114

Implant Device Education Association (IDEA)
P.O. Box 540684
2617 Andjon
Dallas, TX 75354-0684
Phone: (214) 618-0882
FAX: (214) 350-4988
and P.O. Box 826
100 North Main, Suite 401
El Dorado, KS 67042
Phone: (316) 321-9218

Implant Survivors
2425 Parental Home Road
Jacksonville, FL 32216
Phone: (904) 725-5639

La Leche League International
9616 Minneapolis Avenue
P.O. Box 1209
Franklin Park, Illinois 60131-8209
Phone: (708) 455-7730

Lupus Foundation
1717 Massachusetts Ave., N.W.
Washington, DC 20026
Phone: 1-800-558-0121

Mid-Michigan Survivors of Breast Implants
852 Elmwood #222
Lansing, MI 48917-2070
(517) 886-1412

National Alliance of Breast Cancer Organizations
9 East 37th St., 10th Floor
New York, New York 10016

National Chronic Fatigue Syndrome Association
3521 Broadway, Suite 222
Kansas City, MO 64114
Phone: (816) 931-4777

National Women's Health Network
1325 G Street, N.W.
Lower Level
Washington, D.C. 20005
Phone: (202) 347-1140

Public Citizen Health Research Group
2000 "P" St., N.W.
Washington, DC 20036
(To receive the consumer packet on breast implants, send $6.00 to the address listed above.)

Reach to Recover
American Cancer Society
Phone: 1-800-ACS-2345
(Or check your local phone directory for a local office number)

United Scleroderma Federation
One Newbury St.
Peabody, MA 01960
Phone: 1-800-422-1113

Silicone Scene
1050 Cinnamon Lane
Corona, CA 91720
(Please send 9" by 12" self-addressed envelope with 75 cents postage affixed and $4.00 for newsletter and directory information.)

United Scleroderma Foundation
P.O. Box 399
Watsonville, CA 95077-0399
Phone: 1-800-722-HOPE

Y-Me National Organization for Breast Cancer Information
   and Support
18220 Harwood Avenue
Homewood, Illinois 60430
Phone: 1-800-221-2141

Federal Government

National Cancer Institute
Office of Cancer Communications
Building 31, Room 1OA-24
9000 Rockville Pike
Bethesda, Maryland 20892
1-800-4-CANCER (22623,)

U.S. Food and Drug Administration Office of Consumer Affairs
5600 Fishers Lane, Rm. 16-63
Rockville, MD 20857
(301) 443-3170

FDA Breast Implant Information Line: To receive the most recent information package leave your name and address on this Voice-Mail System: 1-800-532-4440

FDA, Center for Devices and Radiological Health (CDRH)
Office of Health and Industry Programs, (HFZ-205)
5600 Fishers Lane
Rockville, MD 20857

FDA, Center for Devices and Radiological Health (CDRH)
Mammography Quality Radiation Programs
1901 Chapman Avenue, Rm. 322
Rockville, MD 20857

Current Bibliographies in Medicine

The National Library of Medicine is pleased to announce the publication of Silicone Implants January 1989 through August 1994, a new bibliography in its Current Bibliographies in Medicine series. Silicone Implants provides citations to hundreds of journal articles, books and book chapters, conference proceedings and papers, and dissertations from August 1992 to the present. It provides a comprehensive look at these implants including beneficial and adverse effects as well as techniques used. All types of implants are covered, such as breast, dental, and skin. It is available from the Superintendent of Documents (see below) for approximately $8.50.

This version of Silicone Implant supplements a 1992 publication titled Silicone Implants which covered the published literature from January 1989 through July 1992. This publication:

> Hunt, Jennie; van de Kamp, Jacqueline. Silicone implants. Bethesda (MD): National Library of Medicine; 1992. 985 citations. (Current Bibliographies in medicine; 92-6).

is available from your local medical library or federal depository library. For those with computer access to the Internet, the national information highway, it may be obtained free-of-charge via FTP (File Transfer Protocol) by addressing nlmpubs.nlm.nih.gov. Call 1-800-272-4787 for any questions on obtaining this earlier publication.

The National Library of Medicine's Current Bibliographies in Medicine series covers topics of wide popular interest. Other recent titles in this series include Ovarian Cancer (CBM 94-2) and Persian Gulf Experience and Health (CBM 94-3). To order the entire series of 10 bibliographies for calendar year 1994, send a check or money order for $60.00 to the Superintendent of Documents, P.O. Box 371954, Pittsburgh, PA 15250-7954 citing GPO List ID; CBM94. Orders for individual bibliographies in the series ($8.50) should also be sent to the Superintendent of Documents citing the title and number (e.g., Ovarian Cancer CBM 94-2). For credit card orders, call 202-783-3238.

FDA Freedom of Information

We sincerely hope that the information in this chapter has been of help to you. If you need more technical information, submit a written request to the FDA Freedom of Information Staff.

The Freedom of Information Act allows anyone to request from FDA records not normally prepared for public distribution.

Your letter should include your name, address and telephone number; and a statement of the records being sought, identified as specifically as possible. A request for specific information that is releasable to the public can be processed much more quickly than a request for all "information" on a particular subject. There is a charge of 10 cents per page. You are billed after your request for information has been filled.

The following documents regarding silicone and saline breast implants are available from FDA and may be obtained by submitting a written request to the following address:

Food and Drug Administration
Freedom of Information Staff (HFI-35)
5600 Fishers Lane
Rockville, MD 20857
FAX: 301-443-1726
Voice Mail Message: 301-443-6310

There are charges for these documents, based on the number of pages and review/search time involved.

- CDRH Toxicology Risk Assessment Committee Report, Potential Carcinogenic Release of 2 4-TDA from the Polyester Polyurethane Foam Covering of Silicone Gel-Filled Breast Implants," July 22, 1991. (21 pages; $2.10)

- Silicone in Medical Devices, Conference Proceedings, February 1-2, 1991, Baltimore, Maryland. (331 pages; hard copy reproduction cost is $33.10; microfiche reproduction cost is $2.00)

- General and Plastic Surgery Devices Panel Meeting, November 12, 13, 14, 1991. (1,283 pages; microfiche cost $7.00)

- General and Plastic Surgery Devices Panel Meeting, February 18, 19, 20, 1992. (1,381 pages; microfiche cost is $7.50)

- Dow Corning Corporation Summary of Scientific Studies and Internal Company Documents Concerning Silicone Breast Implants," February 10, 1992. (867 pages; $86.70 reproduction costs, hard-copy only.)

Journal articles from July 1992 to the present may be found by doing a literature search at your local library.

A custom search of the complaints maintained in the data bases in the FDA Center for Devices and Radiological Health may be requested from the "MDR" (Medical Device Reporting) and "PRP" (Product Reporting Program) systems. Actual charges will be assessed.

- Summary of Safety and Effectiveness for MISTI Single and Double Lumen Silicone Gel-Filled Mammary Prothesis Manufactured by Bioplasty, Inc. (76 pages; $7.60)

- Summary of Safety and Effectiveness for Double-Lumen Silicone Gel-Filled Breast Prosthesis manufactured by Dow Corning Wright. (223 pages; $23.00 reproduction costs, hard-copy)

- Summary of Safety and Effectiveness for Single-Lumen Silicone Gel-Filled Breast Prosthesis (Silastic II Mammary Implant H.P. and Silastic MSI Mammary Implant H.P.) Manufactured by Dow Corning Wright. (210 pages; $21.00 reproduction costs, hard-copy)

DO NOT enclose payment; you will be billed after the documents have been mailed.

If you have questions relating to your Freedom of Information request, please write to:

Freedom of Information Office (HFZ-82)
Center for Devices and Radiological Health
Food and Drug Administration
12720 Twinbrook Parkway
Rockville, Maryland 20857

Other Information

Both FDA and manufacturers of a number of breast implant devices have participated in the creation of a single comprehensive data base of records relating to breast implants. This compendium of over a million pages includes 510K submissions, pre-market approval (PMA) application submissions, and all related documentation. There is a fee for this information. It may be ordered in whole or in part, and may be obtained by contacting the following company:

Docu-Quest
Attn: Joseph King
105 E. 4th Street
Cincinnati, OH 45202
(513) 651-4040

Chapter 22

Breast Reconstruction Trials Using Saline-Filled Implants

Information is available in PDQ concerning two clinical trials using saline-filled implants for breast reconstruction. These trials are being conducted by two saline implant manufacturers at the request of the Food and Drug Administration (FDA).

Saline-filled breast implants are silicone envelopes filled with salt water. These devices were on the market prior to the Medical Device Amendments of 1976, which gave FDA regulatory authority over these products. Like many other pre-amendment devices, saline-filled implants have been allowed, under the law, to remain on the market until FDA systematically requires manufacturers to demonstrate their safety and effectiveness.

Saline implants currently are the only product generally available to women who seek breast implants. Although they have silicone rubber envelopes like silicone gel-filled implants, FDA believes that saline implants present a lower degree of risk than gel-filled implants because leakage or rupture releases only salt water into the body. Since 1992, silicone gel-filled implants for breast reconstruction have been available only for women who cannot use saline-filled implants and who agree to participate in clinical studies.

Manufacturers have agreed to disseminate, through surgeons, updated patient information to prospective patients. FDA is in the process of updating the patient information sheet, with the assistance of health professional groups, consumer groups, and manufacturers.

NCI Cancerfax 208/400077.

Women considering implants should carefully read these patient information sheets, as well as the informed consent form, and discuss the risks with their doctors before undergoing implant surgery. Known risks include rupture, capsular contracture, and infection. Saline implants are also known to interfere with mammography. Special radiographic techniques need to be used for women with implants in order to minimize interference.

Chapter 23

Radiation Therapy: A Treatment for Early Stage Breast Cancer

Radiation therapy as primary treatment for breast cancer is a promising technique for women who have early stage breast cancer. This procedure, which allows a woman to keep her breast, involves removing the lump or cancerous tissue from the breast (lumpectomy) and some or all of the underarm lymph nodes. The breast is then treated with radiation (x-ray).

During the last 20 years, considerable experience has been gained with this form of treatment. Research comparing this treatment with the traditional surgical approach, mastectomy, is continuing. Preliminary research results are encouraging, though data on the long-term effects are still being collected. At present, the survival rates for women with early stage breast cancer who are treated with radiation therapy seem to be equal to those for women treated by mastectomy.

This chapter describes the procedures used in radiation therapy and tells you what to expect from the beginning of your treatment to your recovery at home. After reading this chapter and discussing it with your doctor, you may want to talk with another woman who has had radiation therapy to treat her breast cancer. She may have some practical advice and be able to answer some of your questions.

NIH Pub No. 91-659

Informed Consent: When Treatment Is Recommended

When treatment is recommended, most health care facilities now require patients to sign a form stating their willingness to proceed. This is to certify that you understand what procedures will be done and have consented to have them performed.

Consent to treatment is only meaningful if given by a patient who has had an opportunity to learn about recommended alternatives and to evaluate them. Before consenting to any course of treatment, be sure your doctor lets you know:

- The recommended procedure;
- Its purpose;
- Risks and side effects associated with it;
- Likely consequences with and without treatment;
- Other available alternatives; and
- Advantages and disadvantages of one treatment over another.

Even if you want your doctor to assume full responsibility for all decision making, you are likely to discover that your concerns about treatment decrease as your understanding of breast cancer and its treatment increases.

Questions To Ask Your Doctor

Before Radiation Therapy

- What kind of procedure are you recommending?
- What are the potential risks and benefits?
- Am I a candidate for any other type of procedure?
- What are the risks and benefits of those alternatives?
- How should I expect to look after the treatment?
- How should I expect to feel?

After Radiation Therapy

- When will I be able to get back into my normal routine?
- What can I do to ensure a safe recovery?
- What problems, if any, should I report to you?

Radiation Therapy: A Treatment for Early Stage Breast Cancer

- What type of exercises should I do?
- How frequently should I see you for a checkup?

Treatment Steps

Once the lump has been removed and breast cancer has been diagnosed, radiation treatment usually involves the following steps:

- Surgery to remove some or all of the underarm lymph nodes;
- External radiation therapy to the breast and surrounding area; and
- "Booster" radiation therapy to the biopsy site.

Lymph Node Surgery

Before radiation therapy begins, some or all of the underarm lymph nodes are usually removed to determine if the cancer has spread beyond the breast. If all of the lymph nodes are removed, the surgery is called **axillary dissection**; if only some of the lymph nodes are removed, it is called **axillary sampling**. Other tests such as bone and liver scans may also be done to provide your doctor with valuable information needed to plan further treatment. This process is known as "staging" the disease.

Hospital procedures and policies vary, but there are a number of things you can probably expect to have happen when you check in for lymph node surgery.

In the Hospital. You will probably be admitted the afternoon before your surgery so that some routine tests, such as blood and urine tests and a chest x-ray, can be performed. Shortly before the operation, the surgical area (underarm) will be shaved, and you may be given some medication to help you relax.

When it is time for your surgery, you will be taken to the operating room and an anesthesiologist will put you to sleep. Electrocardiogram sensors will be attached to your arms and legs with adhesive pads to monitor your heart rate during surgery. The surgical area will be cleaned, and sterile sheets will be draped over your body, except for the area around the operation. An axillary dissection usually takes several hours; an axillary sampling about an hour.

When you awaken from surgery, you will be in the recovery room. Your underarm area will be bandaged, and a tube may be in place at the surgical site to drain any fluid that may accumulate. Your throat may be sore from the tube that was placed in it to carry air to your lungs during surgery. You may also feel a little nauseated and have a dry mouth. These are common side effects of anesthesia.

You will spend an hour or so in the recovery room. Oxygen will be available in case you need it to ease your breathing. Wires may be taped to your chest to measure your heartbeat. An intravenous (IV) tube will be in a vein in your arm to give fluid, nourishment, or medication after surgery. The IV tube will probably be removed after you begin to drink and eat.

It's common to feel drowsy for several hours after surgery. You may feel some discomfort under your arm; some women experience numbness, tingling, or pain in the chest, shoulder area, and upper arm. Your doctor will prescribe medication to relieve any discomfort you may have following your surgery. The numbness under your arm will decrease gradually, but total feeling may not return for a long time.

After you return to your room, a nurse will check your temperature, pulse, blood pressure, and bandage. She will ask you to turn, cough, and breathe deeply to keep your lungs clear after the anesthesia. You may also be encouraged to move your feet and legs to improve your blood circulation. Although each woman reacts to surgery differently, you will probably discover that by the next day you will be able to sit up in bed and walk from your bed to a chair in your room. Your doctor will probably encourage you to walk around and eat solid food as soon as possible.

After Surgery. At first you will have to be careful not to move your arm too much. But by the second or third day, you may be ready to begin exercises to ease the tension in your arm and shoulder. Women who have axillary sampling usually recover their arm motion fairly quickly because their surgery is not as extensive as axillary dissection.

You will be taking sponge baths for a few days after surgery until your incision starts to heal. Before you leave the hospital, ask the doctor or nurse for instructions on taking care of your incision. When you have permission to bathe or shower, do so gently and pat, don't rub, the area of your incision.

Radiation Therapy: A Treatment for Early Stage Breast Cancer

The average stay in the hospital for an axillary dissection is 7 to 10 days, and 2 to 4 days for an axillary sampling. Before you leave, the tube that drains fluid from your incision will be removed. Your stitches will be taken out in 1 to 3 weeks at the doctor's office or clinic.

Once you are home, you should continue to exercise until you have regained the full use of your arm. As you increase your exercise and begin to renew your daily activities, you must be careful not to over-exert yourself. Take clues from your body; rest before you become tired.

To keep your skin soft and to promote healing, you may want to massage your incision gently with cocoa butter or vitamin E cream. As time goes by, the redness, bruising, and swelling will disappear. But you should watch for any signs of infection such as inflammation, tenderness, or drainage. If you develop any of these signs or a fever, call your doctor. Although each woman recovers from surgery at her own rate, most women are ready for the next part of their treatment, radiation therapy, about 1 or 2 weeks after their lymph node surgery.

Exercising After Surgery. Exercising will help you ease the tension in your arm and shoulder and will hasten your recovery. It is especially important for women who have had an axillary dissection. You will probably be able to begin exercising within a few days of your operation. Your doctor, nurse, or physical therapist can show you what exercises to do. Ask your doctor if you might begin with these few simple movements:

- Lie in bed with your arm at your side. Raise your arm straight up and back, trying to touch the headboard behind you.

- Raise your shoulders. Rotate them forward, down, and back in a circular motion to loosen your chest, shoulder, and upper back muscles.

- Lying in bed, clasp your hands behind your head and push your elbows into the mattress.

- With your elbow bent and your arm at a 90 degree angle to your body, rotate your shoulder forward until the forearm is down and then backward until it is up.

- With your arm raised, clench and unclench your fist.

- Breathe deeply.

- Rotate your chin to the left and right. Cock your head sideways.

The key is to exercise only to the point of pulling or pain. Don't push yourself.

External Radiation Therapy

During this procedure, high-energy x-rays are aimed at the breast and sometimes at nearby areas that still contain some lymph nodes, such as under the arm (if only a "sampling" was done), above the collarbone, and along the breastbone. The goal of radiation therapy is to destroy any cancer cells that may still remain in the breast or surrounding lymph node areas.

These high-energy x-rays are delivered by a linear accelerator or a cobalt machine. The difference between the two machines is simply that the beams are produced by different energy sources.

Often, a patient's first visit to the radiation department takes 1 to 2 hours and doesn't involve any treatments. You will probably talk with the radiation therapist, a physician with special training in the use of radiation, who will review your records and decide the best way to proceed with your treatment.

You will probably also meet the technician who delivers the treatment, and the radiation therapy nurse, who works closely with the doctor and can answer any questions you have about treatment, potential side effects, and what you can do about them.

During the first visit, ink lines or small tattoo marks will be drawn on your skin around the treatment area to mark exactly where to aim the radiation. The marks are generally made with permanent ink, and you should not attempt to wash them off until treatment is completed. These marks ensure that the area treated is the same every day. Many women wear old underclothes during treatment because the marking may stain clothing.

The radiation therapist will consult with the dosimetrist, who computes the dosages of radiation. The standard treatment for early

Radiation Therapy: A Treatment for Early Stage Breast Cancer

stage breast cancer is almost always 4,400 to 5,000 **Rads** (radiation absorbed dose), A rad refers to the amount of radiation that is absorbed by the breast tissue.

Your actual number of treatments will depend on the total dose you need. Usually, treatments are given 5 days a week, Monday through Friday, for about 5 weeks. To protect normal tissue, it is better to give a little radiation each day than to give a lot of radiation all at once. A single treatment takes about 20 to 25 minutes. Only a few minutes of this time are of exposure to radiation; most of the time is spent putting the patient in position. Most, people continue to work or pursue other activities throughout the treatment period.

It is very important to have all your treatments. However, if you have to miss a treatment, it can be made up. If you do not finish the full course, you may not have gotten enough radiation to destroy the cancer cells.

For more information about what to expect during radiation therapy, contact the National Cancer Institute for a copy of *Radiation Therapy and You: A Guide to Self-Help During Treatment*.

"Booster" Radiation Therapy

About 1 or 2 weeks after the external radiation therapy has been completed, nearly all women will receive a concentrated "booster" dose of radiation to the area where the breast lump was located.

This treatment may be done either externally, using an electron beam, or internally, using an implant of radioactive material. The electron beam "booster" is delivered by a type of linear accelerator machine similar to the one used in external radiation therapy. The treatment procedure is also similar to that of external radiation therapy, with the patient coming to the hospital daily for 5 to 10 days. If you have this type of booster treatment, you may notice an increase in skin redness at the site of the electron beam treatments. This is normal.

The implant procedure requires a short hospital stay of 2 to 3 days. Thin plastic tubes are threaded through the breast tissue where the original lump was removed. This may be done using either a local or general anesthesia. The number and location of the tubes depend on the size and location of the tumor that was removed. The doctor may take an x-ray of your breast after inserting the tubes to make sure they are in the correct position. When you return to your hospital room, radioactive seeds (usually iridium) will be inserted into the tubes. The implant will remain in your breast for 2 to 3 days, during which time it will deliver approximately 2,000 rads to the surrounding tissue.

While the implant is in place, you will stay in a private room because the implant emits small amounts of radiation, which may be a possible risk to those who come in close contact with you. For that reason, visitors and the nursing staff will have to limit their time with you. You may notice some breast sensitivity around the area of the implant, especially if you move around a lot, but you should not have much pain or other discomfort. If you are uncomfortable, ask your nurse for some pain medication. You'll be free to move around your room, sit and read, do needlework or write letters.

The implant will be removed in your room, without anesthesia. The process feels very much like having stitches taken out. Once it is removed there is no risk of radiation exposure to others and you can usually go home.

Side Effects of Radiation Therapy

During Treatment

Many women feel mildly to moderately tired during radiation therapy, especially as treatments progress. Treatment for cancer can be stressful and the daily trips to the hospital take a lot of energy. Try to rest as much as you can and plan your activities at levels that are comfortable for you. Don't push yourself. It is especially important to eat properly while you are having radiation treatments, because your body needs wholesome food to restore its strength and to repair injured cells. It's also important for you to maintain your weight. Even if you are overweight, do not try to lose weight until you have finished all of your treatments.

The skin around the treated area may begin to look reddened, irritated, tanned, or sunburned. In some women the skin becomes quite dry; in others it becomes very moist, especially under the breast fold. These side effects are most likely to occur toward the end of treatment.

Be gentle with your skin. Try not to irritate it. Don't use perfumed or deodorant soaps, ointments, or anything besides lukewarm

Radiation Therapy: A Treatment for Early Stage Breast Cancer

water and plain soap (such as Ivory) on your breast. Some women wear soft cotton bras, without wiring, or go braless whenever possible. Some like to wear a soft T-shirt or other loose clothing.

Your doctor and nurse will be watching you closely as treatment progresses. Be sure to mention any side effects you may have.

After Treatment

You may notice other changes in your breast due to the radiation therapy and changes may continue for 6 to 12 months after treatment. As the redness goes away, you will notice a slight darkening of the skin, much as when a sunburn fades to a suntan. The pores may be enlarged and more noticeable.

You may have some change in skin sensitivity. Some women report increased sensation, others have decreased feeling. The skin and the fatty tissue of the breast may feel thicker, and you may notice that your breast is firmer than it was before your radiation treatment. Some older women have said that their breast feels and looks as it did when they were in their twenties. Others report a change in the size of the treated breast. It may become larger because of fluid buildup or smaller because of development of fibrous tissue, but many women have little or no change at all.

After 10 to 12 months, you should notice few additional changes caused by the radiation therapy. If changes in size, shape, appearance, or texture occur after this time, report them to your doctor at once.

Precautions

A problem that may arise after treatment for breast cancer is swelling of the arm on the side of the treatment. This condition, called lymphedema, is caused by the loss or damage of underarm lymph nodes and their connecting vessels. It occurs because circulation of lymph fluid is slowed in the arm, making it harder to fight infection. You should take special care of your arm to prevent infection.

Follow these simple rules:

- Avoid burns while cooking or smoking;
- Avoid sunburns;
- Have all injections, vaccinations, blood samples, and blood pressure tests done on the other arm whenever possible;

- Use an electric razor with a narrow head for underarm shaving to reduce the risk of nicks or scratches;
- Carry heavy packages or handbags on the other arm;
- Wash cuts promptly, treat them with antibacterial medication, and cover them with a sterile dressing; check often for redness, soreness, or other signs of infection;
- Never cut cuticles; use hand cream or lotion;
- Wear watches or jewelry loosely, if at all, on the operated arm;
- Wear protective gloves when gardening and when using strong detergents, etc.;
- Use a thimble when sewing;
- Avoid harsh chemicals and abrasive compounds;
- Use insect repellent to avoid bites and stings; and
- Avoid elastic cuffs on blouses and nightgowns.

Call your doctor at once if your arm becomes red, swollen, or feels hot. In the meantime, put your arm over your head and alternately squeeze and relax your fist.

Though you should be cautious, it's also important to use your arm normally. Don't favor it or keep it dependent.

Common Questions About Radiation Therapy

Will radiation affect my normal cells?

Radiation is a strong treatment for cancer and can sometimes affect normal cells. However, normal cells are not as sensitive to radiation and will usually recover when treatment is finished.

Will anything be done to protect me from excess radiation?

The x-ray machine with which you'll be treated has special protections built in to limit your radiation to the specific area outlined. If needed, other areas of your body will be covered by special lead shields.

What will radiation feel like during the treatment?

Radiation treatment is like having a regular x-ray; most patients feel no sensation. You may feel warmth or a tingling, but you're not likely to feel any pain or discomfort.

Radiation Therapy: A Treatment for Early Stage Breast Cancer

Will I be radioactive after treatments?

No. The treatment beam is the only thing that is radioactive when you receive external radiation therapy. Neither your normal tissues nor the cancerous tissues are radioactive during or after treatment. If you have a radiation implant, small amounts of radiation will be emitted. However, once the implant is removed, you are no longer radioactive.

What will my breast look like after treatment?

There is no way to predict the cosmetic outcome of this type of treatment for a particular woman. The extent of the initial surgery, the size of the breast, the type of incision, and the effects of radiation on the skin are all factors. However, the breast usually looks quite normal and most women are pleased that they chose this breast-saving treatment.

What is chemotherapy and when is it used?

Chemotherapy is the use of drugs to destroy cancer cells. Anticancer drugs are used to reach areas of the body where cancer cells may be hiding, and to eliminate them before they multiply and hurt the normal cells and organs. More information on this supplementary treatment can be found *Chemotherapy and You; A Guide to Self-Help During Treatment* and *Adjuvant Therapy: Facts for Women With Breast Cancer*, both of which are available from the National Cancer Institute. The first pamphlet is reproduced in Omnigraphics' *The New Cancer Sourcebook* and the second is reprinted in this volume. Please consult the index for page references.

How frequently should I plan to see a doctor after radiation therapy treatment?

Your doctor will tell you when to schedule your first post-treatment exam. The two of you will then decide whether you should continue to make regular visits to him or her or to a medical oncologist, an internist, a gynecologist, or a family practitioner. Most doctors believe that women treated for breast cancer should have professional exams every 3 to 6 months for the first 3 years after surgery. More information on follow-up exams, possible signs of recurrence, and taking care of yourself can be found in *After Breast Cancer: A Guide to Followup Care*, another booklet available from the National Cancer Institute.

Adjusting Emotionally

After you have completed treatment, you'll have a lot of things on your mind. You may think about the fact that you've just been treated for a serious disease and hope this treatment will control your cancer forever. Breast cancer often has a dramatic emotional impact and you may be wondering how it will affect your lifestyle and your personal relationships. You might even be unsure how to act toward your family and friends.

Although every woman reacts to breast cancer differently, these types of concerns are common. Just as you will be taking action to help yourself physically recover from treatment, you can take steps to ease your emotional adjustment as well.

Expressing your feelings to your doctor and the people you love can be important emotional medicine. If you try to handle your problems alone, everyone will lose: you will lose chances to express yourself, your family and friends will lose opportunities to share your difficulties and help you work through them, and your doctor may not understand what you need to fully recover.

Remember, your family and close friends can be your strongest supporters. But chances are, they aren't quite sure how they can show their support. You can help them by being open and honest about the way you feel.

If informal approaches to dealing with your feelings don't work, consider professional help. Psychiatrists, psychologists, social workers, nurses, and religious counselors can help your emotional adjustment.

Others Are Willing To Help

You may also want to talk with other women who have had similar experiences. Reach to Recovery is an American Cancer Society program designed to help breast cancer patients meet the physical, emotional, and cosmetic needs related to cancer and its treatment. Women who have had radiation therapy to treat their breast cancer volunteer to participate in the program by providing practical infor-

Radiation Therapy: A Treatment for Early Stage Breast Cancer

mation and sharing their experiences with others. All volunteers are carefully selected and trained.

Programs vary from city to city. Call your local American Cancer Society unit for more information or contact departments of radiation therapy at major medical centers.

Intimacy

Whether you are single or married, you are likely to wonder how your treatment for breast cancer will affect your intimate relationships. Your partner will also have concerns. You can help each other by expressing them.

Intimate relationships are built on mutual love, trust, attraction, shared interests, common experiences, and a host of other feelings. Breast cancer treatment will not necessarily change these feelings. What it may change is some of the physical aspects of lovemaking, what's pleasurable to you and what's not. It may also temporarily affect your partner's and your attitudes toward intimacy.

Because fatigue often is associated with radiation treatment, you may need additional rest. You can continue to enjoy an intimate relationship by planning special time to spend alone with your partner.

Sometimes a partner is afraid that touching the treated breast will hurt you. Let your partner know what's comfortable to you and what's not. You can bring new closeness to your relationship by talking about your treatment and the way you feel.

Helping Children Cope

Children react to illness in a variety of ways. Some feel angry at their mothers for becoming ill. Others are frightened. Still others worry that they might have caused the illness.

Although you may be tempted to protect your children by not telling them about your disease and its treatment, it's usually better to be honest. Even young children sense when something is wrong. Preschool children often feel deserted when their mother goes to the hospital. And if she returns feeling weak or depressed, they may become frightened. Teenagers sometimes suddenly change their behavior because they fear their mother's illness will keep them from maintaining the independence they have begun to enjoy. If you can avoid imposing too much responsibility on your teenage children, and if you share some of your feelings with them, you may be able to keep their problems to a minimum.

It is a good idea to tell your children the truth as simply and positively as possible. Be careful not to burden them with any more information than is necessary. Encourage their questions, and answer those questions honestly. You will probably find that talking helps your children to accept your illness and the temporary disruption it causes.

Breast Self-Examination

After radiation therapy, breast self-examination (BSE) should continue to be part of your routine. You will want to examine your breasts and your scar (if you had the lymph nodes removed) once a month to note any changes in the way they look or feel. Though you may have been doing BSE before your treatment, you will have to relearn what's considered "normal" for you now.

If you menstruate, the best time to do BSE is 2 or 3 days after your period ends, when your breasts are least likely to be tender or swollen. If you no longer menstruate, pick a day, such as the first day of the month, to do BSE.

Here is how to do BSE (for a narrative with accompanying illustrations, please refer to pages 234-236):

1. Stand before a mirror. Inspect your breast for anything unusual, such as any discharge from the nipple, or puckering, dimpling, or scaling of the skin. Inspect the scar for new swelling, lumps, redness, or color change. Although redness can be a result of irritation from your bra or prosthesis, report it to your physician. The next two steps are designed to emphasize any change in the shape or contour of your breast. As you do them, you should be able to feel your chest muscles tighten.

2. Watching closely in the mirror, clasp your hands behind your head and press your hands forward.

3. Next, press your hands firmly on your hips and bow slightly toward your mirror as you pull your shoulders and elbows forward.

Radiation Therapy: A Treatment for Early Stage Breast Cancer

The next part of the exam is done while standing. Some women do it in the shower because fingers glide over soapy skin, making it easy to concentrate on the texture underneath.

4. Raise your arm on the unoperated side. Using three or four fingers of your other hand, explore your breast firmly, carefully, and thoroughly. Beginning at the outer edge, press the flat part of your fingers in small circles, moving the circles slowly around the breast. Gradually work toward the nipple. Be sure to cover the entire breast. Pay special attention to the area between the breast and the underarm, including the underarm itself. Feel for any unusual lump or mass under the skin.

5. Gently squeeze the nipple and look for a discharge. Raise your arm on the operated side. Use three or four fingers of your opposite hand and begin at the top of the scar from the lymph node surgery. Press gently, using small circular motions, and feel the entire length of the scar. Look for thickenings, lumps, and hard places. As with your breast, familiarity with your scar makes it easier to notice any changes. Lumps, thickening, and inflammation are among changes you should bring to the attention of your doctor.

6. Steps 4 and 5 should be repeated lying down. Lie flat on your back, raise your arm on the unoperated side over your head, and place a pillow or folded towel under your shoulder. This position flattens the breast and makes it easier to examine. Use the same circular motion described earlier.

For More Information

The Cancer Information Service (CIS) is a nationwide toll-free telephone program sponsored by the National Cancer Institute. Trained information specialists are available to answer questions about cancer from the public, cancer patients and their families, and health professionals. By calling the following toll-free number, you will be automatically connected to the CIS office serving your area:

1-800-4-CANCER

Spanish speaking staff members are also available.

The National Cancer Institute also has developed PDQ (Physician Data Query), a computerized database designed to give doctors quick and easy access to:

- The latest treatment information for most types of cancer.
- Descriptions of clinical trials that are open for patient entry.
- Names of organizations and physicians involved in cancer care.

To get access to PDQ, a doctor can use an office computer with a telephone hookup and a PDQ access code or the services of a medical library with online searching capability. Most Cancer Information Service offices (1-800-4-CANCER) provide physicians with free PDQ searches and can tell doctors how to get regular access to the database. Patients may ask their doctor to use PDQ or may call 1-800-4-CANCER themselves. Information specialists at this toll-free number use a variety of sources, including PDQ, to answer questions about cancer prevention, diagnosis, and treatment.

Chapter 24

Adjuvant Therapy: Facts for Women with Breast Cancer

Early in its development, breast cancer may begin to spread beyond the breast to other parts of a woman's body by way of the bloodstream and the lymph system. To control this spread, a form of cancer treatment called adjuvant therapy is sometimes used following primary treatment with either surgery or surgery combined with radiation therapy. In breast cancer, adjuvant therapy involves the use of drugs that either kill cancer cells (chemotherapy) or deprive them of hormones needed for growth (hormone therapy). Adjuvant therapy is being used with increasing success for breast cancer patients who are at risk of having their cancer recur after primary treatment.

Planning Treatment

In deciding if a woman needs adjuvant therapy and what type of treatment would help her the most, doctors must consider several factors. First they must find out if the cancer has spread beyond the breast.

One of the first places breast cancer may spread is to the lymph nodes under the arm. Lymph nodes are bean-shaped structures that filter impurities from the lymph fluid that circulates through the breast and all other parts of the body, during surgery, some or all of the underarm lymph nodes are removed and are examined later under a microscope. Lymph nodes with cancer cells are said to be "positive."

NIH Pub No. 87-2877.

Nodes are described as "negative" when there is no evidence that cancer cells have spread to them. If cancer cells are found in the lymph nodes, there is a strong possibility that other cancer cells are circulating in the body. At the present time, adjuvant therapy is recommended for women with positive underarm lymph nodes and should be considered for other women at high risk of having their cancer recur.

Doctors know that some types of breast cancer depend partly on the female hormones (estrogen and progesterone) for growth. By using certain drugs that block the effects of hormones or lower their levels in the blood, doctors can extend the survival of women whose breast cancer is hormone-dependant.

In addition to examining the lymph nodes when planning treatment, doctors also try to identify women who are most likely to respond to hormone therapy. To do this, they perform tests on a sample of the tumor that was removed during the biopsy. These tests, called hormone receptor assays, show that about two-thirds of all women with breast cancer have tumors that contain estrogen receptors (ER). Women who are ER positive are more likely to respond to hormone therapy than are women who are ER negative (no estrogen receptors). A further way to tell if hormone treatment will be effective is a second test, for progesterone receptors (PR). A woman whose tumor is both ER and PR positive has an 80 percent chance of responding to hormone therapy.

Another factor that is important in planning for adjuvant therapy is a woman's menopausal status. Studies have shown that the effectiveness of different types of adjuvant therapy for breast cancer depends on whether a woman is pre- or postmenopausal. Women who are premenopausal generally respond better to adjuvant chemotherapy. Women who are postmenopausal and ER-positive generally respond to adjuvant hormone therapy. As discussed below, other factors may be considered in deciding treatment for an individual patient.

Options for Treatment

Adjuvant chemotherapy and hormone therapy are both effective treatments for breast cancer patients. While significant advances in treatment research have been made, there is no single best therapy for any group of patients.

Adjuvant Therapy: Facts for Women with Breast Cancer

Premenopausal Women

- For premenopausal breast cancer patients with positive underarm lymph nodes, adjuvant chemotherapy has been shown to be of much benefit, regardless of hormone receptor status. Adjuvant chemotherapy with a combination of drugs is recommended.

- For premenopausal patients with negative lymph nodes, adjuvant therapy is generally not recommended. However, it should be considered for certain high-risk patients. Patients at high risk include those women who have large or aggressive tumors, those who develop breast cancer during pregnancy, or patients who are under age 40. These women have a higher risk of recurrence and may be helped by adjuvant chemotherapy.

Postmenopausal Women

- For postmenopausal patients with positive nodes and positive hormone receptor levels, hormone therapy with a drug called tamoxifen is recommended.

- For postmenopausal patients with positive nodes and negative hormone receptor levels, chemotherapy may be considered.

- For postmenopausal patients with negative nodes, there is no indication for routine adjuvant therapy. For certain high-risk patients, however, adjuvant chemotherapy should be considered.

At this time, scientists are conducting clinical trials (research with patients) using adjuvant therapy. They are evaluating the possible benefits of this type of treatment in women with negative lymph nodes. Other studies are designed to find the most effective adjuvant therapy for women with positive nodes. Breast cancer patients and their doctors are encouraged to participate in such clinical trials. Patients who take part in research make an important contribution to medical science and have the first chance to benefit from improved treatment methods.

At many hospitals throughout the country, the National Cancer Institute supports studies of new treatments for breast cancer. To learn about these clinical trials, your doctor may use PDQ (Physician Data Query), a computer information system. PDQ can give your doctor the latest information on clinical trials for each type and stage of cancer. Doctors have access to PDQ through their personal computers or a library.

Course of Treatment

Drugs commonly used to treat breast cancer include cyclophosphamide (Cytoxan), methotrexate, 5-fluorouracil (5-FU), doxorubicin (Adriamycin), vincristine (Oncovin), L-PAM (also known as mephalan or L-Phenylalanine mustard), and prednisone, given in combinations of two to five drugs. Research indicates that combinations of drugs are generally more effective than single drugs, but no one combination have proved best. Tamoxifen, an anti-estrogen drug, is given to postmenopausal women who are ER-positive.

Chemotherapy is given by mouth or by injection into a vein or muscle on a daily, weekly, or monthly schedule. Therapy generally starts shortly after surgery or radiation therapy and may last from 6 months to a year. Tamoxifen, which is taken orally appears to be more effective when given for a longer period (at least 2 years). However, exactly how long adjuvant therapy should be given for best results has not been determined.

Side Effects

The powerful drugs used in chemotherapy destroy constantly dividing cancer cells. Unfortunately, they also affect healthy dividing cells, causing side effects such as nausea and vomiting, loss of appetite, weakness, mouth ulcers, fatigue, hair loss, weight gain, menstrual changes, and lowered resistance to infections.

Whether a woman will have side effects depends on the drugs she is taking and her own response to them. However, most side effects are temporary and gradually go away once treatment is stopped, although some side effects can be permanent. For example, certain

Adjuvant Therapy: Facts for Women with Breast Cancer

drugs cause sterility or, in case of Adriamycin, injury to the heart. There is even the remote chance that some drugs may cause a second cancer to develop in the future.

Tamoxifen is tolerated well by most patients. However, it does cause short-term side effects related to lowered levels of estrogen such as hot flashes. Long-term side effects of tamoxifen are unknown at present but appear to be minimal.

Side effects can sometimes be prevented and often they can be treated or minimized. Cancer researchers are working to make chemotherapy more effective and to lessen its side effects. Most doctors believe that the overall benefits achieved by adjuvant therapy for breast cancer outweigh the risk of serious side effects. Each woman and her doctor need to evaluate the known and potential side effects of adjuvant therapy when making decisions about treatment. More information on side effects and other aspects of chemotherapy can be found in the National Cancer Institute publication, *Chemotherapy and You: A Guide to Self-Help During Treatment*, which is also reproduced in Omnigraphics' *The Cancer Sourcebook*.

Emotional Concerns

Concerns about breast cancer and its treatment may have a dramatic emotional impact on a woman. The need for chemotherapy and its effect on a woman's life can cause a range of feelings. Fear, anxiety, and depression are common to many breast cancer patients undergoing adjuvant therapy.

When a woman starts chemotherapy, her lifestyle may change. She may have to adjust her routine to fit treatment schedules. And, her overall health may suffer from treatment side effects. These kinds of changes are not pleasant, but they can be handled. It is important for all women who are undergoing treatment for breast cancer to remember that they are not alone. Many other cancer patients have successfully dealt with similar feelings and problems.

During treatment, a woman may wonder what is happening to her, whether the drugs are working, and how she can deal with her stress and anxiety. If a woman doesn't understand the way it is explained, she should keep asking until she does. A woman should also be aware of her emotional well-being, and remember that it is just as important as her physical health. If a woman feels frightened or discouraged, she should seek out help.

Talking with an understanding friend or family member or with another patient may be helpful. She may wish to talk things over with a member of the clergy or a health professional with whom she feels comfortable. She can talk with her doctor, nurse, or social worker, or ask about seeing a mental health professional. Many hospitals have support groups for people undergoing chemotherapy. Everyone needs some support during difficult times and she should not hesitate to ask for help while she's being treated for breast cancer.

Follow-up Care

Any woman who has had cancer in one breast is at an increased risk of developing cancer in her other breast, so breast self-examination (BSE) is very important. No matter what kind of treatment a woman has had, she needs to do BSE once a month. Her doctor can tell her how to do BSE if she doesn't already know. Nurses are also trained to teach BSE. The method is described in this sourcebook. Please consult the index for page references.

Most doctors believe that women treated for breast cancer should have regular exams every 3 to 6 months for the first 3 years after treatment, and once or twice a year thereafter. During some visits, the doctor will perform a physical exam of the breast tissue, chest area, underarms, and neck. Other visits may include a mammogram of the breast, X-rays, blood tests, and bone scans.

These tests will help the doctor to check for reappearance of cancer cells in the original site and elsewhere in the body. After 3 years, these exams my be done once or twice a year. However, a woman should always remain under a doctor's care for her breast disease. More information about follow-up care can be found in the National Cancer Institute booklet, *After Breast Cancer: A Guide to Followup Care.*

Chapter 25

Delivering Cancer-Fighting Drugs

Glass Models of Arteries Show How Drugs Flow to Tumor Sites

Standing next to an intricate apparatus made of graceful, curving glass tubes, Dr. Robert J. Lutz pushes a button and a thin stream of red liquid begins to wind its way through the clear fluid-filled network. As the researcher watches intently, the stream curves left at one fork, moves past two more offshoots, and ultimately bypasses the most important branch, the branch that represents the artery leading to the uterus and cervix.

This experiment, one of dozens to be conducted over the next several months, will help scientists better understand how drugs flow through blood vessels and whether various injection methods deliver adequate and uniform concentrations of medication to targeted sites. Once the studies are completed, Dr. Lutz's findings will be applied in a prospective clinical trial for treating cancer of the cervix, which kills about 4,500 women in the United States each year.

The glass model research is expected to help physicians at the National Institutes of Health (NIH) find the best way to deliver toxic anticancer drugs to cervical tumors while avoiding sensitive tissues around the bladder and rectum. Dr. Alan H. Epstein, senior investigator in the radiation oncology branch of the National Cancer Institute in Bethesda, Maryland, will head the clinical study.

NCRR *Reporter* July/August 1993.

The basic laws of fluid dynamics, which allow engineers to predict how fluid will flow through pipes, also apply to studies of blood and drug flow in arteries, says Dr. Lutz, a senior scientist in the Biomedical Engineering and Instrumentation Program (BEIP) of the National Center for Research Resources in Bethesda. Using the transparent models, he and his associates can evaluate a multitude of drug infusion sites and delivery techniques without experimenting on humans or animals.

Last year technicians in the BEIP glass unit built a model of the major blood vessels that surround the human uterus and cervix, based on drawings and photographs from anatomy textbooks. "In addition to the structural details, there are other important aspects of the modeling that must not be overlooked. This is where traditional engineering comes into play," says Dr. Lutz. For example, the glass tubing is filled with a transparent mixture of glycerine and water that has the viscosity of blood, and a pulsating flow pump mimics the beating of the heart.

By monitoring the flow of dye in the model, the scientists can estimate how infused drugs are likely to flow in the body. The experimental infusions are recorded on videotape, and fluid is collected at various points along the artificial arteries to determine the concentration of dye at different locations.

The glass model does not mimic real arteries in every detail- for example, the rigid tubing does not expand and contract as blood vessels do–but it is a close enough match for fluid mechanics studies, says Dr. Lutz. "Studies have shown that elasticity is an important–but not critical–factor when looking at fluid flow and drug delivery in arterial systems. Changes in the radius of the arteries can be as small as 15 or 20 percent," he says. "Our data represent a good first approximation of the flow system." Indeed, additional studies at NIH in both animals and humans have verified many of Dr. Lutz's findings.

The prospective cervical cancer study will not be the first clinical trial to be aided by studies in BEIP-built models of arteries. In a series of experiments conducted over more than a decade, Dr. Lutz, Dr. Robert L. Dedrick, chief of the BEIP chemical engineering section, and their colleagues have used transparent models of the blood vessels in and around the brain and the liver to assess potential drug infusion sites, catheter designs, and injection procedures. This research was conducted in collaboration with scientists at the National Cancer Institute and the National Institute of Neurological Disorders and Stroke.

The models have shown that conventional, slow infusions of drugs into arteries often allow the medication to remain in a separate stream that may bypass the targeted blood vessel and tumor instead of uniformly mixing with the blood. This streaming phenomenon may lead to harmful accumulation of drugs in healthy tissues and leave diseased regions unaffected. In the case of malignant brain tumors, the streaming phenomenon helped to explain why conventional intra-arterial infusions sometimes caused severe eye pain or blindness: the toxic drug apparently could remain in a separate stream and concentrate in arteries that lead to the eye instead of mixing with the blood and reaching the brain tumor.

To overcome the streaming problem, BEIP engineers developed a drug-delivery pump that eliminated or reduced streaming not only in the glass models but also in patients in clinical trials. In three recent studies at NIH, patients who had malignant brain tumors received intra-arterial anticancer medication that was pumped in pulses synchronous with the heartbeat. Compared to slow, continuous intra-arterial infusions, the pump produced greater mixing and better drug delivery to the cancerous regions of the brain.

Because of the BEIP engineers' earlier successes, Dr. Epstein and his colleagues at the National Cancer Institute decided to enlist their help when planning the cervical cancer trials. "We got in touch with Drs. Dedrick and Lutz and the group at BEIP because they are renowned for their expertise in regional drug delivery," says Dr. Epstein.

The cancer researchers are working with the experimental drug iododeoxyuridine (IUDR), which is incorporated into the DNA of tumor cells and makes them more susceptible to the killing effects of radiation. In a phase I clinical trial now under way at NIH, the scientists plan to administer varying doses of IUDR to 24 women who have inoperable cervical cancer. The study will help to establish the most effective and least toxic dosage that can be used in conjunction with radiation therapy.

The drug will be infused intravenously over a period of 7 days, and pellets of radioactive material will be inserted into the cervix to kill the cancerous cells. "However, because of IUDR's sensitizing effect, tissues such as the bladder and the rectum, which lie close to the cervix, might also be damaged," says Dr. Epstein.

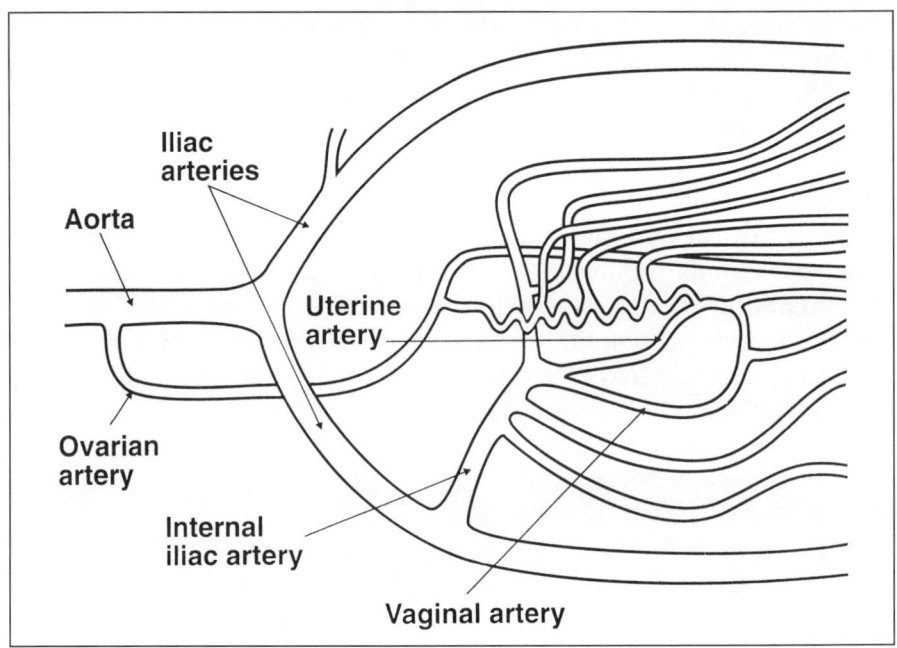

Figure 25.1. The glass model of the female pelvic arteries is positioned as if the patient were lying on her left side. The aorta, the body's main artery, branches out into the two iliac arteries, which supply blood to the legs. Dr. Robert J. Lutz and his colleagues are analyzing different drug delivery techniques and injection sites along the internal iliac artery and its branches. The scientists hope to deliver therapeutic and uniform concentrations of anticancer drugs to the uterine and vaginal arteries which supply blood to cervical tissue.

Once the phase I study is completed, possibly within 1-2 years, Dr. Epstein plans to begin a second trial in which IUDR is injected directly into the arteries that lead to the cervix. More focused administration of IUDR should prevent sensitization of neighboring tissues. "We hope that intra-arterial infusions will deliver more of the drug to the tumor with less risk of toxicity elsewhere," says Dr. Epstein. "Unfortunately the distribution of the drug when given intra-arterially is very unpredictable. We don't yet understand how the drug will be distributed in the pelvic arterial system, but that's what Dr. Lutz's research is all about." Selection of the drug infusion sites and delivery techniques will be guided by the glass model research.

So far Dr. Lutz's experiments suggest that the streaming phenomenon can occur in uterine arteries just as it did in the brain and liver studies. "In fact, the model shows that if the catheter is not placed properly, IUDR could be delivered to tissue regions that are undesirable for radiation sensitization, like the bladder or rectal tissues," says Dr. Lutz. "The question we have to address is: How do we deliver the drug locally and get it well mixed in the cervical tissue?"

Options include using the pulsed infusion pump that was employed in the brain studies or a novel catheter design that was developed in conjunction with the BEIP liver studies. "The catheter contains a partially inflated balloon that disturbs the blood flow pattern when inserted in any artery and may enhance mixing when the drug is delivered," says Dr. Lutz. Although the catheter was effective in models of liver arteries, it has not yet been used clinically.

Dr. Epstein is hopeful that the glass model research will offer insights into regional drug delivery that reach beyond applications to cervical cancer. "If this model can be refined, and as we gain more experience, it will have a more general applicability to intra-arterial infusion of drugs, a procedure that is commonly used in many types of cancer," he says.

Dr. Epstein is still accepting patients in the clinical trial of intravenous IUDR infusions to treat inoperable cervical cancer. Physicians should contact him at the NCI Radiation Oncology Branch, Building 10, Room B3B69, National Institutes of Health, Bethesda, MD 20892; Telephone: 301-496-5457; FAX: 301-480-5439.

Additional Reading

> Saris, S. C., Blasberg, R. G., Carson, R. E., et al., Intravascular streaming during carotid artery infusions. Journal of Neurosurgery 74:763-772, 1991.
> Lutz, R. J. and Miller, D. L., Mixing studies during hepatic artery infusion in an in vitro model. Cancer 62:106&1073, 1988.
> Lutz, R. J., Dedrick, R. L., Boretos, J. W., et al., Mixing studies during intracarotid artery infusions in an in vitro model. Journal of Neurosurgery 64:277-283, 1986.

This research is supported by the Biomedical Engineering and Instrumentation Program of the National Center for Research Resources and the National Cancer Institute.

— *by Victoria L. Contie*

Chapter 26

"The Queen of Neurosis" Gilda Radner's Experience with Ovarian Cancer

She crowned herself "the Queen of Neurosis," but this time, it was not simply an overactive imagination that made her fear for her health. It was symptoms of the ovarian cancer that eventually claimed her life.

Gilda Radner, one of the original Not Ready for Prime Time Players of television's "Saturday Night Live," claimed in her book *It's Always Something* that she could get neurotic over any health problem. "I hated to be sick and I had an imagination that could turn a stomachache into the plague."

So, she wrote, when a complete physical examination in January 1986 failed to explain the overwhelming fatigue and general malaise she was feeling, she agreed with the doctor that her symptoms might just be from depression; she had, after all, been going through a rough period in both her personal and professional life. It was not until October—10 months and several symptoms, diagnoses, and failed therapies later—that cancer of the ovaries was confirmed.

Delay in diagnosing ovarian cancer is not unusual. Early detection is difficult because disease confined to the ovary seldom produces symptoms. When symptoms do surface, they are often vague and easily mistaken for other, often minor, ailments.

Radner's cancer was not discovered until it had spread to her bowel and liver. She suffered from fatigue, low-grade fever, pelvic cramping, abdominal bloating, gas, and aches and pains in her upper

---

FDA Consumer Reprint May 1993 Pub No. FDA 93-1206.

thighs and legs. Loss of appetite and a feeling of fullness, indigestion, nausea, weight loss, and, less often, vaginal bleeding and low back pain are other symptoms.

As the tumor grows, it may press on the bowel and bladder, causing constipation and frequent urination. Malignant cells can break away from the tumor and spread directly to other organs in the abdomen, such as the stomach, colon and diaphragm (muscle separating the chest cavity from the abdomen), causing a fluid buildup that results in swelling and discomfort. The cells can also enter the bloodstream or lymph system and spread to other parts of the body.

Radner wrote that her complaints had been variously attributed to Epstein-Barr virus infection, depression, stress, and anxiety. She had undergone blood tests, a barium enema, and ultrasound (pelvic sonogram). According to Radner, the sonogram, done in the summer of 1986, showed "congestion" and the "ovaries weren't exactly in the place they were supposed to be, but that wasn't serious." There was no sign of tumor or bowel obstruction.

Aspirin to Acupuncture

Attempting to combat her ills through both mainstream and holistic medicine, Radner tried remedies that ran the gamut from aspirin, anti-inflammatories and anti-depressants to health foods, vitamins, acupuncture, and colonics (unconventional type enemas).

"Suddenly, I began to wonder how to please so many people," she wrote. "Do I take the magnesium citrate? What about the coffee enema? Do I do both? Do I do the abdominal massage or the colonic? Do I tell the doctors about each other?"

Then, late in October, an abnormal liver function test prompted more exams. A CAT scan and analysis of fluid from the abdomen confirmed ovarian cancer.

Diagnosed at age 40, Radner was younger than most women with the disease. The chance of developing ovarian cancer increases with age; most cases are found in women 55 to 75 years old. As was true with Radner, however, women with a family history of the disease generally are diagnosed at a younger age.

Each year in the United States, ovarian cancer is diagnosed in 22,000 women and claims more than 13,000 lives. It is most common in women living in Europe and North America; Asian women have a relatively low incidence. Although Chinese and Japanese women living in the United States have higher rates of ovarian cancer than their counterparts in Asia, the disease is still less common among this group than among the native white population in the United States. Rates among black women in all parts of the world are low.

Certain factors are associated with an increased risk of getting ovarian cancer. Although the lifetime risk for most women is 1 in 70, it doubles for women who have never been pregnant and women who have had breast cancer.

Women with close relatives who have had ovarian cancer are also at greater risk, reaching perhaps a 50 percent chance in women who have at least two first-degree relatives (mother, sister or daughter) with the disease. This compares with a 1.4 percent chance in women without a family history. Radner wrote that her mother had breast cancer and a cousin had both breast and ovarian cancer. Later, it was learned that other of her relatives had ovarian cancer as well.

The Familial Ovarian Cancer Registry, established in 1981 at Roswell Park Cancer Institute in Buffalo, N.Y., included 2,144 cases of ovarian cancer in 899 families as of April 1992. Despite the familial nature of some cases, familial ovarian cancer is estimated to account for only 5 to 10 percent of the total cases.

Evidence suggests that hormones may influence development of the disease. The risk of ovarian cancer is reduced in women who have had multiple pregnancies and in those who used birth control pills. The Cancer and Steroid Hormone Study by the national Centers for Disease Control and the National Institute of Child Health and Human Services found that use of oral contraceptives for even a few months reduced the risk of ovarian cancer by 40 percent in women 20 to 54 years old.

The study, published in the March 12, 1987, New England Journal of Medicine, also found that the longer a woman used birth control pills, the lower her risk of ovarian cancer, and that the protective effect persisted long after stopping the pill. Based on these data, since 1989, the labeling for oral contraceptives has included decreased incidence of ovarian cancer among the non-contraceptive health benefits of the pill.

On the reverse side of the coin, in January 1993, FDA requested that drug firms revise fertility drug labels to include ovarian cancer as a potential adverse drug reaction. The action was in response to a report in the November 1992 issue of the *American Journal of Epidemiology* suggesting a possible relationship between use of fertility-enhancing drugs and ovarian cancer. The analysis was based on data from 12 studies comparing women with ovarian cancer to those without the disease. Only three of the studies, however, contained data on the use of fertility drugs and risk of ovarian cancer. (A 1987 article in the same journal reported no association between the drugs and ovarian cancer.)

FDA urged caution in interpreting the findings of the 1992 report because the analysis only included small numbers of women and because the article gave no information about the fertility drugs prescribed, reasons for the infertility, or tumor size or stage of disease at diagnosis.

Search for a Screening Test

According to the registry, more than 90 percent of women diagnosed with ovarian cancer while it's still confined to the ovary are alive five years after diagnosis. Among women whose cancer has spread beyond the ovary by the time it's diagnosed, only 25 percent survive five years. However, unlike cervical or breast cancer (which may be detected early by a Pap test or mammogram, respectively), ovarian cancer has no reliable screening test.

"The traditional routine pelvic examination, now relied on as the only screening measure available, is largely ineffective for early detection," says Grant Bagley, M.D., an obstetrician/gynecologist in the Food and Drug Administration's Office of Health Affairs. "Often you can't feel a normal-sized ovary. And even if you can, it's hard to tell if it's enlarged because ovaries vary in size from person to person and day to day. Ovarian cancers start very small, and by the time they're large enough to feel, the cancer is most likely already advanced." The problem with ovarian cancer, he says, is that "you have to detect very small changes, and these are hard to detect on a pelvic exam because it's a very indirect examination."

Researchers are looking for tumor markers—substances that may appear in abnormal amounts in the blood or urine—that may prove useful in developing a screening test.

One marker that has received much attention recently is CA 125, a substance in the blood that is elevated in patients with advanced ovarian tumors. Doctors now measure CA 125 levels in patients treated for advanced disease to determine if the tumor has shrunk or if disease has recurred. Its value in monitoring treatment prompted

"The Queen of Neurosis"—Guilda Radner's Experience

scientists to study its potential for early detection. Its use for screening, however, is investigational.

Transvaginal ultrasound is also being studied as a screening tool. With ultrasound, high-frequency sound waves are projected into the body, and the echoes produced are converted by computer into a picture. Unlike abdominal ultrasound, in which the sound wave-emitting device is placed on the outside of the belly, transvaginal ultrasound uses a probe placed in the vagina that can reach within millimeters of the ovaries, producing more detailed images.

"There is uncertainty as to the value of these tools as screening tests and their ultimate impact on mortality," says John Gohagan, Ph.D., chief of the National Cancer Institute's Early Detection Branch in the Division of Cancer Prevention and Control. NCI is conducting a clinical trial including 74,000 women aged 60 to 74 to clarify the issue. The trial is designed to assess the value of CA 125 and transvaginal ultrasound for early detection of ovarian cancer and to measure their impact on mortality.

Women in the trial are randomly assigned to either a screening group or a control group of 37,000 women each. The screening group will have periodic pelvic examinations along with CA 125 and transvaginal ultrasound tests. The control group will have routine medical care.

Diagnostic Procedures

If a woman or her doctor suspects ovarian cancer, diagnosis begins with a medical history of the patient, review of her symptoms, and complete physical examination, including a pelvic exam, in which the physician feels the vagina, ovaries, fallopian tubes, bladder, and rectum to check for any growths. A Pap test may also be done because, even though it cannot reliably detect ovarian cancer, it may detect cancer cells that have migrated to the uterine cervix from the ovaries.

Blood and urine tests may also be done, as well other procedures, depending on the woman's symptoms and results of her physical exam. These procedures include:

- **abdominal or transvaginal ultrasound.** Helps distinguish fluid-filled cysts from a solid tumor

- **CAT scan.** Produces x-ray images of cross-sections of body tissues

- **lower GI series (barium enema).** Visualizes the bowel on x-ray to detect abnormal areas that may be caused by ovarian cancer

- **intravenouspyelogram (IVP).** Produces x-ray pictures of the kidneys, bladder and ureters (tubes carrying urine from the kidneys to the bladder). Often, ovarian cysts or tumors can cause pressure on these organs, which may show up on an IVP.

The only sure way to diagnose ovarian cancer, however, is through microscopic examination by a pathologist of abnormal-looking fluid or tissue. While fluid can sometimes be obtained by needle aspiration or other techniques, more commonly a laparotomy or laparoscopy is done. Laparotomy is an exploratory operation in which the surgeon examines the abdomen thoroughly and removes fluid or tissue for examination. In laparoscopy, a flexible, lighted tube is passed through a small incision in the abdomen, allowing the surgeon to examine the area and extract tissue for a biopsy.

If cancer is suspected, the surgeon usually removes the entire affected ovary to avoid cutting through the outer layer, which might cause the tumor to spread.

The tissue is sent to the pathologist for immediate evaluation, and if cancer is confirmed, the surgeon nearly always removes the second ovary, the uterus, and the fallopian tubes. Samples are taken of nearby lymph nodes, the diaphragm, the omentum (a fold of membranous lining in the abdominal cavity), and fluid from the abdomen to see whether the cancer has spread. If no fluid is found, several "washings" are taken: A saline solution is put into the abdomen and then removed to be examined for cancer cells. If there are suspicious lesions, tissue samples are also taken from the liver, small intestine, and large intestine.

Early Treatment Crucial

Trusting her instincts may have saved Jessica Marsh's life. Due in part to her own vigilance and persistence, Marsh (not her real name), a secretary in Rockville, Md., was diagnosed before her cancer had spread beyond the ovary, affording her a brighter prognosis.

"The Queen of Neurosis"—Guilda Radner's Experience

For three months in the fall of 1985, Marsh, then 36 years old, had noticed pains in her right side around the time of her menstrual periods. Although the pains were brief and not severe, she decided to have her doctor check it out. A week or so before her appointment, however, a very sharp pain prompted her to call the doctor again. Her gynecologist was out of town, but the doctor on call had her come in.

"He told me that my stomach was distended, gave me a pelvic exam, and then congratulated me, telling me I was three months pregnant," Marsh recalls. "I told him I wasn't pregnant, that I already had two children and knew what it was like to be pregnant, and this was not a pregnancy."

At Marsh's insistence, the physician arranged for her to have a pelvic sonogram that day at a local hospital.

"I had the sonogram and the next thing I knew, the doctor who had examined me at the office came in, repeated the sonogram, and told me there was a mass and he wanted to do some more tests. The next morning, I had surgery to remove my ovaries, uterus, and fallopian tubes."

Although Marsh's experience may not be typical, it illustrates again the difficulty in correctly diagnosing the disease early. Yet, early detection and treatment can mean the difference between life and death. According to the Familial Ovarian Cancer Registry, more than 90 percent of women diagnosed with ovarian cancer while it's still confined to the ovary are alive five years after diagnosis. Among women whose cancer has spread beyond the ovary by the time it's diagnosed, only 25 percent survive five years.

Treatment Options

Ovarian cancer is always treated surgically, removing as much tumor as is feasible. Chemotherapy (drug treatment) or radiation therapy, or both, may also be given, depending on the extent of disease. Ovarian tumors usually grow outward, with an irregular, cauliflower-like shape. When the cancer spreads, parts of the tumor break off and attach to nearby organs. Cells may then spread to lymph nodes and distant organs.

Cancer limited to the ovaries may be successfully treated with surgery alone, removing the ovaries, fallopian tubes, omentum (a fold of tissue attached to organs in the abdominal cavity), and uterus.

Some patients may also receive chemotherapy or radiation therapy to kill any cancer cells remaining after surgery.

Disease that has spread beyond the ovaries almost always requires chemotherapy or radiation therapy in addition to surgery. Radiation therapy may be given by placing a radioactive solution into the pelvis and abdomen through a thin tube, coating the organs and total abdominal contents. Less commonly, external radiation using high-energy x-rays directed to the pelvis and abdomen may be prescribed.

The type of drugs used in chemotherapy depends not only on the extent of disease, but also on the type of cancer. About 85 to 90 percent of ovarian cancers arise from epithelial cells, which form the outer layer of the ovary. The rest derive from other cell types that make up the organ.

FDA has approved several drugs to treat ovarian cancer. "Outside of a clinical trial, the first-line therapy is usually cyclophosphamide [Cytoxan, Neosar] in combination with carboplatin [Paraplatin] or cisplatin [Platinol]," says Robert Justice, M.D., a medical oncologist with FDA's division of oncology and pulmonary drug products in the Center for Drug Evaluation and Research. "Other commonly used drugs approved to treat the disease are doxorubicin [Adriamycin, Doxorubicin HCl], altretamine [Hexalen], and paclitaxel [Taxol], and several more are being studied," he says.

The newest drug, Taxol, was approved Dec. 29, 1992, for advanced cases of ovarian cancer that have not responded to other therapies or have progressed after treatment.

NCI and FDA scientists cooperated in studies to evaluate the safety and effectiveness of taxol. FDA's research role in drug development is a fairly new concept, designed to help speed the approval process for drugs for life-threatening diseases.

"It's a commitment by the agency to do more than just wait for packages of data to come in [from the drug's sponsor] and review them for approval," says Jerry M. Collins, PhD., director of the Office of Research Resources in the Center for Drug Evaluation and Research. "We can't do this for every new drug in every therapeutic area," he says, "but for AIDS and cancer, we have done similar research before."

The goal of Collins' taxol studies is to see if there's a relationship between blood levels of the drug and the clinical response, which could be tumor shrinkage or toxicity.

The healing properties of Taxol were known to at least one community long before Western medicine recognized the drug's potential.

"The Queen of Neurosis"—Guilda Radner's Experience

According to an article in the Sept.4, 1991, *Journal of the American Medical Association*, around the turn of the century, a British official in the Indian subcontinent noted that parts of the European yew, *Taxus baccata*, were used in an Indian clarified butter preparation for treating cancer.

It wasn't until 1962, however, that the U.S. Forest Service delivered crude bark extracts of the Pacific yew, *Taxus brevifola*, to the National Cancer Institute. A series of NCI experiments showed the extract was effective against several kinds of cancer in mice.

In 1971, researchers at the Research Triangle Institute in Durham, N.C., isolated taxol from the extract, but interest in the compound waned until the mid-1970s. In 1979, a researcher at Albert Einstein College of Medicine in New York described how taxol works to defeat cancer by inhibiting cell division.

Today, Taxol—alone or in combination with other drugs—is being studied for a wide variety of adult and childhood cancers. In July 1992, FDA authorized use of the drug for ovarian cancer under a "treatment IND." Treatment INDs permit earlier and wider access to experimental drugs by patients with life-threatening conditions for which there is no satisfactory treatment.

In December 1992, Taxol was approved for advanced disease unresponsive to other therapies. The drug was approved in a record five months.

Side Effects of Cancer Treatments

Surgery, the first-line treatment for ovarian cancer, requires several days' hospitalization and a recuperative period of from four to six weeks. Removing the ovaries, which are the main source of the female hormones estrogen and progesterone, causes immediate menopause, and the symptomatic hot flashes are more severe than when menopause occurs more gradually, as it usually does naturally.

Radiation therapy can cause mild skin reactions, such as redness and drying in treated areas, urinary discomfort, diarrhea, and vaginal dryness. (Menopause can also cause vaginal dryness.) A small percent of patients may develop bowel obstruction, sometimes requiring surgical correction.

Other possible side effects of radiation therapy, commonly experienced with chemotherapy as well, include loss of energy and appetite, nausea, and vomiting.

Chemotherapy may also cause mouth sores, hair loss, and reduced platelet and blood cell counts that can lead to infections, anemia or bleeding. The drugs used to treat ovarian cancer may also have neurologic effects, causing hearing loss, ringing in the ears, nerve damage, and numbness or tingling in the face, fingers and toes. There may also be kidney damage.

Most side effects are temporary, and sometimes dietary changes or medicines can ease the symptoms. In 1991, FDA approved Zofran (ondansetron hydrochloride) to counter nausea and vomiting associated with chemotherapy.

"Ondansetron represents a real breakthrough in cancer treatment," says Roger B. Cohen, M.D., medical oncologist with the division of cytokine biology in FDA's Center for Biologics Evaluation and Research. "Nausea from chemotherapy is often abolished with minimal side effects, leading to dramatic improvements in patients' sense of well-being and quality of life," he says.

Other drugs previously approved for the same use are Reglan (metocloparamide) and Marinol (dronabinol).

Transfusions can correct red blood cell and platelet deficiencies. Hematopoietic growth factors such as G-CSF, approved in 1991, stimulate production of infection-fighting white blood cells. GM-CSF, which received FDA approval in 1991 to increase white cell counts after bone marrow transplantation, is now being studied for its effectiveness in stimulating white cells after cancer chemotherapy. Among other drugs now under study for their ability to increase white cell counts, and perhaps platelets as well, are stem cell factor and PIXY 321. PIXY 321 is a genetically engineered product consisting of GM-CSF and another hematopoietic growth factor, interleukin-3.

When therapy is completed, the woman continues to have regular checkups that include pelvic examinations and laboratory tests to measure blood levels of tumor markers such as CA 125. The doctor may recommend a laparotomy or laparoscopy after completion of chemotherapy to inspect the abdomen and pelvis and take multiple tissue biopsies. This "secondlook surgery" helps evaluate the effectiveness of chemotherapy and determine whether treatment should be continued or stopped. Often a laparotomy or laparoscopy has been done previously to diagnose ovarian cancer.

Cause and Prevention Elusive

Although several risk factors for ovarian cancer have been identified, its cause eludes scientists. Hypotheses have been advanced, but none proven, and so there is no rationale on which to base effective prevention strategies.

The Familial Ovarian Cancer Registry, however, urges that women with a family history of the disease receive genetic counseling, beginning in their early 20s, and undergo physical surveillance (pelvic and abdominal examination, CA 125, and pelvic or transvaginal ultrasound) every six months beginning in their early 30s. It also recommends they have prophylactic removal of the ovaries by age 35 if they have completed their families.

These recommendations apply to women in whom two or more of the following family members have ovarian cancer: mother, sister, daughter, grandmother, aunt.

Before her own ordeal with ovarian cancer began, Gilda Radner was unaware that several members of her family suffered from the disease. After a lengthy illness, she died in May 1989.

Jessica Marsh, seven years after her diagnosis, is today free of cancer and feeling fine. "I've become a much more positive person since my cancer," she says. "Life is too short to worry about little things. If life deals me lemons, I'll make lemonade."

—by Marian Segal

Marian Segal is a member of FDA's public affairs staff.

Chapter 27

When the Woman You Love Has Breast Cancer

If your wife or partner has been diagnosed with breast cancer, it's important that you become an integral part of her healing. Of course, your partner must make the final decisions regarding her treatment with her doctor. However, it is important that you listen to her feelings and fears, learn about treatment options, and become involved in her care.

You may feel a lot of conflicting emotions right now. The traditional male role-solving problems and acting knowledgeable, protective and in charge—may be causing you turmoil. You may even be experiencing guilt over worrying about your own emotional pain.

These feelings are normal, as you and your partner try to come to terms with the diagnosis of breast cancer. This chapter will guide you through the stages of breast cancer, from initial doctor's appointments and diagnosis to treatment and your future together. For each stage, the chapter discusses potential trouble spots and provides some helpful suggestions. You'll learn more about your partner's feelings, your own feelings, how your relationship may be affected, and ways to improve your communication, physical closeness and sexual intimacy.

Throughout this chapter, terms such as "partner" and "wife" will be used interchangeably, but we understand the range of possible relationships in which you may be involved. The term "wife" is not meant to disparage any relationship. We hope that this chapter can

---

©1994 by Y-ME National Breast Cancer Organization Inc. Used by permission.

help you better discover, understand and communicate what is important to you and your loved one as the first step in the healing process.

Initial Doctor's Visit Diagnosis

What She May Be Feeling

> "At the time of the diagnosis, we were shocked. When we learned that five positive nodes were discovered, we knew that severe treatment would be required. I shifted my business responsibilities so that I could spend time with her. I took her to each doctor's visit."

When first confronted with a breast cancer diagnosis, your wife may experience fear, denial, frustration, isolation, confusion, guilt, anxiety and a sense of betrayal. Many women understandably change their everyday priorities, putting themselves first. This new attitude may be confusing or disturbing to you.

Your partner may distance herself from you, physically and emotionally, to protect you from potential loss.

Her feelings of helplessness, hopelessness or despair may be compounded by her need to change from being the family caretaker to becoming the one who needs care. She may be afraid of becoming a burden on you and your children. She will also fear changes in appearance and sexuality. Some suggestions: cry together, encourage her.

What You May be Feeling

> "The first thing the hotline counselor said to my wife was that breast cancer is not an automatic death sentence, and that there are many, many survivors out there. We both felt better and could begin to think more clearly. Because when you hear 'cancer' all sorts of things go through your head; I've had schoolmates whose wives died. I don't care how well you're put together, you never imagine the best, you always imagine the worst. So you're immediately devastated. You feel hopeless; you don't even have time to think reasonably."

When the Woman You Love Has Breast Cancer

You may also be feeling fear, anger, denial and a sense of betrayal. You may feel that you have to adopt the strong role which has stereotypically been associated with men. And as a man, you may not be oriented toward your deepest feelings. Critical issues for you are likely to be anxiety over the future and the possible loss of your wife. Such thoughts may trigger fears regarding your own mortality. Many men feel guilty over this, so it's important to recognize that your fears and feelings of guilt are normal and common.

It's also normal for you to worry. Studies conducted with husbands of breast cancer patients found that the husbands went through a variety of emotional and psychosomatic problems—including eating and sleeping disorders. They also had a significant amount of anxiety before and after their wives' surgery.

You may feel overwhelmed, that the news comes so quickly that you have no time to prepare. You may be in great pain and not want your loved ones to see you this way; you may even want to seek counseling without your wife. Support groups for men, though still relatively rare, are available.

You may also have strong needs at this point for information as well as for choice and control. State openly what you need, and give yourself permission to experience these feelings fully.

Sometimes a journal may help to give you a sense of control. This may be especially useful during treatment and subsequent doctor's visits. You can write down every doctor's visit, the date and time, anything else that needs to be checked later, and every procedure suggested or performed. Write down what you're feeling as well.

At this point, you may also want to tape record consultations, request photographs of mastectomies (to help prepare you and your wife), prepare questions, and request printed information regarding treatment options (see the next section on "Treatment Options").

During treatment, you can be supportive in a number of important roles: coordinator of social support, monitor of normal functioning, patient advocate, and even physician's assistant

How This Could Affect Your Relationship

Whenever one partner gets sick, a couple's usual pattern of give and take, dependence and independence, is altered. Serious illness can bring a couple closer together. However, like any crisis, it can also disclose shortcomings in your relationship.

Communication

> "You really need outside support that can function like an anchor, to stop the drift—someone who can say, 'This is what you can expect, these are A, B and C, and A is going to be like this, etc.' That stops the drift; puts everything on hold. Immediately after talking to a counselor, my wife felt better, and when she felt better, I felt better—because I hadn't known anything about breast cancer up to that point."

Once your partner is diagnosed with cancer, your relationship will very likely change. With open, trusting communication, that change can be positive.

Tell your wife what you're feeling. Establish clear and open communication: avoid mind reading and don't make assumptions.

Talk in specifics, and attempt to feel comfortable with a free exchange of ideas. Express your feelings and "own" them; that is, use "I" messages. When your wife tells you something, listen to what is expressed without becoming defensive. Make sure you understand her message. Give feedback so that your wife knows how you feel about what was said—express your viewpoint during the conversation, not three days later.

Communication can also be physical—as simple as holding your wife's hand. Comforting your partner in this manner may make you feel better.

Build on the strong, positive areas of your relationship to help feel closer and enjoy each other. Strive for cooperation coupled with independence, and place a high value on flexibility:

- demonstrate mutual love, respect and understanding

- maintain independent identities and accept each other as separate individuals

- give each other privacy

- trust each other

- make a commitment to tough it out together.

Direct, open communication should also be extended to the family, so that you and your wife have as large a support system as possible. Family and friends cannot offer help if they don't know you're in a crisis. If children are not told, they will sense that something is wrong, and confusion will be added to their concern.

Physical Closeness and Sexual Intimacy

Cancer is not contagious, and sexual activity will not make cancer worse. You cannot "catch" cancer by kissing, hugging or having intercourse; a cancer cell from one person's body cannot take root and grow in someone else.

Treatment Options

What You Both May Be Feeling

You and your wife may feel pressured to decide on a course of treatment in a brief period of time. This can make you feel powerless and confused.

How This Could Affect Your Relationship

> "Husbands or partners of women with breast cancer do not know others in the same situation, because it is not something that is discussed. Men are supposed to be strong. We have often been brought up to believe that we are capable of handling setbacks, that 'real men don't cry.'"

Give your wife the opportunity to communicate her feelings and fears. Become involved with her doctors and nurses. Take an interest in her treatments as well. Such support can help your wife better tolerate her necessary treatments.

Communication

> "My primary concern was proving my support for my wife. I told my grown sons to call their mother more often, because I thought it would be helpful for her to have someone to talk to."

Become informed: read and talk with your wife and her doctors about all possible therapies. Sometimes you and your partner will interpret what you read or hear differently. This very difference can become the basis of careful, intelligent decision-making. By becoming informed, you and your loved one can make important decisions together with confidence. Information is available at the library, doctors' offices, Cancer Information Service, and the Y-ME National Breast Cancer Organization.

Surgery (Mastectomy/lumpectomy)

"I learned a long, long time ago that when they are small children have a unique sense of being able to determine when something's wrong. Children are just like adults. You have to approach things directly and explain what's happened, what we've found, where we are, what we known, what we don't know, and what is scaring us. This is important, because then the family can give you the support you need; then they're giving the support from an equal knowledgeable level."

What She May Be Feeling

After mastectomy or lumpectomy, your wife may have feelings of embarrassment or low self-esteem, as well as physical discomfort.

Though your wife needs emotional support at this point she may find it tiring to deal with too many well-meaning friends. She may have to conserve her energy and screen out those individuals whose interaction is not helpful. You may have to mediate between your wife and her friends and relatives: when she's tired, explain to them that your wife appreciates their concern but is not up to seeing them that day.

Try to be at the hospital as much as possible. Be optimistic, but don't promise miracles. Reinforce genuine hopes and promise her what you can guarantee: for example, let her know that you won't abandon her. Acknowledge her anger, confusion, and frustration. And because a positive attitude may help your wife fight cancer help her keep an optimistic frame of mind.

When the Woman You Love Has Breast Cancer

What You May Be Feeling

> *"My sister and brother-in-law went with us to the hospital. The family came together. It wasn't just me alone—there was somebody else, some people that I could talk to, so that I wasn't sitting there alone. One of the options people have is to seek family help, to let the family know what's going on. You can just say 'I need you to take a day off and come with me.'"*

Many men have trouble acting as a support system for their partner while coping with their own emotions. While you need to be strong for your wife, you may be feeling guilty, lonely or abandoned. You may be afraid of what would happen if you were to become ill now, since everyone depends on you.

You may have feelings of fear and even repulsion—these are natural. Generally, however, it is not your partner's superficial change in appearance that affects you so strongly, but rather its psychological significance to you. The fear of losing your wife may cause you to withdraw affection and sexual intimacy as part of a larger, more harmful process of withdrawal. In other words, if you cannot look at your wife's scar, you may be expressing deeper feelings—perhaps anger over suddenly being responsible for the children and other household chores, or fear at being reminded of your own vulnerability.

Many men also feel a real sense of loss. It is unrealistic to expect a man to have no reaction whatsoever when his lover loses her breast. For these reasons, you may have to make as many adjustments as your wife.

Communication

Couples should go through the entire process—diagnosis, treatment and recovery—as partners. Communication is important: silence may be misinterpreted as a lack of interest.

During recovery, men may feel cut off from the information flow, leaving them isolated and angry. However, just as you helped your partner gather information before treatment, you can continue to take a proactive role during treatment, especially with physicians. This can be very valuable, as your wife may forget to bring up an important point. For example, one man whose wife has kidney disease questioned the doctor about the use of chemotherapy drugs, which are metabolized through the kidneys. He worked to get her oncologist and kidney specialist to talk to one another, and a modified chemotherapy program was used.

Communication and information is also very important for sexual health after cancer treatment. When you know what to expect, it is easier to have a meaningful discussion about potential challenges to this aspect of your relationship.

Physical Closeness and Sexual Intimacy

Perhaps nothing can prepare your wife (and you) for the shock of what her chest may look like. Acknowledging that the loss of a breast is very sad for both of you begins the grieving and promotes the healing process.

Looking at the scar together with your wife will help you both adjust to the physical changes. The sooner a couple can look at the scar—preferably before leaving the hospital—the sooner they can deal with the fact that the breast is gone. (Or in the case of a lumpectomy, that a scar is present.) Remember that most scars are at first red and raw, but with time they fade and are much less frightening.

Sexual issues can arise after surgery, because the loss of a breast can damage a woman's sense of attractiveness and self-esteem. She may be embarrassed in certain sexual positions, such as the woman on top, since the scar is more noticeable in that position. Or she may have pain or stiffness in her arms and shoulders, especially after axillary dissection (surgery involving her armpit area). You may want to avoid positions which put weight on her shoulders or arm. It can be helpful to support these areas with pillows during intercourse.

Sexual activity is usually safe during and after cancer treatment. Check with your doctor if you have questions.

> *"Ask every question that crosses your mind. Do not be intimidated by a doctor. If you don't understand the answer, ask your question again. Tell the doctor, 'I don't understand what you're saying,' or 'Can you explain that to me again?' Every time any doctor says, 'We're going to do such-and-such,' you need to ask the question, 'Why?'"*

Coming Home

What She May Be Feeling

Coming home after surgery, your wife may suddenly feel lonely or disoriented because her extensive medical and psychological support team at the hospital is not immediately available. Discuss these concerns with her. Help her develop new support resources such as family and friends. Many women find it helpful to develop a buddy system with another breast cancer survivor at this time.

She may be emotionally distant: her body mobilizes all of its resources to combat infections and restore strength, and her mind focuses on how badly she feels and what she must do to get better. These things can change the way she feels about her body, herself, or her sexual activity.

What You May Be Feeling

> "By going through these monumental concerns one after the other—discussing my wife's breast cancer with Y-ME and with doctors—the whole thing was put in a better perspective I realized that it's something ,you can handle—it isn't beyond you, it isn't bigger than you"

You may feel overwhelmed by the changes in your partner and in your own household responsibilities. You cannot do everything; do what you can. Help your wife with household chores, but encourage her to do what she can, because a regular schedule can be very therapeutic.

It is very important to let your partner know that you accept her because of who she is. Be understanding. Love her. Reassure her. Be kind and sympathetic. Help change dressings and give back rubs. And encourage your wife to begin or maintain an exercise routine. Regular exercise is very helpful both physically and emotionally.

How This Could Affect Your Relationship

Contrary to myths, only 7% of marriages in which the wife had breast cancer end in divorce, and most of these are due to pre-existing problems. Typically, relationships that were strong before the diagnosis of breast cancer remain strong after surgery and treatment.

However, expect a shift in her priorities and a change in your roles. Very likely, nothing will be as it was. You may find yourself less attracted to your wife, yet still so in love that it hurts. Perhaps you will find yourself treating her too delicately. In some cases, the adjustments you have to make—both sexual and in daily life—may disturb or annoy you.

Be ready to make changes. Examine what is important. Relax housekeeping standards, prepare simpler meals, and have children take on additional chores. Other family members can also help. Sort out necessary tasks from those that can go undone.

Communication

Be honest with your wife. Tell her that while she may have changed physically, your love for her has not. Share how you would feel if you lost her.

Communication should also extend to sexual intimacy. Both of you should talk about your sexual feelings and desires. Your wife may feel that her sexuality has been diminished, and she may think that you feel that way too. She may have trouble communicating her fears, and if you wait for signals from her to talk about it, no one will take that first, necessary step. Communication can overcome feelings of isolation and rejection.

Physical Closeness and Sexual Intimacy

Re-establishing a sexual relationship is essential to your relationship and to your wife's healing process. Remember that what is normal for you and your wife is whatever gives you pleasure together. One-fourth to one—third of couples have sexual difficulties following surgery, so re-establishing a sexual relationship may take time.

After your wife has come home, increase non-sexual intimacy. Physical contact in general—a hug, a touch, holding hands, kissing your wife's lips—can take place for its own sake, not as a prelude to sex.

A woman's sexual feelings may be changed by her perception of her altered body image, as well as by overt depression or even unconscious mood changes. Women say that their most pressing need at this time is to be held and hugged, but they are concerned that their husband will be offended if this is not an invitation to lovemaking.

Typically, a man will be relieved to discover that his partner is not rejecting him. And he is often pleased and proud that he can offer something of value to his wife—by showing affection, he can make her feel more secure, loved and protected. When you spend intimate time together, try to put day-to-day problems on hold.

You may have a fear of hurting your wife during lovemaking. In that case, you should talk with her about sexual positions which are more comfortable for her.

Follow-up Treatment (Chemotherapy/Hormone Therapy and Radiation)

> *"I think that, on the whole, men do the right thing. There are stories of men who have walked out, but I would like to think that's rare. I think basically, if a man loves the woman, he knows what he's going to do."*

What She May Be Feeling

Chemotherapy. Chemotherapy is given in cycles; a recipe repeated every few weeks. Each chemotherapy agent has its own side effects most of which are temporary—lasting hours to days. Some women will have none, others many. This does not reflect the severity of the disease, only the individual's tolerance to these drugs.

There are medications that can relieve some of these side effects, but some doctors do not routinely prescribe them. If your partner's side effects seem particularly severe, ask the doctor whether intervention is available to relieve the symptoms.

Many women feel fatigue. Encourage your wife to be active to see friends, to work if possible, but allow her extra time to rest. Let her know you understand how she feels by volunteering to do tasks she normally does without making her feel guilty. Nausea can make her even less active. Medications can help. Changing diet often helps.

Not all chemotherapy causes hair loss, and some women experience only partial baldness. Ask the doctor what you can expect on her particular drug regimen. Hair loss, when it occurs, is devastating to most women. With breast cancer, personal body image concerns are already present—but baldness lets the world know. Remind your wife that her hair will grow back, that she is beautiful to you, and that she is still very much loved. Participate in wig shopping with her.

Subtle side effects can occur with chemotherapy: dry skin, cracked nails and mouth sores. All are temporary, but these small inconveniences can become a major irritant. Remind your wife that hair loss and other chemotherapy side effects are generally temporary.

If your wife develops menopausal symptoms, loss of menses, hot flashes or vaginal dryness, she is dealing with one more issue-loss of femininity. Hot flashes come unexpectedly and can disturb sleep and normal activities.

Your wife can reduce the nausea from chemotherapy by learning relaxation skills. By making sure that the house doesn't smell like food when she walks in, you can help her reduce nausea brought on by chemotherapy. You might also want to have herbal teas and crackers available.

Radiation Therapy

> *"Every time she looks in the mirror, goes into the bath, holds her children, is in bed with her husband, cancer faces her. The woman sees the reaction in the faces of her family members. Nothing but love and understanding can help"*

Radiation therapy can be fatiguing—it is given every day for five to seven weeks after lumpectomy. Every treatment is a reminder to your wife of her diagnosis and her mortality, making this a stressful time.

Often, radiation therapy is easier than chemotherapy, because the immediate side effects are milder. Most women have a skin reaction, which is sometimes like a bad burn which constantly aches. The breast can swell and may hurt and feel heavy. Sexual breast play can be very uncomfortable at this time.

Radiation therapy or surgery can also cause lymphedema, which is a swelling around the breast, or under and down the arm, caused by a buildup of lymphatic fluid. Lymphedema may occur suddenly after radiation, or it may be brought on by physical exertion following treatment.

For some women, especially those with severe cases, lymphedema can be devastating: their arms may not fit into their clothes, and they may have to wear a special elastic sleeve. To keep swelling to a minimum, encourage your wife to perform appropriate exercises and to avoid heavy lifting and working long hours near a hot oven.

Severe lymphedema should be discussed with the doctor, because there are certain procedures that can help relieve symptoms.

What You May Be Feeling

You may be feeling frustrated and helpless, especially since chemotherapy can go on for months. Support your wife by accompanying her to her chemotherapy or radiation therapy appointments. Accompany her to a wig shop. Help pick out some interesting hats. If she comes home with a novel scarf or turban, compliment her on it. Dare her to be different!

Physical Closeness and Sexual Intimacy

Chemotherapy may leave your lover tired, nauseous, anxious or depressed for periods of time. Radiation therapy can cause irritation or swelling in her breast or arm. As a result, she may not be interested in intercourse. During this time, you can be physically intimate in other ways—through kissing, touching, stroking, cuddling, hugging, massage, or loving words.

Chemotherapy can also bring about changes that directly affect your partner's interest in sex. It can directly or indirectly induce the development of menopause, even if she is quite young. Your wife may experience hot flashes, vaginal dryness and thinning of the vaginal walls—which can result in painful intercourse and postcoital bleeding.

Some of these changes can be addressed directly. For example, vaginal dryness can be reduced with a vaginal lubricating jelly, which can be purchased over the counter. A gynecologist may recommend other products to help. Remember that sexual activity does not expose you to the effects of chemotherapy or radiation.

What She May Be Feeling

> *"During my wife's illness we became closer mentally and less close physically. She was embarrassed. She did not want to be touched in a sexual way. We held each other, we talked, we watched TV, listened to music . . . as close friends."*

After treatment, your loved one will always wonder whether the cancer is going to come back. (You may remain just as worried.) She may interpret every little ache and pain as new cancer.

Such fears can linger indefinitely and intensify. Your wife may also show a dependence on doctors and experience "anniversary" symptoms around the date of the original diagnosis. You should understand which symptoms are significant and make sure she checks them with her doctor.

Even in the most loving relationship, your wife or partner may reach out to other women with breast cancer through a hotline or support group, so that she can share common concerns.

Do not think that she is moving away from you. There are times when a woman needs reassurance and solace from someone who has been there—someone to whom she can reveal her innermost thoughts. This is healthy. When talking with other survivors, your partner need not be overly concerned with their feelings, as she may be with yours.

How This Could Affect Your Relationship

For most couples, changes are generally positive. Many feel that the experience of breast cancer brought them closer to each other.

Physical Closeness and Sexual Intimacy

After your wife has completed her chemotherapy or radiation treatments, sexual desire can bounce back for both of you. So add romance to your life: have special dinners together, leave each other notes, send cards or give gifts.

If your wife has had breast reconstruction, she may enjoy sex more because of the boost that her "new" body gives to her feelings of attractiveness and self-esteem. However, reconstruction will probably not completely restore the pleasure she used to feel from having her breast caressed.

While we are making great strides in plastic surgery, it is important to realize that a reconstructed breast is not identical to the breast which has been lost. A reconstructed breast may be harder, parts of it may be numb, and the shape may be different. Massaging, squeezing or caressing a reconstructed breast will not cause any harm, but there is generally a lack of sensation in the area, so the breast may no longer be a great source of sexual stimulation. However, most women are pleased with the reconstructed breast, especially when they are realistic about the surgical outcome.

Conclusion

> *"We adjusted positions for sexual intercourse, and I accepted her decreased interest in sexual activity. She likes hugging, and that's okay with me."*

Many who have not only survived breast cancer but have turned it into a positive, even enriching, experience have done so because they had an ally in their partner.

In fact, most couples are drawn closer together by the experience.

We encourage you to continue learning about the medical and psychological effects of breast cancer. If you and your wife make a commitment to go through diagnosis, treatment and recovery as partners, her recovery may occur more quickly.

Now is the time to learn more about the disease, so that you can do all you can to support your wife or partner's recovery.

> *"Support, participation and discussion are needed during these times. Women have told me that they could face the hair loss, the skin changes, and all the other side effects, if they just knew that their loved ones would stand by them."*

Chapter 28

Cosmetic Help for Cancer Patients

Sometimes the 36-year-old cancer patient lets herself remember when she had the energy to "run around with her kids like a maniac" and stay up until the early hours of the morning. That was before a recurrence of Hodgkin's disease forced her to begin the chemotherapy treatment that left her nauseated, fatigued, somewhat dispirited, and bald.

Before chemotherapy, Sharon (who asked that her last name not be used) had beautiful, jet-black hair. Now she keeps a strawberry blond wig handy for those times she says she "needs a good laugh" to help her "escape" from the side effects of chemotherapy, as well as the reality of having cancer.

"The wig has bangs coming down. I never used to wear bangs," she says. "Sometimes I put on long, dangling earrings with the wig and some of the cosmetics that they gave me when the hospital made me up. It's pretty funny because I'm not the kind of person that used to use all this stuff."

Her mother, Dorothy (who also asked that her last name not be used), helped coax Sharon from her hospital room to the "Look Good . . . Feel Better" workshop at North Shore University Hospital, Manahasset, N.Y., where she was receiving her treatment. Dorothy says her daughter was quite skeptical and felt she didn't want to be bothered with having anyone teach her individualized skin care and makeup techniques, or how to work with wigs, turbans and scarves.

FDA Consumer July/August 1992.

But once they started working on her, "Sharon got such a kick out of it and laughed for hours afterwards. The thing a mother looks for is her child's happiness," says Dorothy. "While having your child have cancer is not a happy thing, for those moments, Sharon's smile was my smile, too."

The notion that it's hard to weather going through an arduous course of radiation or chemotherapy treatment without looking good and feeling good about oneself has gained scientific respect, according to Julia Rowland, Ph.D., director of psycho-oncology research, Georgetown University Medical Center, Washington, D.C.

"Looking good despite what we may be going through can help one take control again and can be a critical component to the healing process by providing powerful psychological benefits," says Rowland.

Course Available. The "Look Good . . . Feel Better" course, available to Sharon and others around the country, was developed jointly for national use by the Cosmetic, Toiletry, and Fragrance Association (CTFA) Foundation, the National Cosmetology Association, and the American Cancer Society nearly three years ago. It's an attempt to help patients learn to minimize the side effects of cancer drugs and radiation treatment, which can cause changes in hair, complexion and nails.

"Look Good . . . Feel Better" teaches hands-on beauty techniques in group or one-on-one makeover workshops conducted by specially trained, volunteer cosmetologists in hospitals, community centers, and salons.

According to Carolyn Deaver, vice president, CTFA Foundation, the program is also operating in Australia and will be launched in Canada this year. Though the current program is geared for women, a similar program for men undergoing cancer treatment is expected to be developed.

If a patient is unable to attend a makeover workshop, there is a video and brochure available free of charge, which can be used at home.

Here are some of the problems that these programs and pamphlets tackle:

Hair Loss Hard to Take

Drugs capable of killing cancer cells can also attack normal cells. This accounts for many of chemotherapy's unpleasant side effects.

Cosmetic Help for Cancer Patients

Hair loss, although temporary, and not always a side effect of chemotherapy, is often cited by patients who experience it as the most devastating cosmetic side effect of chemotherapy.

"Every time I pass a mirror and look at my bald head," says 43-year-old Corrine Wenze of South Farmingdale, N.Y., "it's a constant reminder of my disease. Even when I look at babies I cringe because they remind me I have only about six loyal strands of my own hair."

Wenze says that when she first found out she had breast cancer she "wallowed very well by playing video games for nearly a month. I wanted to fall into a hole and disappear. I didn't believe I could have cancer."

She continues, "You know the surgeon sent me home without my breast and then sent me through cancer treatment. It wasn't until I went to the "Look Good . . . Feel Better" program that I picked up. They made me feel more cared for by caring for me and then showing me how to care for myself."

Rowland says losing one's hair is often the first overwhelming confrontation patients have with their illness. Until that point, they might have easily hidden their disease from everyone, including themselves.

According to cosmetologists, the best time to start looking for a wig is before the first chemotherapy treatment. Synthetic wigs are the easiest to maintain because they don't need to be set and are not affected by humidity like natural hair. They're also less costly than natural hair wigs.

Bijan Safai, M.D., chief of Memorial Sloan-Kettering Cancer Center's dermatology service in New York City, says that in most cases, patients' hair begins to grow back within a few weeks after their chemotherapy treatment ends. But if a wig does not fit right and exerts excessive pressure at certain points; the hair follicles at those points will die and hair will never grow back. So he recommends wigs that don't need to be glued or taped down, and that don't require elastic bands that hold them tightly against the scalp.

Frequently, the cost of a wig is reimbursable by third-party payers if it is prescribed as a "cranial prosthesis" by a physician. Other options cancer patients can consider are brightly colored scarves, turbans or hats.

William Cahan, M.D., senior attending surgeon at Memorial Sloan-Kettering, says many of his male cancer patients choose to wear hairpieces close to their natural hair color and style while undergoing cancer treatment. However, some prefer to have fun wearing hats such as French berets and beanies with propellers. Like Sharon choosing to wear a strawberry blond wig, these men seem to get through their treatment by self-kidding.

Chemotherapy Dries Skin

Chemotherapy is easier on the skin than on the hair. Even so, whatever a person skin type, chemotherapy will make skin drier because the drugs interfere with oil and sweat glands. Keeping skin as moist as possible during treatment is important to keep it looking young and healthy. Moisture can also prevent cracking and chapping, which can lead to infection in the cancer patient, whose immune system is suppressed.

Cancer patients are advised never to pull, tug or scrub the face too hard. Overzealous cleansing can strip away the remaining natural oils. Soap-free face cleansers that gently cleanse makeup and oil without drying skin are preferable. Safai recommends using an anti-microbial soap, however, to effectively clean areas like the armpits and genitals, which are prone to infection.

Moisturizing day and night can slow down the skin's loss of moisture by leaving behind a filmy deposit of oil. The oil not only helps retard moisture evaporation, but also makes the surface of the skin softer and more pliable. This may be especially important for hands and soles of the feet, which may become sore and blistered. Rubber gloves should be used when doing household chores.

Cancer patients are advised to moisturize with products containing sunscreens with a sun protection factor (SPF) of at least 15 because people undergoing chemotherapy may be more sensitive to harmful ultraviolet rays. (For more on sunscreens, see "Cool Tips for Summer Safety" in the June 1992 FDA Consumer and "No Safe Tan" in the May 1991 FDA Consumer). Dry, chapped lips can be helped with non-pigmented lip balms or petrolatum-based products, according to Harley Haynes, M.D., a dermatologist with Brigham and Women's Hospital and Harvard Medical School. He recommends using lipstick only when the lips are in good condition. Chemotherapy may also affect the nails, retarding their growth and, in many cases, causing them to become thin and brittle and develop horizontal grooves.

It's not a good idea to cover the nails with acrylics or other types of wraps, says Haynes, since these materials can trap bacteria that may cause infection. Instead, the nails can be clipped short and moisturized with lotions. A light-color nail polish will camouflage any nail imperfections. But to prevent nails from drying out, only nonacetone-based nail polish remover should be used.

Cancer patients who have professional manicures should bring their own implements to guard against infection. Cuticles should be pushed back rather than cut.

Skin Reactions to Radiation

Radiation treatment, unlike chemotherapy, affects only the skin that is irradiated or close to the point of irradiation. Its most common effect is a brief, intense sunburn-like reaction that causes blistering, says Alan Lorincz, M.D., professor of dermatology, University of Chicago, Pritzer School of Medicine.

Sometimes, however, a chronic skin condition may occur in which the treated skin thins and loses elasticity and may become lighter or darken. This skin needs to be treated especially gently with emollients and sunscreen products with a high sun protection factor. It can be expected to be more susceptible than the rest of the person's skin to chronic irritation and breakdown.

During chemotherapy and radiation treatment skin will, in general, become more sensitive to allergens or irritants. So cancer patients are advised not to share any of their hygiene products with anyone else and not to use old products that have changed in appearance, odor or texture.

Not a Time to Experiment

In general, it's not a good time to experiment with new brands of products, unless products usually used become irritating. Some cancer patients, however, want to experiment with cosmetics to try to camouflage certain facial effects of cancer treatment, such as skin discolorations, blotchiness, dark circles under the eyes, or loss of eyebrows and lashes. Experts advise trying out only one product at a time for several days before starting a second new product.

After taking the necessary precautions noted below, cancer patients will find that cosmetics can be important tools, says Rita Davies, a volunteer cosmetologist with the American Cancer Society.

Foundation and concealer are good for evening out skin tone. Eye crayons applied in a feathery motion can give the appearance of lashes, and brow powders can create natural-looking eyebrows. Mascara that has a wand with a small comb can help give body to remaining eyelashes.

Cosmetics can give a lift not only to the face, but to a cancer patient's outlook on life. As Rowland says, "I think we underestimate the impact of outward appearances. If we put on a costume we feel differently about ourselves. If we put on special clothes we feel differently about ourselves. Similarly, cosmetics are a way to fortify the self during chemotherapy or radiation."

Where To Find a Program

For help locating a "Look Good . . . Feel Better" program, call the local chapter of the American Cancer Society or 1-800-395-LOOK.

Shopping for Cosmetics

Though cosmetics generally have a lengthy safety record, this does not mean that a consumer should assume that the products they're using are absolutely free from risk, says John Bailey, Ph.D., of FDA's division of colors and cosmetics technology. He reminds shoppers that the law does not require pre-market approval of cosmetic products by the agency, although "untested" products must be labeled as such.

Individual cosmetic companies are responsible for ensuring that their products are safe for use by the consumer and have a great deal of freedom in how they formulate their products. (See "Cosmetic Safety: More Complex Than at First Blush" in the November 1991 issue of FDA Consumer.)

When purchasing cosmetics, he says, it is very important to read the label for a description of the product, including its ingredients, and any warning statements about the use of the product. Besides reading the product label. Bailey advises consumers to exercise good judgment in purchasing and using cosmetic products. For example, old products, or products that are inadequately preserved, may become contaminated with microorganisms. Never purchase a product that doesn't look or smell right and don't share cosmetics with other people or "wet" products with saliva.

Cosmetic Help for Cancer Patients

Persons undergoing medical treatment, such as chemotherapy, should consult their physicians if they have experienced allergic reactions to cosmetics in the past, or if they notice any unusual reaction after use.

—by Cheryl Platzman Weinstock

Cheryl Platzman Weinstock is a freelance writer in Long Island, N.Y.

Chapter 29

Ovarian Cancer: Screening, Treatment, and Followup

Introduction

Ovarian cancer is the leading cause of death from gynecologic malignancies in the United States. In 1994, approximately 24,000 new cases of ovarian cancer will be diagnosed, and 13,600 women will die of the disease. Over the past several years, significant new information has been generated regarding the epidemiology, biology, risk reduction, screening, treatment, and follow-up of ovarian cancer.

On April 97, 1994, the National Cancer Institute, together with the Office of Medical Applications of Research of the National Institutes of Health, convened a Consensus Development Conference on Ovarian Cancer: Screening, Treatment, and Followup. The purpose of this conference was to identify the issues for which there are currently sufficient confirmed data, so that health care providers will have these data available to them and so that all women can benefit from this information. Second, for issues that are important but for which there are not sufficient data, the panel was charged with recommending directions for important avenues of future research.

At the consensus conference, members of an independent, non-Federal, scientific panel with public and patient representation heard and discussed the current data pertinent to these issues. The panel

---

National Institutes of Health Consensus Development Conference Statement, August 15, 1994, 11 AM—Final.

then weighed the scientific evidence and drafted answers to the following key questions:

- What is the current status of screening and prevention of ovarian cancer?

- What is the appropriate management of early-stage ovarian cancer?

- What is the appropriate management of advanced epithelial ovarian cancer?

- What is appropriate followup after primary therapy?

- What are important directions for future research?

What Is the Current Status of Screening and Prevention of Ovarian Cancer?

Recent events have brought ovarian cancer under close scrutiny in the lay press and have increased demand for early detection of this devastating disease. The survival rate of women with early-stage ovarian cancer is significantly higher than that of women with advanced-stage disease. Unfortunately, the vast majority of women with ovarian cancer are diagnosed with advanced disease. Although sometimes women with early ovarian cancer have symptoms such as vague gastrointestinal discomfort, pelvic pressure, and pain, more often women with early ovarian cancer have no symptoms, or very mild and nonspecific symptoms. By the time symptoms are present, women with ovarian cancer usually have advanced disease. The advent of the CA 125 serum tumor marker and improvements in pelvic ultrasound, along with newer techniques of color Doppler imaging (CDI) studies of ovarian vessels, have led some to advocate the use of these modalities in the attempt to detect early-stage ovarian cancer. To place the disease in perspective, its prevalence is 30-50/100,000, with the lifetime incidence being 1 in 70 women.

Risk Factors. Although the cause is unknown, some women are at higher risk of developing ovarian cancer than others. Risk factors include advancing age; nulliparity; North American or Northern European descent; a personal history of endometrial, colon, or breast cancer; and a family history of ovarian cancer. The evidence is inconsistent regarding the use of fertility drugs as a risk factor. Less than 0.05 percent of women are at significantly increased risk because of three hereditary ovarian cancer syndromes: breast-ovarian cancer syndrome; site-specific ovarian cancer syndrome; and hereditary nonpolyposis colorectal cancer or Lynch syndrome II, which includes early-onset nonpolyposis colorectal cancer, endometrial cancer, cancer of the upper gastrointestinal system (including biliary ducts, pancreas, and possibly small bowel), urothelial carcinomas of the renal pelvis and ureter, and ovarian cancer.

Screening for Ovarian Cancer. To be suitable for screening, a disease must have a significant prevalence and be a significant cause of mortality. There must be a pre-clinical phase that can be detected, and the disease must be amenable to therapy. The screening test itself must have sufficient specificity, sensitivity, and positive predictive value (PPV) to be effective, and it must be cost-effective. In ovarian cancer, if one assumes a prevalence of 50/100,000, a test with 99 percent specificity and 100 percent sensitivity would yield only 1 in 21 women with a positive screen actually having the disease (i.e., PPV = 4.8 percent). It must be noted that currently available tests do not attain the aforementioned high level of sensitivity.

Three screening tests are in general use: bimanual rectovaginal pelvic examination, CA 125, and transvaginal ultrasonography (TVS). CDI is also being investigated in some centers regarding its role as an adjunct to TVS. Historically, rectovaginal pelvic examination has been the only method used to detect ovarian cancer at any stage. (See Table 27.1 for description of stages.) Although pelvic exam is an important part of routine gynecologic care, it has inadequate sensitivity and specificity as a screening test for ovarian cancer.

CA 125 is an antigenic determinant detected by radioimmunoassay. It is elevated in 80 percent of epithelial ovarian cancers. However, only half of the patients with stage I cancers have elevated levels. Because detecting early disease is the goal of screening, CA 125 alone is not an adequate screening test. In addition, a significant proportion of healthy women and women with benign disease have elevations in CA 125 resulting in an unacceptably low specificity for this test.

Transabdominal ultrasound and TVS have been studied as noninvasive screening tools. TVS is currently the preferred modality. However, specificity of ultrasonography is not adequate for use as a single screening modality. For example, in a representative study, 5,479 women, 96 percent of whom were 45 years of age or older, were screened using abdominal ultrasound, and there were 338 positive screens. This resulted in exploratory laparotomy in 326 women, and five stage I ovarian cancers were found. Three had borderline histology, and therefore, diagnosis at a later date may not have affected survival. Sixty-five laparotomies were performed for each case of ovarian cancer detected. In a similar screening study of women with a family history of ovarian cancer, 1,601 pre- and postmenopausal women were screened using TVS. Sixty-one operations detected five stage I ovarian cancers, three of which were of borderline histology. The combination of CA 125 screening and TVS significantly improves the specificity of screening and has reduced the proportion of women requiring unnecessary surgical intervention. However, there is a potential for significant anxiety related to abnormal screening test results as well as morbidity and even mortality from resultant surgical procedures in women with no significant pathology, which may outweigh any potential benefits.

Recommendations for Screening. All women should have a comprehensive family history taken by a physician knowledgeable in the risks associated with ovarian cancer and should continue to undergo annual rectovaginal pelvic examination as part of routine medical care. The lifetime risk of ovarian cancer in a woman with no affected relatives is 1 in 70, and in a woman with one first-degree relative with ovarian cancer, the risk is 5 percent. With current knowledge and technology, the benefits of screening a woman who has one or no first-degree relatives with ovarian cancer are unproven. The risks may outweigh the benefits, particularly in women with no family history or other high risk factors. There is currently no evidence to support routine screening in these women. However, participation in clinical screening trials is an appropriate option and is important in helping to ultimately define the potential benefits and risks of screening. If a woman has one first-degree relative with ovarian cancer (making her lifetime risk of developing the disease 5 percent) but no clinical trials are available to her, she may feel that despite the absence of prospec-

Stage	Characteristic
I	Growth limited to the ovaries
IA	Growth limited to one ovary; no ascites; no tumor on the external surfaces, capsule intact
IB	Growth limited to both ovaries; no ascites; no tumor on the external surfaces, capsule intact
IC	Tumor either stage IA or stage IB but with tumor on the surface of one or both ovaries, or with capsule ruptured, or with ascites containing malignant cells or with positive peritoneal washings
II	Growth involving one or both ovaries on pelvic extension
IIA	Extension or metastases to the uterus or rubes
IIB	Extension to other pelvic tissues
IIC	Tumor either stage IIA or IIB with tumor on the surface of one or both ovaries, or with capsule(s) ruptured, or with ascites containing malignant cells or with positive peritoneal washings
III	Tumor involving one or both ovaries with peritoneal implants outside the pelvis or positive retroperitoneal or inguinal nodes; superficial liver metastases equals stage III; tumor is limited to the true pelvis but with histologically verified malignant extension to small bowel or omentum
IIIA	Tumor grossly limited to the true pelvis with negative nodes but with histologically confirmed microscopic seeding of abdominal peritoneal surfaces
IIIB	Tumor of one or both ovaries; histologically confirmed implants of abdominal peritoneal surface, none exceeding 2 cm in diameter; nodes negative
IIIC	Abdominal implants greater than 2 cm in diameter or positive retroperitoneal or inguinal nodes
IV	Growth involving one or both ovaries with distant metastases; if pleural effusion is present, there must be positive cytologic test results to allot a case to stage IV; parenchymal liver metastases equals stage IV

Figure 29.1. FIGO (1986) Staging System for Ovarian Cancer. Source: Staging Announcement: FIGO Cancer Committee. Gynecol Oncol 25:383, 1986.

tive data, this is sufficient risk for her to be screened. This alternative and opportunity should be available to the woman and her physician.

With two or more first-degree relatives, a woman's lifetime risk rises to 7 percent. There are no conclusive data that screening benefits these women. However, women with two or more family members affected by ovarian cancer have a 3 percent chance of having a hereditary ovarian cancer syndrome and should be counseled by a gynecologic oncologist or other qualified specialist regarding their individual risk.

For patients with a hereditary ovarian cancer syndrome (assuming autosomal dominant inheritance with 80 percent penetrance), the lifetime risk of ovarian cancer is approximately 40 percent. There are no data demonstrating that screening these high-risk women reduces their mortality from ovarian cancer. Nonetheless, at least annual rectovaginal pelvic examination, CA 125 determinations, and TVS are recommended in these women. When childbearing is completed, or at least by age 35, prophylactic bilateral oophorectomy is recommended to reduce this significant risk. Prophylactic oophorectomy does not preclude a small risk of developing peritoneal carcinomatosis, which is clinically similar to advanced ovarian cancer.

Protective Factors and Prophylactic Bilateral Oophorectomy. Clearly established protective factors include greater than one full-term pregnancy, oral contraceptive use, and breast-feeding, all of which reduce incessant ovulation. Tubal ligation has also been described as a possible protective factor. The risk reduction associated with greater than 5 years of oral contraceptive use is estimated in one study to be 37 percent. Relatively short duration of use may be beneficial, but prolonged use appears to extend this benefit.

A woman with one first-degree relative with ovarian cancer has a lifetime risk of ovarian cancer of 5 percent. This is probably not high enough to warrant prophylactic oophorectomy as an independent operative procedure with its attendant risks. The probability of a hereditary ovarian cancer syndrome in a family pedigree increases with the number of affected relatives, with the number of affected generations, and with young age of onset of disease. Therefore, prophylactic oophorectomy should be considered in these settings with careful weighing of the risks and potential benefits. The risk of ovarian cancer in women from families with hereditary ovarian cancer syndromes (as discussed above) is sufficiently high to recommend prophylactic oophorectomy in these women at age 35 or after childbearing is completed.

Prophylactic oophorectomy performed in women undergoing abdominal surgery for other indications such as benign uterine disease is also associated with a significant reduction in the risk of ovarian cancer. However, estrogen replacement therapy should be discussed with the patient prior to the procedure.

Although prophylactic oophorectomy lowers the risk of ovarian cancer in both pre- and postmenopausal women, non-compliance with estrogen replacement therapy may result in a significant reduction in life expectancy due to cardiovascular disease and osteoporosis in premenopausal women who have bilateral oophorectomy, compared with women with retained ovaries. Therefore, premenopausal women who cannot comply with estrogen replacement therapy should be advised regarding these risks as well as the benefits of prophylactic oophorectomy.

What is the Appropriate Management of Early-Stage Ovarian Cancer?

Management of the Adnexal Mass. It is estimated that 5 to 10 percent of women in the United States will undergo a surgical procedure for a suspected ovarian neoplasm during their lifetime, and 13 to 21 percent of these women will be found to have an ovarian malignancy. Since the majority of adnexal masses are benign, it is important to try to determine preoperatively whether a patient is at high risk for ovarian malignancy, in order to ensure proper management. To determine whether an adnexal mass requires surgery, and what the appropriate preparation and intervention should be, preoperative evaluation must include a complete history and physical examination (including bimanual and rectovaginal examination). TVS examination can help to further evaluate a suspected ovarian mass. CA 125 may aid in the evaluation in postmenopausal women, but can confound it in premenopausal women because of the many benign conditions associated with an elevated serum CA 125 level.

Once an adnexal mass has been documented, management depends on a combination of many predictive factors including:

- Age and menopausal status
- Size of the mass

- Ultrasonographic features
- Presence or absence of symptoms
- Level of CA 125
- Unilaterality versus bilaterality

A woman's age is an important factor in predicting whether an ovarian mass is malignant. Despite the fact that ovarian cancer is more common in older women, it occurs in young women as well. In premenopausal, asymptomatic women with simple cystic adnexal masses less than 6-10 cm, expectant management is a reasonable approach, since 70 percent of these masses will resolve without therapy. The common practice of ovarian suppression with oral contraceptives in these women is unproven. Expectant management should include a repeat physical and pelvic examination and TVS. Changes in clinical or ultrasonographic findings to those more characteristic of malignancy, or persistence of a significant mass, are indications for surgery. Most ovarian masses in postmenopausal women will require surgical evaluation. The possible exception may be in those women with a subclinical cyst detected on ultrasound, which is unilocular, less than 5 cm in diameter, and associated with normal serum CA 125 levels. Although a variety of clinical and laboratory parameters are extremely useful in both pre- and postmenopausal women, no combination of factors can be considered 100 percent accurate in predicting malignancy.

Surgical Therapy. Once surgical removal is indicated, the question of which surgical approach to use (laparoscopy versus laparotomy) must be addressed. Large numbers of laparoscopic procedures are being performed in this country for adnexal masses. However, data are lacking as to the efficacy and safety of this approach in the management of possible ovarian malignancy. If an unsuspected ovarian malignancy is detected at the time of diagnostic laparoscopy, staging and debulking by laparotomy should be undertaken without delay, and is ideally performed by a gynecologic oncologist.

Management of Early-Stage Epithelial Ovarian Cancer (Stage I). Approximately 25 percent of women with newly diagnosed ovarian cancer present with stage I disease. Outcomes for these women are much better than those of their counterparts with advanced-stage disease. Nevertheless, a significant proportion of women

Ovarian Cancer: Screening, Treatment, and Followup

with stage I disease die from their malignancies. Much attention has been focused on identifying the subsets of women at highest risk of relapse who may benefit from adjuvant therapy. Precise definition of these subsets on the basis of surgical findings and histologic grade is not agreed upon. However, the following recommendations are made based on existing data:

- Patients with stage IA grade 1 and most IB grade 1 tumors do not require adjuvant therapy.

- All patients with grade 3 tumors require adjuvant therapy.

- Patients with clear cell carcinoma require adjuvant therapy.

- Many but not all women with stage IC disease require adjuvant therapy.

- Consensus on the need for postoperative adjuvant therapy in the remaining subsets of patients with stage I epithelial ovarian cancer could not be reached.

- Although it is clearly acknowledged that many subsets of women with stage I ovarian cancer have a substantial likelihood for recurrence and mortality, the most effective adjuvant therapy has not been established. Ideally, patients with these high-risk stage I cancers should be enrolled in clinical trials to identify adjuvant therapy that will optimally improve survival.

All women who have ovarian cancer should have meticulously performed surgical staging. Most women who have stage I ovarian cancer will have a total abdominal hysterectomy/bilateral salpingo-oophorectomy (TAH-BSO). However, since some of these women are young and are interested in maintaining reproductive capability, after complete surgical staging has been done, there is an option to preserve their reproductive potential. For instance, some young women with stage IA tumors may be able to have the option of preservation of the uterus and contralateral adnexa, and some young women with stage IB tumors may have preservation of the uterus.

Low Malignant Potential Tumors. The recommended treatment for patients with low malignant potential (LMP) ovarian tumors who have completed childbearing is TAH/BSO and optimal staging and debulking. There is no evidence that adjuvant therapy improves disease-free survival or overall survival in these women. Although no prospective study has compared the efficacy of TAH/BSO with more conservative therapy in stage IA disease, data from retrospective studies of conservative therapy in young women suggest that the risk of recurrence is not significantly different than in patients treated with TAH/BSO.

Although repeat staging laparotomy may possibly result in upstaging in those patients who were incompletely staged at the time of their initial surgery, the therapeutic benefit of re-exploration is of questionable value if no evidence of gross residual disease existed at the time of the initial surgery.

Germ Cell Cancers. Ovarian germ cell cancers account for less than 5 percent of all ovarian malignancies. They typically occur in girls and young women. Although no prospective randomized studies exist comparing unilateral with bilateral adnexectomy, retrospective analyses demonstrate equivalent cure rates with either surgical procedure, with or without hysterectomy. Since ovarian germ cell cancers are mostly unilateral, with the exception of dysgerminomas, it seems prudent to avoid biopsy of a normal-appearing contralateral ovary.

Complete surgical staging is necessary to determine the extent of disease and guide postoperative treatment, which most patients require. Current data indicate that the most active adjuvant chemotherapy for germ cell cancers of the ovary is the combination of bleomycin, etoposide, and cis-platinum.

Sex Cord Stromal Cancers. Sex cord stromal cancers are rare and are characterized by somewhat unpredictable biologic behavior. Most are unilateral and can be treated with adnexectomy and staging in young women. In women who have completed childbearing, surgical staging and TAH/BSO are appropriate. Optimal adjuvant therapy has not yet been determined.

Pathology. In cases of unusual histologic subtypes (e.g., LMP tumors), an additional independent review of the pathologic specimen should be sought.

What Is the Appropriate Management of Advanced Epithelial Ovarian Cancer?

Postoperative Evaluation. For the purpose of this report, anything other than stage I ovarian cancer represents advanced disease. Ovarian cancer is diagnosed at an advanced stage in approximately 75 percent of patients. The ability to accurately identify advanced-stage ovarian cancer preoperatively is of particular importance in the community setting since availability of appropriate technical expertise for staging and debulking may require additional preparation or referral. It is critical to avoid unnecessary delay of the primary surgical procedure. A careful history and physical examination, including bimanual rectovaginal pelvic examination, is the first step in patient evaluation. A chest x-ray is part of routine preoperative evaluation in patients suspected of having ovarian cancer. Extensive imaging studies often do not add valuable information to careful diagnostic ultrasound unless symptoms suggest particular organ involvement. CT scans, MRIs, IVPs, and barium enemas may have a role in preoperative evaluation, and this should be determined on a case-by-case basis. Ultrasound is well suited for evaluation of a pelvic mass and assessment of ascites. Sonographic features of pelvic masses are amenable to quantitative grading and have been shown in various studies to be helpful in predicting malignancy. CDI may enhance ultrasound specificity for predicting malignancy of an adnexal mass, but its use in this situation is investigational. CA 125 is elevated in approximately 80 percent of patients with ovarian cancer and is a useful reflection of disease status during and after therapy in those patients. Although not completely diagnostic, combining CA 125 with sonographic morphologic features and menopausal status may assist in assessing the potential for ovarian cancer.

In patients with suspected ovarian cancer, other pre-operative studies should include assessment of hematologic, hepatic, and renal function. Pre-operative bowel preparation should be utilized because the potential for bowel resection exists and is poorly predicted by available pre-operative studies.

Prognostic Factors. Reproducible independent factors that prolong survival include younger age, early stage, low tumor grade, low residual tumor volume, and rapid rate of tumor response. Other prognostic factors include initial tumor volume and para-aortic lymph node involvement. A serum CA 125 level obtained 4 weeks after surgical debulking appears to be helpful; however, it may not be an independent prognostic factor.

Surgery. Adequate and complete surgical intervention is mandatory primary therapy for ovarian carcinoma, permitting precise staging, accurate diagnosis, and optimal cytoreduction. The procedure is best conducted by a qualified gynecologic oncologist when there is high probability of ovarian carcinoma. In situations when a mass is most probably benign, a qualified gynecologic surgeon can provide operative intervention. Consultative backup by a gynecologic oncologist may be advantageous.

The surgical procedure requires an adequate vertical incision, assessment of peritoneal fluid volume, and fluid cytology. For staging purposes, when a patient appears to have early disease, biopsies should be taken from the pelvic side walls, cul-de-sac, and pericolic gutters. The infradiaphragmatic surface should be evaluated by cytology or biopsy. Bowel serosa and mesentery should be evaluated for tumor. The infracolic omentum should be removed. Following biopsies, an extrafascial TAH/BSO should be completed. Pelvic and para-aortic lymph node sampling is a part of surgical staging. Aggressive efforts at maximal cytoreduction are important since minimal residual tumor is associated with improved survival.

In selected patients who have not had the opportunity for adequate staging and debulking at the time of initial surgery, a definitive operative procedure as previously described should be completed expeditiously before further therapy is undertaken. If it is impossible to achieve optional debulking despite maximum effort, interval cytoreduction (surgery performed midway through a chemotherapy regimen) may play a role and is under investigation.

Second-look operations outside of clinical trials should only be undertaken if the anticipated findings will alter subsequent management. Given the fact that many patients with negative second-look laparotomies will develop recurrent cancer, protocols should be developed to evaluate the benefits of consolidation therapy in the context of clinical trials.

Ovarian Cancer: Screening, Treatment, and Followup

Chemotherapy. Systemic chemotherapy following the appropriate surgical procedure is the cornerstone of first-line treatment of advanced epithelial ovarian malignancy. Chemotherapy is most effective in patients who have undergone maximal cytoreductive surgery or who present with a low volume of disease. At the consensus conference, important new data from a randomized trial (in suboptimal stage III and IV) comparing a combination of cis-platinum and paclitaxel (administered over 24 hours) with a combination of cis-platinum and cyclophosphamide were presented and reviewed by the panel. Preliminary results strongly suggested superiority for the paclitaxel-based regimen. Based on these new data, some but not all clinicians and investigators consider the combination of platinum and paclitaxel the treatment of choice for advanced epithelial ovarian cancer. No consensus could be reached on unqualified endorsement of this recommendation pending the availability of long-term results from this trial. In addition, the optimal dose and schedule of paclitaxel is the subject of ongoing clinical trials.

Data from mature randomized clinical trials have indicated that the combination of carboplatin and cyclophosphamide is effective therapy. Other mature trials have shown equal activity for the combination of cis-platinum and cyclophosphamide, but the substitution of carboplatin leads to more acceptable toxicity. Six cycles of chemotherapy have become the standard and yield clinical response rates of approximately 60 to 70 percent and 5-year survivals of 10 to 20 percent.

Currently available data do not in general support the routine addition of doxorubicin to the combination of platinum compounds and cyclophosphamide. In the treatment of ovarian cancer, hematologic toxicity is usually not of sufficient grade to warrant the routine use of hematopoietic growth factors when standard doses of chemotherapy are employed. In addition, high-dose chemotherapy with hematopoietic growth factors or bone marrow transplantation is experimental, and its use should be limited to research settings.

The role of intraperitoneal chemotherapy in the treatment of ovarian cancer remains to be defined.

Radiotherapy. The role of radiotherapy in advanced epithelial ovarian cancer is controversial. Long-term, relapse-free survivals have been demonstrated for stages II and III after optimal debulking and postoperative radiotherapy. No recent prospective trials of whole abdominal irradiation compared with chemotherapy have been performed.

What Is Appropriate Follow-up After Primary Therapy?

The ideal followup of asymptomatic women who have completed primary debulking surgery and chemotherapy and have no clinical evidence of disease is unclear. Second-look laparotomy has been used to assess response to therapy. As indicated above, the role of this procedure is controversial. The followup of asymptomatic patients after primary therapy should include routine complete history, physical, rectovaginal pelvic exam, and CA 125. Although optimal intervals for monitoring have not been determined, current practice is to follow the patient every 3 or 4 months. After 2 years, less frequent followup intervals can be considered. CA 125 has been shown to be a reliable method of monitoring for early detection of recurrence in women whose CA 125 was elevated pre-operatively. A rising CA 125 is a predictor of relapse; however, a negative CA 125 does not exclude the presence of disease. A combination of CA 125 and general physical and pelvic exam has been shown to detect progression of disease in 90 percent of patients with recurrent epithelial ovarian cancer. Radiological exams done on a routine basis have not been shown to improve the detection of recurrence. Their use should be individualized.

Management of Patients at Relapse. In the overwhelming majority of patients who relapse, presently available salvage therapy for ovarian cancer is not curative. Therefore, the goals of follow-up and treatment of relapsed patients need to incorporate quality-of-life considerations as an integral part of treatment. Patients who have relapsed after primary chemotherapy with platinum can be divided into two groups based on interval to relapse. Patients who relapse within 6 months have a poor subsequent response to platinum-containing regimens. Those who relapse after 6 months have a higher likelihood of response to platinum-containing regimens. Paclitaxel is currently the most active single agent for treatment of relapsed ovarian cancer even in patients refractory to platinum. It has an overall response rate of approximately 35 percent. Despite this response rate, there is no evidence yet that this salvage therapy prolongs survival.

Repeat surgical debulking in relapsed patients will probably only benefit a small subset of highly selected patients. These include patients with a long disease-free survival interval (greater than 2 years) who had optimal primary debulking surgery. However, surgery may be important for palliation, such as for the treatment of bowel obstruction in a patient whose quality of life stands to benefit from this intervention. Radiation therapy may be used for the palliation of specific localized symptoms.

When a patient relapses for the second time, there is almost no possibility of cure. Temporary response rates of approximately 15 percent have been achieved by several different chemotherapeutic regimens. After paclitaxel and platinum compounds are no longer effective, agents that may produce response include ifosfamide, hexamethylmelamine, tamoxifen, 5-FU, etoposide, and others. No survival benefit has been demonstrated by any of these regimens.

Given the rigors of chemotherapy, patient quality of life is a major concern. It is important for the physician and patient to discuss the various treatment options; patient preference for either vigorous treatment or no treatment should be respected. In presenting treatment options, physiologic status, not chronological age, should influence the physician's treatment suggestions. The patient should not be given unrealistic expectations. Appropriate psychological support is an important component of care, and patients must receive this. In addition, research should be conducted to determine whether psychological factors affect prognosis, response, and survival.

In patients with refractory ovarian cancer there is no indication for the use of high-dose chemotherapy followed by bone marrow or peripheral blood stem cell rescue other than in the setting of clinical trials.

What Are Important Directions for Future Research?

- Currently available imaging techniques and tumor markers should be utilized in clinical trials to determine whether ovarian cancer can be identified at an earlier stage, whether this can reduce mortality from ovarian cancer, and whether this can be done without increasing morbidity and mortality for those women who have abnormal screening results but do not have ovarian cancer. Study of this question should include both pre- and postmenopausal women.

- New serum markers (e.g., OVX-1, M-CSF7) and imaging techniques should be investigated to see if a more sensitive and specific panel of screening parameters can be identified.

- Researchers should more clearly evaluate and quantify the benefits of currently used oral contraceptives in reducing the risk of ovarian cancer, evaluate the necessary duration of use and the benefits of prolonged use, and evaluate the other benefits and risks and long-term outcome.

- A national serum and tissue bank should be established.

- Identification of women at increased risk for ovarian cancer should be improved. Studies should focus on genetic research, such as BRCA-1. In addition, environmental and epidemiologic research should be continued.

- The safety and efficacy of laparoscopy for women with ovarian cancer should be studied.

- The combination of platinum compounds and paclitaxel should be further investigated in earlier stage disease. In addition, the ideal dose and schedule of paclitaxel must be evaluated in clinical trials.

- A prospective randomized study is needed to identify optimal treatment of various subsets of stage I ovarian cancer.

- Whole abdominal radiation should be re-evaluated and newer radiation techniques evaluated in the treatment of optimally debulked stage II and III disease.

- Innovative approaches to the treatment of advanced primary as well as recurrent ovarian cancer must be identified and studied. Examples include new molecular targets, agents to overcome resistance, and drugs that inhibit signal transduction pathways.

- Clinical trials exploring the role of consolidation therapy in patients with a complete response to primary therapy should be given high priority.

Ovarian Cancer: Screening, Treatment, and Followup

- Measures of the quality of life in women with ovarian cancer must be identified, evaluated, and then utilized in optimizing the care of patients.

Conclusions

Although the number of women dying from ovarian cancer in the United States has continued to rise, the application of available recent information may be able to contribute to the reduction in incidence of and morbidity and mortality from this disease.

1. The risk of ovarian cancer can be reduced by the use of oral contraceptives. However, the other risks and benefits of the birth control pill must be considered.

2. Women who have no family members with ovarian cancer have a 1 in 70 lifetime risk of developing the disease. Women who have one first-degree relative with ovarian cancer have a 5 percent risk, and women with two first-degree relatives have a 7 percent risk. A very small subset of these women (3 percent of the women with two relatives) have an autosomal dominant syndrome with 80 percent penetrance, which places them at very high risk for ovarian cancer. The three known hereditary syndromes that may place a women at exceedingly high risk are familial site-specific ovarian cancer syndrome, breast-ovarian cancer syndrome, and Lynch syndrome II.

3. All women should have a careful family history taken by their primary care physician. Women who are presumed to have one of the syndromes mentioned above, which would place them at exceedingly high risk, should have at least an annual physical exam and a bimanual rectovaginal examination, CA 125 determinations, and TVS. When childbearing is completed, or at least by age 35, prophylactic bilateral oophorectomy is recommended.

4. There is no evidence available yet that the current screening modalities of CA 125 and TVS can be effectively used for widespread screening to reduce mortality from ovarian can-

cer or that their use will result in decreased rather than increased morbidity and mortality. Routine screening has resulted in unnecessary surgery with its attendant potential risks. Clearly, it is important to identify and validate effective screening modalities. Currently available technology for screening should be employed in the context of clinical trials to determine the efficacy of these modalities and their impact on ovarian cancer mortality. In addition, research must be continued to identify additional markers and imaging techniques that will be useful. If a woman has one first-degree relative with ovarian cancer (making her lifetime risk of developing the disease 5 percent) but no clinical trials are available to her, she may feel that despite the absence of prospective data, this is sufficient risk for her to be screened. This alternative and opportunity should be available to the woman and her physician.

5. If a woman is undergoing pelvic surgery, removal of her ovaries at that time will almost fully eliminate her risk of ovarian cancer (although there remains a minimal risk of peritoneal carcinomatosis). If the woman is premenopausal, discussion of estrogen replacement therapy is important prior to removal of the ovaries, since for some younger women, if estrogen replacement is not utilized, the risk of premature menopause and the potential for cardiovascular disease and osteoporosis may outweigh the risk of ovarian conservation and the potential for ovarian cancer.

6. Although laparoscopic management of the ovarian mass is being utilized, there is no current evidence that if the mass is malignant the patient's opportunity for cure is comparable to that with a more traditional approach. Studies should be done to evaluate the risks and benefits of laparoscopic surgery for these women.

7. Women with ovarian masses who have been identified preoperatively as having a significant risk of ovarian cancer should be given the option of having their surgery performed by a gynecologic oncologist.

Ovarian Cancer: Screening, Treatment, and Followup

8. Aggressive attempts at cytoreductive surgery as the primary management of ovarian cancer will improve the patient's opportunity for long-term survival.

9. Women with stage IA grade 1 and most IB grade 1 ovarian cancer do not require postoperative adjuvant therapy. Many remaining stage I patients do require adjuvant therapy. Subsets of stage I must be fully defined and ideal treatment determined.

10. Women with stages II, III, and IV epithelial ovarian cancer (other than LMP tumors) should receive post-operative chemotherapy.

11. One American study concluded that platinum and paclitaxel are the optimal first-line chemotherapy following primary debulking surgery, and most oncologists in the United States are using this regimen. No consensus could be reached on unqualified endorsement of this recommendation pending maturation of the data.

12. Second-look laparotomy should be done only for patients in clinical trials or for those patients in whom the surgery will affect clinical decision-making and clinical course. It should not be employed as routine care for all patients.

13. For women who have completed primary therapy for ovarian cancer, there is no evidence regarding ideal followup. Studies are needed to identify additional second-line therapies and to define how they can best be utilized to prolong survival, improve quality of life, and potentially provide the possibility for cure. Clearly, women with a symptomatic recurrence should receive whatever modalities will improve their symptoms and quality of life.

14. For a woman with recurrent ovarian cancer resistant to platinum who has not received paclitaxel, paclitaxel is the best salvage therapy currently available.

15. Physicians must be encouraged to discuss clinical trial participation with women, and women should be encouraged to participate.

16. All women should have access to accurate and complete information regarding ovarian cancer. Furthermore, there must be no barriers to women's access to qualified specialists, optimal therapy, and protocols.

About the NIH Consensus Development Program

NIH Consensus Development Conferences are convened to evaluate available scientific information and resolve safety and efficacy issues related to a biomedical technology. The resultant NIH Consensus Statements are intended to advance understanding of the technology or issue in question and to be useful to health professionals and the public.

NIH Consensus Statements are prepared by a non-advocate, non-Federal panel of experts, based on (1) presentations by investigators working in areas relevant to the consensus questions during a 2-day public session; (2) questions and statements from conference attendees during open discussion periods that are part of the public session; and (3) closed deliberations by the panel during the remainder of the second day and morning of the third. This statement is an independent report of the panel and is not a policy statement of the NIH or the Federal Government.

Free copies of this statement and bibliographies prepared by the National Library of Medicine are available from the NIH Consensus Program Information Service by 24-hour voice mail at 1-800-NIH-OMAR (644-6627) or from the Office of Medical Applications of Research, National Institutes of Health, Federal Building, Room 618, 7550 Wisconsin Avenue MSC 9120, Bethesda, MD 20892-9120.

Part Three

Prevention

Chapter 30

Implementation of the Breast and Cervical Cancer Mortality Prevention Act

The Burden of Breast and Cervical Cancers

Congress recognized the lifesaving potential offered by early detection of these cancers when it passed the Breast and Cervical Cancer Mortality Prevention Act (Public Law 101-354) in 1990.

Although breast and cervical cancers exhibit different patterns of disease, early detection and prompt treatment can alter the natural progression of both of these diseases and can reduce mortality. Currently, the value of breast cancer screening for women over age 50 is widely accepted, and the benefits of mammography have been demonstrated in a number of clinical trials. The efficacy of cervical cancer screening using the Papanicolaou (Pap) test has not been evaluated in clinical trials; however, evidence from numerous observational studies and the marked decline in cervical cancer incidence and mortality rates in the United States since the large-scale introduction of the Pap test 40 years ago, testify to the impact of this screening test

In fiscal years 1991 and 1992, the Centers for Disease Control and Prevention (CDC) awarded funds to 12 States to establish comprehensive breast and cervical cancer screening programs. This extract from the report provides background information on national trends in both incidence and mortality from these malignancies as well as on screening practices. This information will prove useful in future evaluation of the national impact of this program.

DHHS/CDC Extracted from the 1992 Progress Report to Congress.

Data on disease incidence (the rate of newly diagnosed cancers) and mortality were obtained from CDC's National Center for Health Statistics and the National Cancer Institute's (NCI) Surveillance, Epidemiology, and End Results (SEER) program. These data can readily be used to estimate the magnitude of the problem of breast and cervical cancers and to analyze trends over time. However, rates obtained from small population units and over short time periods should be interpreted with caution.

The use of current data sources presents three limitations:

- **Timeliness.** At least a 3-year delay separates any given year of clinical events and the year when national data are available for review and analysis. Rates reported in this section are from 1989.

- **Lack of national and statewide data on cancer incidence.** The SEER program covers only about 10 percent of the U.S. population. Unfortunately, many States do not have central cancer registries, and those that do vary in population coverage and in the type and quality of data collected. The American Association of Central Cancer Registries is developing standards so that existing State registries can compile high-quality population-based data and use them to evaluate the effectiveness of cancer control efforts.

- Limited information on race/ethnicity and small numbers. This limitation results in a lack of precision of intercensal estimates for various diverse racial/ethnic groups and, as a consequence, of rates of cancer in these groups. Cancer rates for many minority groups are not nationally reported, making it difficult to determine the extent of disease in these populations. For example, rates for Mexican Americans are often based on data from New Mexico and are thus not nationally representative of this group. Rates reported in this section for several racial/ ethnic groups come from previously published sources, including the Report of the Secretary's Task Force on Black and Minority Health, the Indian Health Service's Cancer Mortality Among Native Americans in the United States, and the American Cancer Society's (ACS) Cancer Facts and Figures for Minority Americans.

Breast and Cervical Cancer Mortality Prevention Act

Breast Cancer

Breast cancer is the most common cancer in American women and is second only to lung cancer as a cause of premature mortality. The potential for decreasing mortality rates from breast cancer currently rests with increases in screening and the subsequent detection of the disease at an early stage, when a greater number of treatment options are available and survival rates are improved. ACS estimates that 180,000 new cases of female breast cancer and 46,000 breast cancer deaths will occur in 1992 (Table 30.1). In 1989, this malignancy took the lives of approximately 43,000 women—or about 28 out of every 100,000 women. For the same year, SEER reports that the overall incidence of breast cancer was 104.6 per 100,000 women—a 23-percent increase in occurrence since 1980 and a slight decrease (4.6 percent) in overall incidence from 1988 (Figure 30.1). Both black and white women experienced similar percent increases in overall incidence since 1980.

In general, white women experienced higher incidence rates for breast cancer than black women, but lower mortality rates (Figure 30.2). However, these black/white differences vary by age. Age-specific rates for the years 1985 to 1989 indicate that white women 65 years and over experience higher mortality than black women in that age group and that black women under age 40 experience slightly higher incidence than white women in this group—a relationship that has been relatively consistent since 1973. For both races, incidence rates drop in the oldest age group. Breast cancer rates vary greatly across several racial/ ethnic groups. Figure 30.3 compares annual incidence and mortality rates for the years 1977 to 1983 for whites, blacks, Chinese, Japanese, Filipinos, Native Americans, Mexican Americans from New Mexico, and native Hawaiians. Because these data obtained from SEER reporting centers do not include all cultural groups within each minority and are based on small numbers, they must be interpreted cautiously. The data indicate that white and black women have much higher incidence and mortality rates for breast cancer than the other ethnic/racial groups, with the exception of native Hawaiians. Native Americans have lower rates of this malignancy than the other groups shown.

Beside varying by race, breast cancer mortality rates also vary by State. Age-adjusted breast cancer mortality rates for all races, for whites, and for blacks are presented in Table 30.2. No rate is pre-

Table 30.1.

Estimated Number of New Breast Cancer Cases and Deaths, by State: United States, 1992

State	New Cases	Deaths
Alabama	2700	700
Alaska	175	50
Arizona	2400	600
Arkansas	1700	425
California	18000	4500
Colorado	1800	475
Connecticut	2700	700
Delaware	600	175
District of Columbia	600	150
Florida	11200	2900
Georgia	4400	1100
Hawaii	425	125
Idaho	500	125
Illinois	8600	2200
Indiana	4100	1100
Iowa	2300	600
Kansas	1800	450
Kentucky	2400	650
Louisiana	2600	650
Maine	850	225
Maryland	3500	900
Massachusetts	5400	1400
Michigan	6600	1700
Minnesota	3200	800
Mississippi	1700	425
Missouri	3900	1000
Montana	450	125
Nebraska	1200	300
Nevada	750	200
New Hampshire	900	225
New Jersey	6700	1700
New Mexico	900	225
New York	15900	4000
North Carolina	5100	1300
North Dakota	425	100
Ohio	8600	2200
Oklahoma	2100	550
Oregon	2100	550
Pennsylvania	10700	2800
Rhode Island	1000	250
South Carolina	2300	550
South Dakota	550	150
Tennessee	3600	900
Texas	8700	2200
Utah	700	200
Vermont	475	125
Virginia	4300	1100
Washington	3200	800
West Virginia	1400	350
Wisconsin	3500	900
Wyoming	300	75
Total	**180000**	**46000**

Source: American Cancer Society

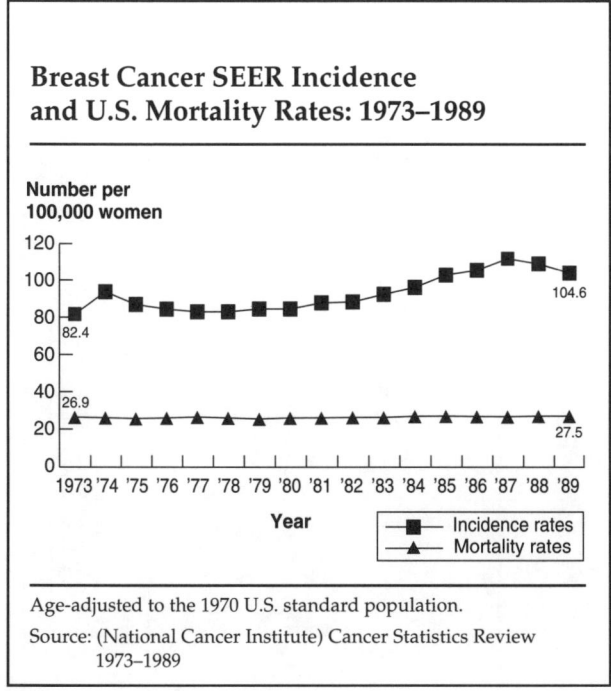

Figure 30.1.

sented for States whose black or white female population was less than 100,000. Overall mortality ranges from 16.8 per 100,000 in Hawaii to 35.2 per 100,000 in the District of Columbia. Differences between rates in the category "all races" may reflect differences in the States' racial/ethnic compositions and the corresponding differences in rates of disease in various racial/ethnic groups.

In the 1980s, rates of *in situ* and localized breast cancer increased in this country, while rates for distant and regional disease remained relatively stable (Figure 30.4). Both whites and blacks have exhibited an increase in *in situ* disease rates, probably attributable to increased use of screening mammography.

A reduction in incidence of advanced disease and an increase in the incidence of early-stage breast cancer are important indicators of an effective cancer control program and will precede a reduction in cancer mortality by several years.

Figure 30.2.

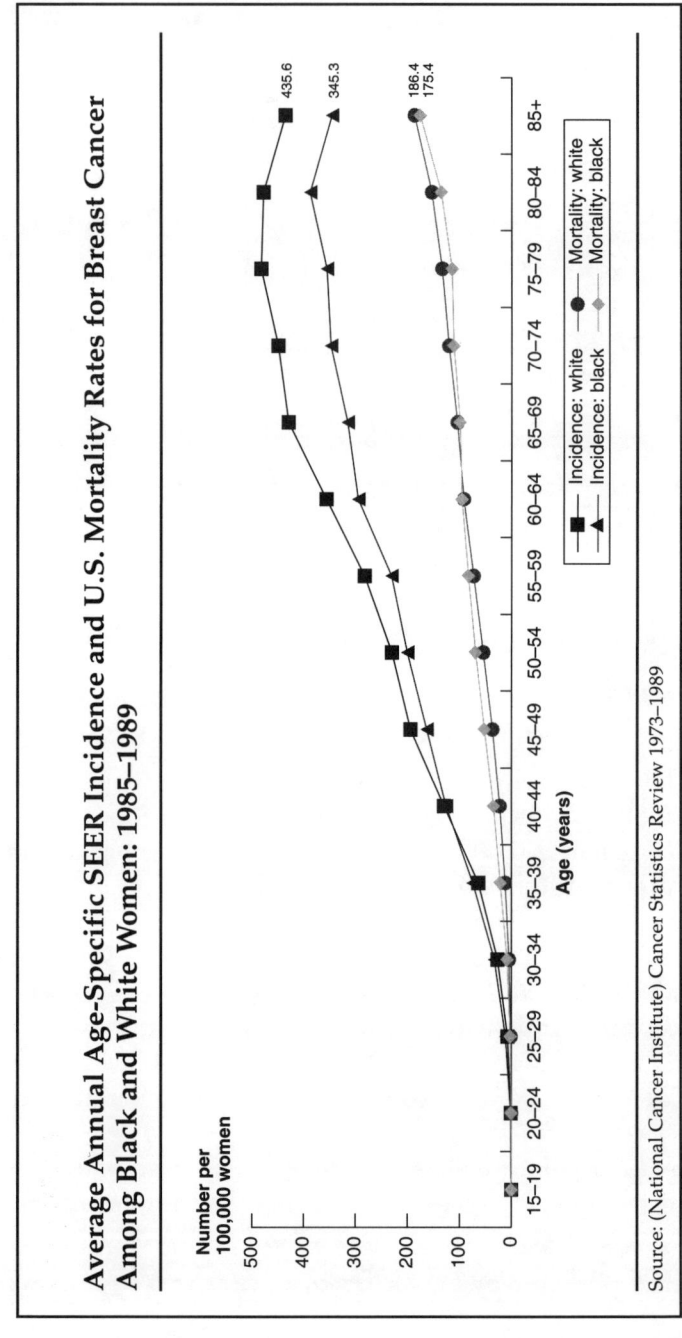

Breast and Cervical Cancer Mortality Prevention Act

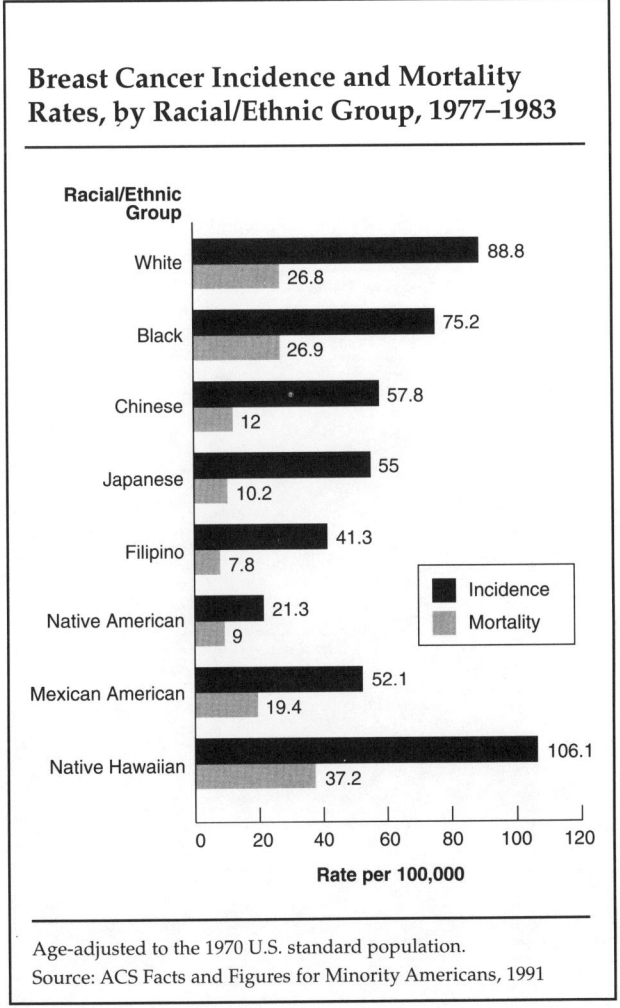

Figure 30.3.

Table 30.2.

Breast Cancer Deaths[#] and Average Annual Age-Adjusted Mortality Rates,[@] by State and Race: United States, 1988–1989

State	Total No. Deaths 1988–1989			Average Annual Rate		
	All Races	White	Black	All Races	White	Black
Alabama	1305	974	330	25.4	24.2	30.3
Alaska	78	67	3	25.6	29.7	—+
Arizona	1023	972	35	23.7	23.9	44.4
Arkansas	779	658	118	23.9	23.0	30.8
California	8388	7466	613	26.8	27.7	32.1
Colorado	873	838	27	24.6	24.8	26.7
Connecticut	1280	1206	70	28.0	27.9	29.7
Delaware	277	233	42	34.6	33.3	41.4
District of Columbia	289	92	196	35.2	33.1	36.3
Florida	5075	4620	449	25.9	25.5	29.6
Georgia	1822	1349	469	25.8	24.9	29.5
Hawaii	190	54	0	16.8	16.4	—+
Idaho	269	268	0	23.8	24.1	—+
Illinois	4245	3713	516	29.3	29.3	31.9
Indiana	1980	1825	152	28.3	27.8	37.0
Iowa	1097	1087	9	26.8	26.9	—+
Kansas	895	846	44	27.4	27.1	35.9
Kentucky	1232	1129	99	26.3	25.7	35.6
Louisiana	1324	932	385	26.9	25.5	30.8
Maine	449	448	0	27.5	27.7	—+
Maryland	1582	1265	308	28.6	28.5	29.9
Massachusetts	2504	2418	76	30.0	30.1	30.4
Michigan	3234	2809	413	28.8	28.3	33.7
Minnesota	1481	1464	8	27.3	27.6	—+
Mississippi	742	510	232	23.7	23.2	25.2
Missouri	1913	1744	166	27.1	26.9	30.4
Montana	236	232	1	24.0	24.4	—+
Nebraska	589	579	10	27.2	27.5	—+
Nevada	318	291	18	26.8	26.5	—+
New Hampshire	408	405	2	31.3	31.3	—+
New Jersey	3354	3007	326	32.0	32.0	32.2
New Mexico	390	373	6	23.8	24.6	—+
New York	7613	6675	883	31.3	32.1	29.2
North Carolina	2191	1726	452	26.9	26.2	31.0
North Dakota	232	229	0	27.6	27.9	—+
Ohio	4150	3738	406	29.3	28.9	33.8
Oklahoma	985	902	57	24.1	24.9	26.4
Oregon	932	909	14	25.9	26.0	—+
Pennsylvania	5206	4796	398	29.8	29.6	32.2
Rhode Island	459	448	9	32.4	32.7	—+
South Carolina	1060	782	278	26.4	26.0	28.4
South Dakota	251	243	0	27.5	27.5	—+
Tennessee	1558	1291	263	24.8	23.6	32.5
Texas	4141	3623	501	22.9	22.6	27.5
Utah	349	342	2	23.7	23.8	—+
Vermont	199	199	0	29.3	29.5	—+
Virginia	1971	1567	396	28.1	27.3	35.0
Washington	1556	1512	19	28.1	28.9	20.2
West Virginia	656	635	20	25.2	25.2	—+
Wisconsin	1753	1700	48	27.7	27.7	31.9
Wyoming	122	120	1	25.1	25.3	—+
Total	**85005**	**75311**	**8870**	**27.5**	**27.5**	**30.9**

[#]From NCHS death tapes, underlying cause of death. [@]Adjusted to the 1970 U.S. population. [+]Fewer than 100,000 in the denominator or less than 5 deaths.

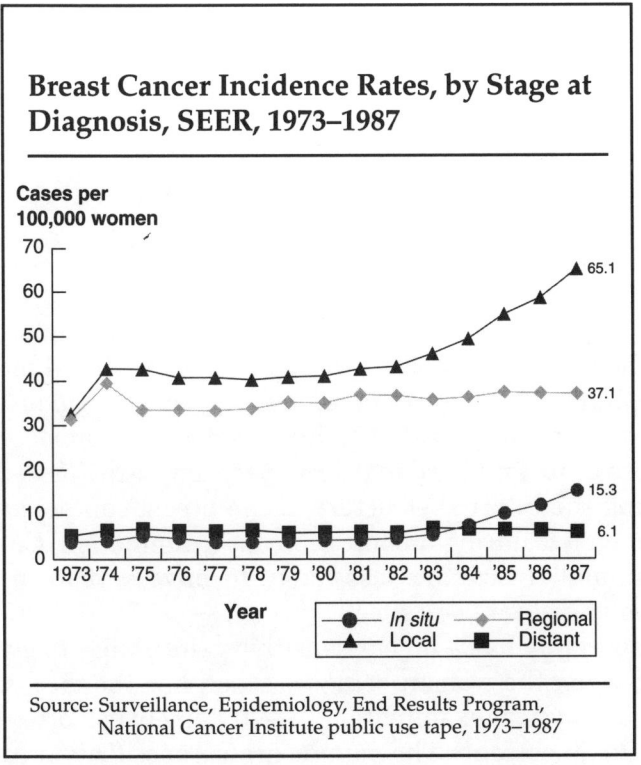

Figure 30.4.

Risk Factors for Developing Breast Cancer

In general, breast cancer is not considered a disease amenable to primary prevention. Established risk factors for the disease include:

- Family history of breast cancer.
- Increasing age.
- Early age at menarche.
- Late age at menopause.
- Late age at first live birth.
- Low parity.
- History of benign breast disease.

- Prior history of breast cancer.
- Exposure to ionizing radiation.
- Caucasian race
- High socioeconomic status.

At present, the early detection of cancer is the key to its control.

The Lifesaving Value of Early Detection

Breast cancer screening by mammography is the single most effective method to detect breast cancer in its earliest and most treatable form. Mammography can detect cancer an average of 1.7 years before the woman can palpate the lump herself. Mammography is a low-dose (less than 4 milliard to 0.4 rad per view) x-ray procedure that by visualizing the internal structure of the breast can detect cancers too small to be felt during a clinical breast examination. Cancers detected at a smaller size are less likely to have spread to regional lymph nodes or distant body sites.

Mammography has a higher sensitivity (its ability to give a positive finding when the woman being screened has the disease) (76-94 percent) than physical examination (57-70 percent) or breast self-examination (20-30 percent). The mammogram's specificity (its ability to give a negative finding when the woman being screened does not have the disease) is greater than 90 percent. Widespread use of this procedure, alone or together with a clinical breast examination performed by a trained health-care provider, reduces risk of breast cancer by 25-30 percent among women 40-70 years of age.

Approximately 92 percent of women diagnosed with localized disease can expect a 5-year relative survival. (Relative survival represents the likelihood that a patient diagnosed with cancer will not die from causes associated specifically with that disease.) A 10-year relative survival is realized by 75-80 percent of women. However, for women with disease that has spread to body sites beyond regional lymph nodes, 5-year relative survival drops dramatically to 19 percent. Treatment at this late stage is not only much less effective, but also more debilitating.

Comparing a current mammogram to an earlier one can reveal subtle changes in the breast that may signal the presence of cancer or other breast abnormalities. The Economic Impact of Breast Cancer Estimates of the cost-effectiveness of mammography vary widely and are extremely sensitive to differences in methodologies, measures, assumptions, and the programs and policies evaluated. For example, estimates of cost per life year saved fall in a range from $22,000 per life year (U.S. Breast Cancer Detection Demonstration Project) for screening of women aged 55-65 years with physical breast examination and mammography to as high as $135,000 per life year saved among women aged 40-49 years. Additional factors affecting the estimates of cost effectiveness include the proportion of high-risk women screened, the sensitivity and specificity of the mammography technique, the interval between examinations, and the cost of each mammogram.

The results of the studies, conducted in the United States and other countries, indicate that the cost-effectiveness of screening for breast cancer generally compares favorably with other expenditures in the health-care field. For example, in 1991 dollars, mild hypertension cost-effectiveness analyses yield a cost of $32,600 per life year saved or gained; and, for liver transplants, a cost of $225,000 per life year saved or gained.

The estimated annual cost of illness for breast cancer is $3.8 billion, including $1.8 billion for medical-care costs (converted to 1987 dollars). During the 1980s, in place of radical mastectomies, modified radical mastectomy and breast-preservation techniques were increasingly performed and contributed to a reduction in the average number of hospital days associated with the treatment of breast cancer (in 1982, an average of 10.0 days compared with 4.6 days during 1990).

Further research and intervention is necessary to clarify cost effectiveness in the context of breast and cervical cancer early detection.

Guidelines for Breast Cancer Screening

In 1989, in an effort to standardize screening processes, the following 11 national organizations reached a consensus on recommendations for the early detection of breast cancer:

- American Academy of Family Physicians.
- American Association of Women Radiologists.
- American Cancer Society.
- American College of Radiology.
- American Medical Association.
- American Osteopathic College of Radiology.
- American Society for Therapeutic Radiology and Oncology.

- American Society of Internal Medicine.
- College of American Pathologists.
- National Cancer Institute.
- National Medical Association.

Consensus Recommendations for Frequency of Breast Cancer Screening

In 1989, 11 national organizations developed standardized breast cancer screening guidelines for women over age 40:

- Clinical examination of the breast and mammography are the basic detection methods. The examinations are complementary, and both are necessary to achieve maximum detection rates.

- The screening process should begin at age 40 and consist of an annual clinical examination with screening mammography performed on 1- to 2-year intervals.

- Beginning at age 50, both clinical examination and mammography should be performed annually.

These recommendations apply only to women without signs or symptoms of breast cancer; the frequency and type of examination will vary for the individual with symptoms and should be determined by the responsible physician.

According to the consensus guidelines, women without breast cancer symptoms should have an annual clinical breast exam and mammographic screening every 1 to 2 years beginning at age 40. Beginning at age 50, both the clinical examination and mammography should be performed every year. These screening guidelines apply only to asymptomatic women, and the frequency and type of examination for women with breast symptoms will vary and should be determined by the responsible physician.

The American Society of Clinical Oncology has since endorsed the above guidelines, and the American College of Obstetricians and Gynecologists has endorsed similar recommendations, which include an

Breast and Cervical Cancer Mortality Prevention Act

annual clinical breast examination beginning at age 18 and one baseline mammogram between the ages of 35 and 40.

In its public education programs, ACS recommends a comprehensive, three-step approach, including screening mammography, clinical breast examination, and monthly breast self-examination. ACS also recommends that women under the age of 40 perform a monthly breast self-examination and obtain a clinical breast examination every 3 years.

The U.S. Preventive Services Task Force recommends that all women over age 40 receive an annual clinical breast examination. Screening mammography every 1 to 2 years is recommended for all women beginning at age 50 and concluding at approximately age 75, unless pathology has been detected.

Prevalence of Breast Cancer Screening

National health promotion and disease prevention objectives, stated in the U.S. Department of Health and Human Services' publication *Healthy People 2000*, propose to:

> Increase to at least 80 percent the proportion of women aged 40 and older who have ever received a clinical breast examination and a mammogram, and to at least 60 percent those aged 50 and older who have received them within the preceding 1 to 2 years.

Baseline estimates in 1987 indicated that 36 percent of women aged 40 and older had ever been screened and that 25 percent of women aged 50 and older had been screened within the preceding 2 years. More recent data from the 1991 Behavioral Risk Factor Surveillance System (BRFSS) indicate that among women surveyed in 45 States and the District of Columbia who were aged 40 and older, about 70 percent had ever had a mammogram and a clinical breast exam. Among women aged 50 and older, about 58 percent reported having a mammogram and clinical breast exam within the past 2 years. Progress is being made toward the year 2000 goals.

Cervical Cancer

In recent decades, cervical cancer has declined in incidence and mortality. Since 1950, the incidence of invasive cervical cancer has decreased 76 percent and mortality from the disease has decreased 74 percent. Much of this decrease has been attributed to widespread use of the Pap test. Since the early 1980s, however, the rate of decline of invasive cervical cancer has slowed and appears to have leveled off in recent years (Figure 30.5). ACS estimates for 1992 predict that 13,500 cases of invasive cervical cancer will be diagnosed and that 4,400 deaths will occur in this year alone. Data from 1989 indicate that 3 cervical cancer deaths occurred per 100,000 women, while the incidence rate at SEER sites was 8.7 per 100,000.

As was seen with breast cancer, rates of cervical cancer vary among selected racial/ethnic groups (Figure 30.6). Blacks experience the highest mortality rates. In 1989, 2.8 times more black women than white women died from this malignancy (7.1 per 100,000 vs. 2.5 per

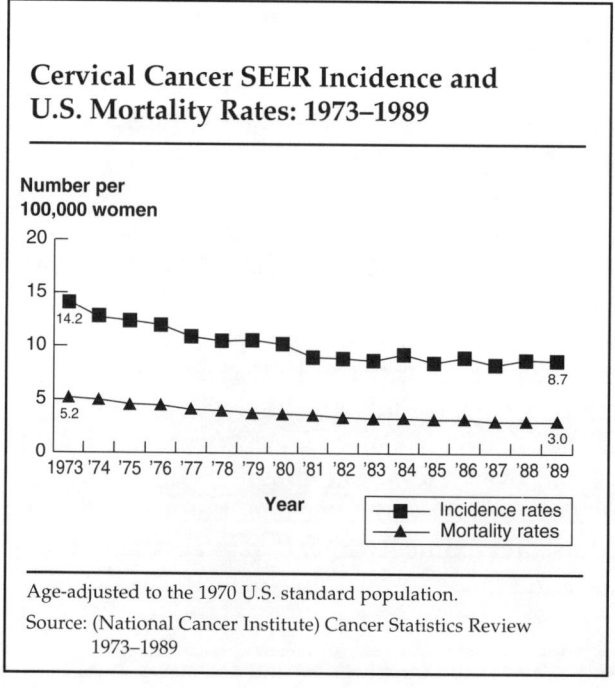

Figure 30.5.

Breast and Cervical Cancer Mortality Prevention Act

100,000). Incidence of the disease was 50 percent higher among blacks as well (12.8 per 100,000 vs. 8.2 per 100,000). The disparity between these two races has been attributed to a number of factors, such as differences in the prevalence of risk factors for the disease; differences in screening, follow-up, and treatment; and differences in the stage of the disease at diagnosis.

In contrast, for the period 1977 to 1983, average annual mortality among Native Americans was 36 percent lower than that among blacks, despite the fact that Native Americans have a slightly higher incidence of invasive cervical cancer. In fact, of the U.S. racial/ethnic groups included in Figure 30.6, Native Americans have the highest incidence of this disease. Mexican Americans and native Hawaiians also experience high incidence of this malignancy. Lowest incidence rates are seen among Japanese Americans.

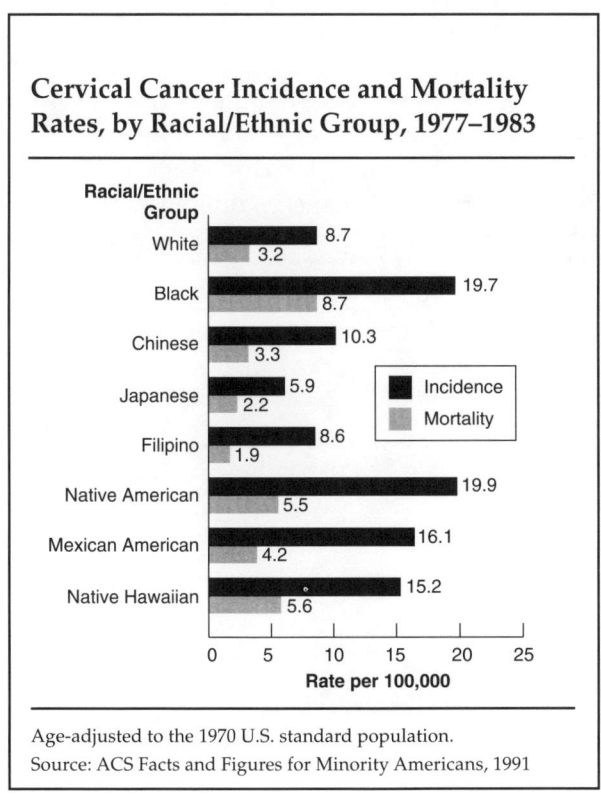

Figure 30.6.

Differences in incidence and mortality also vary by age (Figure 30.7). Both white and black women under age 35 experienced similar rates of invasive disease. However, after this age, incidence rates among white women tended to stabilize. whereas rates among black women increased overall. Mortality from cervical cancer increased with increasing age among both whites and blacks. For both races, about 70 percent of all cervical cancer deaths during the period 1985 to 1989 occurred among women 50 years of age or older. This number is not surprising, given the lower prevalence of cervical cancer screening in older women.

Cervical cancer mortality not only varies by race and age but by State as well (Table 30.3). Overall mortality rates range from 1.6 per 100,000 in Minnesota to 6.2 per 100,000 in the District of Columbia. The incidence of preinvasive carcinoma (*in situ*) of the uterine cervix increased between the 1940s and the 1970s. This rate decreased after the mid-1970s (Figure 30.8). For both white and black women, *in situ* disease was highest in young women and decreased rapidly with age: 88 percent of all cervical cancers (invasive and *in situ*) diagnosed in women under 50 in 1987 were staged as *in situ*. (This number likely underestimates the actual number of *in situ* diagnoses, because case ascertainment may be incomplete for this stage of disease.) In contrast, only 46 percent of cervical cancers diagnosed in women 50 and older are staged as *in situ*. Clearly, screening needs to increase among older women.

Figure 30.7.

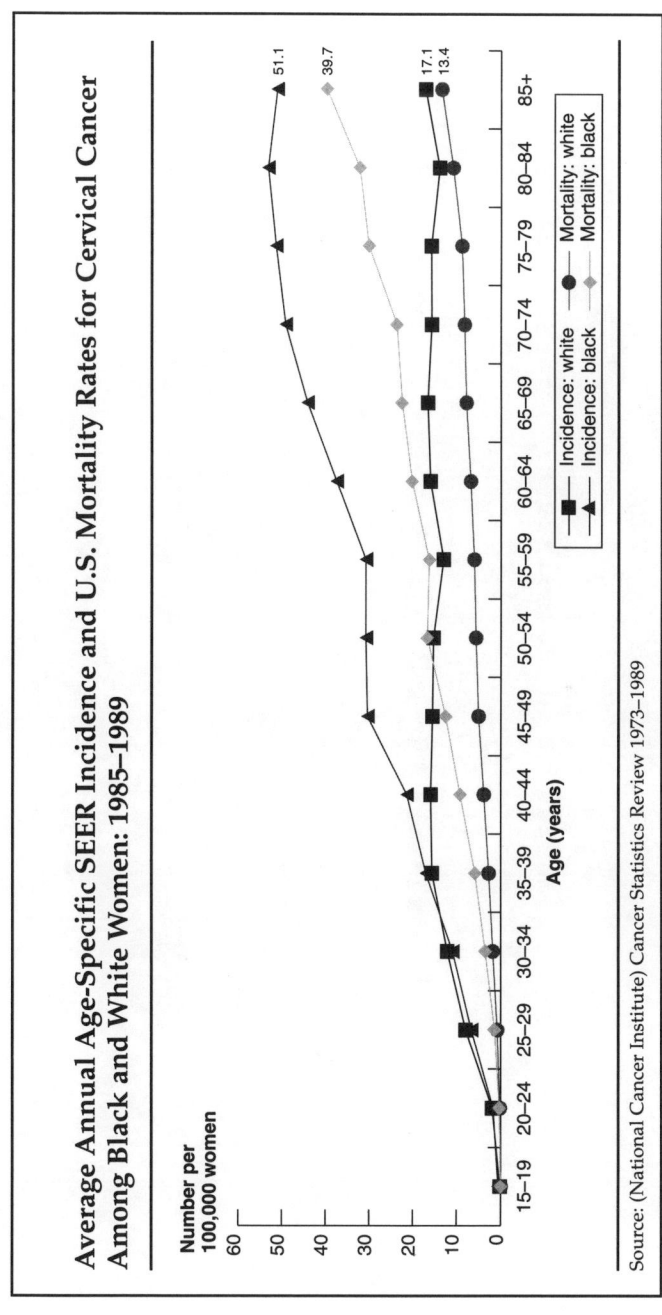

Table 30.3.

Cervical Cancer Deaths[#] and Average Annual Age-Adjusted Mortality Rates,[@] by State and Race: United States, 1988–1989

State	Total No. Deaths 1988–1989			Average Annual Rate		
	All Races	White	Black	All Races	White	Black
Alabama	231	115	113	4.5	2.8	10.4
Alaska	14	9	1	3.1	2.4	—+
Arizona	93	81	5	2.2	2.1	6.3
Arkansas	122	85	36	3.9	3.2	8.7
California	877	680	117	2.8	2.5	5.8
Colorado	91	83	4	2.5	2.4	—+
Connecticut	104	85	17	2.3	2.0	7.4
Delaware	27	20	5	3.7	3.2	5.0
District of Columbia	48	5	43	6.2	2.0	8.3
Florida	517	385	130	3.1	2.6	8.7
Georgia	241	134	106	3.3	2.4	6.7
Hawaii	23	8	0	2.0	1.9	—+
Idaho	23	23	0	2.0	2.0	—+
Illinois	448	308	137	3.3	2.6	8.1
Indiana	214	187	27	3.0	2.9	6.0
Iowa	97	95	1	2.6	2.6	—+
Kansas	91	82	8	3.0	2.9	6.6
Kentucky	194	171	22	4.3	4.0	7.8
Louisiana	154	82	72	3.1	2.3	5.6
Maine	40	40	0	2.7	2.7	—+
Maryland	164	105	57	2.8	2.3	5.4
Massachusetts	191	175	12	2.6	2.5	5.1
Michigan	325	250	71	2.9	2.6	5.7
Minnesota	88	81	2	1.6	1.5	—+
Mississippi	126	49	77	3.9	2.1	8.2
Missouri	205	157	47	3.1	2.7	8.3
Montana	33	30	0	3.4	3.2	—+
Nebraska	42	35	6	2.1	1.8	—+
Nevada	40	34	2	3.3	2.9	—+
New Hampshire	49	48	1	3.8	3.8	—+
New Jersey	325	229	92	3.4	2.7	9.0
New Mexico	53	41	0	3.4	2.9	—+
New York	726	504	209	3.1	2.6	6.8
North Carolina	285	153	126	3.5	2.3	8.2
North Dakota	14	13	0	1.7	1.6	—+
Ohio	387	330	55	2.8	2.6	4.6
Oklahoma	123	98	15	3.1	2.8	6.5
Oregon	92	86	1	2.8	2.7	—+
Pennsylvania	445	372	68	2.7	2.4	5.6
Rhode Island	26	25	0	2.1	2.1	—+
South Carolina	154	70	83	3.9	2.4	8.5
South Dakota	19	15	0	2.4	1.9	—+
Tennessee	208	156	51	3.3	2.9	6.3
Texas	525	396	118	2.9	2.5	6.4
Utah	27	26	0	1.8	1.8	—+
Vermont	17	17	0	2.6	2.6	—+
Virginia	240	160	76	3.4	2.8	6.3
Washington	124	114	1	2.3	2.2	—+
West Virginia	87	85	2	3.6	3.6	—+
Wisconsin	128	119	7	2.0	1.9	4.6
Wyoming	13	13	0	2.6	2.6	—+
Total	**8930**	**6664**	**2023**	**3.0**	**2.5**	**6.9**

[#]From NCHS death tapes, underlying cause of death. [@]Adjusted to the 1970 U.S. population. [+]Fewer than 100,000 in the denominator or less than 5 deaths.

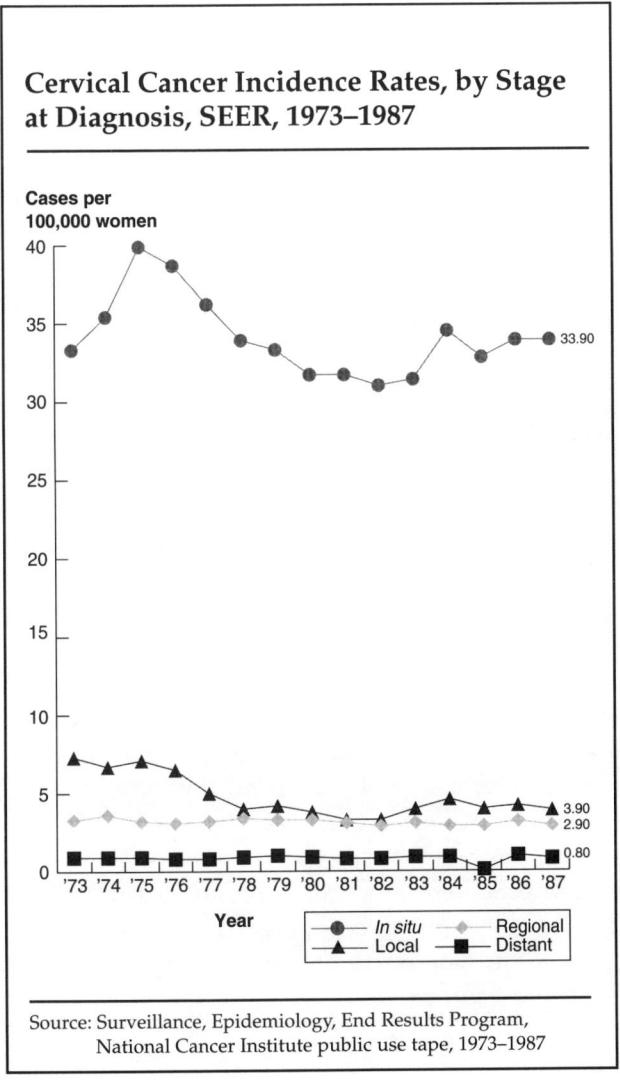

Figure 30.8.

Risk Factors for Developing Cervical Cancer

Cancer of the cervix has been associated with several factors, including:

- Early age at first intercourse.
- A history of multiple male sex partners.
- A history of sexually transmitted diseases.
- Infection with certain genotypes of human papilloma virus.
- Smoking.
- Black, Hispanic, or Native American racial/ethnic background.
- Low socioeconomic status.

Although some behavioral factors may be modified, control of cervical cancer primarily depends on early detection through the use of the Pap test.

The Lifesaving Value of Early Detection

Detection and treatment of precancerous cervical lesions (dysplasia) identified by Pap screening can actually prevent invasive cervical cancer. For women diagnosed with dysplastic lesions or carcinoma *in situ*, the likelihood of survival is almost 100 percent if they receive appropriate follow-up and treatment. For patients with invasive but localized cervical cancer, the 5-year relative survival rate falls slightly, to 89 percent. Five-year relative survival is only about 14 percent, however, for patients in whom the invasive cervical cancer has spread to distant sites in the body.

Guidelines for Cervical Cancer Screening

An annual Pap test and pelvic examination are recommended for all women who are or who have been sexually active or who have reached the age of 18. After a woman has had normal results from three or more consecutive annual examinations, the Pap test may be performed less frequently, at the discretion of the woman's health-care provider.

Breast and Cervical Cancer Mortality Prevention Act

Recommended Frequency for Cervical Cancer Screening in Asymptomatic Women

- An annual Papanicolaou test and pelvic examination in all women who are or have been sexually active or who have reached the age of 18.

- After three or more consecutive, satisfactory, normal annual examinations, the Papanicolaou test may be performed less frequently, at the discretion of the health-care provider.

Prevalence of Cervical Cancer Screening

Baseline estimates in 1987 indicated that 88 percent of women had had a Pap test and that 75 percent had had one within the preceding 3 years. The 1991 BRFSS found that 92.4 percent of women aged 18 and older with uterine cervix reported ever having had a Pap test. About 78 percent had had a Pap test within the previous 2 years.

National health promotion and disease prevention objectives, as stated in *Healthy People 2000*, propose to:

> Increase to at least 95 percent the proportion of women aged 18 and older with uterine cervix who have ever received a Pap test, and to at least 85 percent those who have received a Pap test within the preceding 1 to 3 years.

The key elements essential to the success of early detection and control programs for breast and cervical cancers currently exist in the United States. The elements, however, may vary in extensiveness, in location, and for different population groups. Few comprehensive programs are in place. The need for such programs is urgent, as Dr. Harold P. Freeman, Director of Harlem Hospital Center's Department of Surgery, stressed in a testimony before a congressional subcommittee:

> "There are pockets of disaster all over this country where poor, uninsured, and underinsured Americans are dying of cancer and other illnesses because of lack of information about and access to quality health-care services. Action must

be taken immediately to correct the appalling health conditions reflected in these communities."

Conclusion

The National Breast and Cervical Cancer Early Detection Program was initiated to be in the vanguard of endeavors to reach underserved populations and to assume responsibility for coordinating comprehensive public health screening programs to reduce mortality from these two cancers.

Chapter 31

Results from the National Breast and Cervical Cancer Early Detection Program

To reduce the burden of morbidity and mortality from breast and cervical cancers among U.S. women, Congress enacted the Breast and Cervical Cancer Mortality Prevention Act (Public Law 101-354) in August 1990. This legislation authorized CDC to establish the National Breast and Cervical Cancer Early Detection Program (NBCCEDP), which provides state health agencies with grants to increase breast and cervical cancer screening among women[1]. Most funds pay for screening and follow-up services for under-served women, particularly women who are elderly, have low incomes, are under-insured or uninsured, or are members of racial/ethnic minority groups[2]. This report presents age- and race-specific cancer screening (i.e., mammography and Papanicolaou [Pap] smear) results for women who received these services through the NBCCEDP from October 1, 1991, to September 30, 1993.

During this period, eleven states, (California, Colorado, Maryland, Michigan, Minnesota, Missouri, Nebraska, New Mexico, North Carolina, South Carolina, and Texas,) with NBCCEDP-funded cancer screening programs reported data to CDC. For each woman who received a cancer screening examination, data were obtained about demographics, screening location and results, diagnostic procedures and outcomes, and treatment information. The forms used for data collection varied among local sites and states; state program officials stan-

Morbidity and Mortality Weekly Report July 29, 1994 43:29.

dardized data formats before transmitting files electronically to CDC. CDC requests that radiologists report mammography results using categories specified in the Breast Imaging Reporting and Data System (BIRADS) of the American College of Radiology[3] and that laboratories report Pap smear results using categories from the Bethesda System[4]. This analysis presents results from initial mammography screening examinations and excludes results from women who may have undergone subsequent screening examinations. Results were adjusted for state and age using all women undergoing screening through the NBCCEDP as the standard population.

From October 1, 1991, through September 30, 1993, approximately 67,000 women, 40 years old and older, had a mammogram through the NBCCEDP; of these women, 7.2 percent had abnormal results (i.e., suspicious abnormality, highly suggestive of malignancy, or assessment incomplete§) (Table 31. 1). Overall, the proportion of women who had abnormal results declined with increasing age, from 7.8 percent for women aged 40–49 years to 5.3 percent for women aged 70 or older. However, for results highly suggestive of malignancy (the most serious result) the opposite trend was observed. The proportion of abnormal mammography results was highest for non-Hispanic whites (7.9 percent) and non-Hispanic blacks (7.8 percent) and lowest for Asians/Pacific Islanders (4.1 percent).

During the same period, approximately 100,500 women had Pap smears; of these, 5.1 percent had abnormal results (i.e., low-grade squamous intraepithelial lesion [SIL], high-grade SIL, or squamous cell carcinoma) (Table 31.2). The proportion of women with abnormal results declined sharply with increasing age, from 11.5 percent for women more than 30 years old to 1.9 percent for women more than 70 years old. The proportion of abnormal Pap smear results varied slightly among racial/ethnic groups (except Asians/Pacific Islanders) ranging from 4.2 percent for Hispanics to 4.7 percent for American Indians/Alaskan Natives; the proportion was lowest for Asians/Pacific Islanders (2.0 percent).

Reported by: Epidemiology and Statistics Branch and Office of the Director, Division of Cancer Prevention and Control, National Center for Chronic Disease Prevention and Health Promotion, CDC.

Results from the Early Detection Program

Table 31.1. Percentage distribution of mammography screening results* among women aged 40 or more years, by age group and race/ethnicity—National Breast and Cervical Cancer Early Detection Program (NBCCEDP), October 1, 1991—September 30, 1993†.

Characteristic	No. examined	Negative or benign	Probably benign	Abnormal results				Total	Unsatisfactory examination
				Suspicious abnormality	Highly suggestive of malignancy	Assessment incomplete§			
Age group (yrs)									
40–49	29,316	83.5%	8.6%	1.7%	0.2%	5.9%		7.8%	0.1%
50–59	20,449	84.1%	8.5%	1.9%	0.3%	5.1%		7.3%	0.1%
60–69	12,536	86.0%	7.6%	1.5%	0.3%	4.6%		6.4%	<0.1%
≥70	4,529	87.8%	6.8%	1.9%	0.4%	3.0%		5.3%	0.1%
Race/Ethnicity									
White, non-Hispanic	23,712	83.9%	8.1%	2.0%	0.4%	5.5%		7.9%	0.1%
Black, non-Hispanic	10,827	83.8%	8.4%	1.8%	0.3%	5.7%		7.8%	0.1%
Hispanic¶	18,385	84.0%	9.0%	1.3%	0.2%	5.4%		6.9%	0.1%
Asian/Pacific Islander	1,666	88.8%	7.1%	1.7%	<0.1%	2.4%		4.1%	<0.1%
American Indian/Alaskan Native	8,179	87.2%	6.2%	1.4%	0.4%	4.8%		6.6%	<0.1%
Other/Unknown**	4,061	85.9%	7.4%	1.7%	0.3%	4.7%		6.7%	<0.1%
Overall	66,830	84.4%	8.3%	1.7%	0.3%	5.2%		7.2%	0.1%

*Results are from initial screening examinations and exclude results for women who may have undergone subsequent screening examinations. Result categories are from the Breast Imaging Reporting and Data System (3). Data were adjusted for state and age using all women undergoing screening through the NBCCEDP as the standard population.
† Data were reported to CDC from 11 states with NBCCEDP-funded cancer screening programs (California, Colorado, Maryland, Michigan, Minnesota, Missouri, Nebraska, New Mexico, North Carolina, South Carolina, and Texas).
§ A mammography finding that requires additional radiologic evaluation (3).
¶ May be of any race.
**Includes 2,079 white women and 437 black women of unknown ethnicity.

Table 31.2. Percentage distribution of Papanicolaou smear screening results*, by age group and race/ethnicity—National Breast and Cervical Cancer Early Detection Program (NBCCEDP), October 1, 1991—September 30, 1993.†

Characteristic	No. examined	Negative or benign§	ASCUS¶	Low-grade SIL**	High-grade SIL	Squamous cell cancer	Total	Other	Unsatisfactory examination
Age group (yrs)									
<30	31,569	78.3%	8.0%	9.4%	2.1%	<0.1%	11.5%	0.6%	1.5%
30-39	18,359	86.9%	5.4%	4.2%	1.4%	0.1%	5.7%	0.5%	1.6%
40-49	23,455	89.5%	5.2%	2.4%	0.7%	<0.1%	3.1%	0.5%	1.8%
50-59	14,897	91.5%	4.3%	1.6%	0.7%	<0.1%	2.4%	0.4%	1.4%
60-69	8,889	93.0%	3.3%	1.2%	0.3%	0.1%	1.6%	0.5%	1.6%
≥70	3,245	92.5%	4.0%	1.3%	0.6%	<0.1%	1.9%	0.5%	1.1%
Race/Ethnicity									
White, non-Hispanic	38,754	88.9%	4.4%	3.6%	1.0%	<0.1%	4.6%	0.4%	1.7%
Black, non-Hispanic	12,971	89.5%	4.2%	3.8%	0.7%	0.1%	4.6%	0.3%	1.3%
Hispanic††	26,886	88.1%	5.7%	3.4%	0.8%	<0.1%	4.2%	0.4%	1.4%
Asian/Pacific Islander	2,008	92.6%	4.2%	1.3%	0.7%	<0.1%	2.0%	0.2%	0.9%
American Indian/ Alaskan Native	13,544	85.6%	7.6%	3.9%	0.8%	<0.1%	4.7%	0.4%	1.8%
Other/Unknown§§	6,251	84.4%	7.7%	4.7%	0.9%	<0.1%	5.6%	0.3%	1.9%
Overall	100,414	87.3%	5.4%	4.0%	1.1%	<0.1%	5.1%	0.5%	1.7%

* Result categories are from the Bethesda System (4). Data were adjusted for state and age using all women undergoing screening through the NBCCEDP as the standard population.
† Data were reported to CDC from 11 states with NBCCEDP-funded cancer screening programs (California, Colorado, Maryland, Michigan, Minnesota, Missouri, Nebraska, New Mexico, North Carolina, South Carolina, and Texas).
§ Includes infection and reactive changes.
¶ Atypical squamous cells of uncertain significance.
** Squamous intraepithelial lesions.
†† May be of any race.
§§ Includes 3,083 white women and 389 black women of unknown ethnicity.

Results from the Early Detection Program

Editorial Note. Despite the proven effectiveness of mammography and Pap smears in detecting breast and cervical cancers in early, more treatable stages, not all women have access to necessary screening and follow-up services. The NBCCEDP is mandated to detect cancer and pre-cancerous lesions in women who are at high risk for not being screened and therefore at higher risk for having cancer diagnosed at a later stage. This report represents one of the largest case studies on screening services targeting under-served women.

The overall proportion of abnormal mammograms reported by NBCCEDP during 1991–1993 is consistent with findings in a previous study[5], although these two studies used different result categories. The overall decline with increasing age in the proportion of abnormal mammography results is attributable primarily to results categorized as assessment incomplete—an outcome more common among younger women, whose dense breast tissue make radiologic assessment more difficult. The percentage of findings categorized as highly suggestive of malignancy increases with age, reflecting the increasing incidence of breast cancer with increasing age[6]. The higher proportion of abnormal results among white and black women reflects the higher reported incidence of breast cancer in these groups than in other racial/ethnic groups. Reasons for these differences in incidence are unclear.

Most of the Pap smear results reported by NBCCEDP during 1991–1993 are similar to findings in previous studies[7,8]. The steady decline with increasing age in the proportion of abnormal Pap smear results is attributable primarily to the increase in results categorized as low-grade SIL.

The findings in this report are subject to at least two limitations. First, NBCCEDP results are derived from screening tests and therefore do not represent the final diagnoses. Some abnormal results classified as cancer may not be confirmed as such on biopsy, and some results classified as non-cancerous may be found to be cancer. Because states have had difficulty tracking the diagnostic results of women with abnormal screening examinations, complete information is not yet available to analyze diagnostic outcomes. Second, because use of the BIRADS reporting categories was initiated in NBCCEDP in 1991 (before BIRADS was officially disseminated to U.S. radiologists by the American College of Radiologists), the categories for reporting results of mammography screening probably have not been used uniformly among the participating states, particularly during the first year of the program. However, as radiologists become more familiar with BIRADS, its use in different program sites probably will become more uniform.

CDC's NBCCEDP increases cancer screening among women by increasing access to screening and follow-up services, increasing education programs for women and health-care providers, and improving measures to assure quality of mammography and Pap smear testing. These activities are implemented through partnerships with state health agencies; 45 states are participating in NBCCEDP at different levels. These efforts should increase detection and treatment of precancerous cervical lesions and early-stage breast cancer and ultimately reduce the incidence of cervical cancer and morbidity and mortality from breast cancer among under-served women.

References

1. CDC. Implementation of the Breast and Cervical Cancer Mortality Prevention Act: 1992 progress report to Congress. Atlanta: US Department of Health and Human Services, Public Health Service, 1993 (in press).

2. CDC. Update: National Breast and Cervical Cancer Early Detection Program, July 1991–July 1992. MMWR 1992;41:739-43.

3. Kopans DB, D'Orsi CJ, Adler DD, et al. Breast Imaging Reporting and Data System. Reston, Virginia; American College of Radiology 1993.

4. Broder S. Rapid communication: the Bethesda System for reporting cervical/vaginal cytologic diagnoses report of the 1991 Bethesda Workshop. JAMA 1992;267:1892.

5. Sickles EA, Ominsky SH, Sollitto RA, Galvin HB, Monticciolo DL. Medical audit of a rapid throughput mammography screening practice: methodology and results of 27,114 examinations. Radiology 1990;175:323-7.

6. Hankey BF, Brinton LA, Kessler LG, Abrams J. Section IV: breast. In: Miller BA, Reis LAG, Hankey BF, et al, eds. SEER cancer statistics review, 1973–1990. Bethesda, Maryland: US Department of Health and Human Services, Public Health Service, National Institutes of Health, National Cancer Institute, 1993:1V.1–IV.24; DHHS publication no. (NIH)93-2789.

7. Bottles K, Reiter RC, Steiner AL, Zaleski S, Bedrossian CW, Johnson SR. Problems encountered with the Bethesda System: the University of Iowa experience. Obstet Gynecol 1991;78:410-4.

8. Sadeghi SB, Hsieh EW, Gunn SW. Prevalence of cervical intraepithelial neoplasia in sexually active teenagers and adults. Am J Obstet Gynecol 1984;148:726-9.

Chapter 32

Preventive Mastectomy

Preventive mastectomy (also called prophylactic mastectomy) is surgery to remove one or both breasts of women who have strong risk factors for breast cancer but no evidence of the disease. The surgery may involve removing the entire breast (total mastectomy) or removing just the breast tissue but not the skin and nipple (subcutaneous mastectomy). After either procedure, the patient may decide to have breast reconstruction, plastic surgery to restore the shape of the breast.

Preventive mastectomy is a controversial subject. This procedure may be appropriate for women who have had certain types of breast cancer because they are at risk of developing breast cancer again—in the same and/or the opposite breast. It also may be recommended for women whose breast tissue is so dense that physical examination or mammography is difficult, necessitating multiple biopsies, which in turn cause tissue scarring and further complicate examination of the breast tissue. However, doctors do not always agree on the most effective way to manage the care of women who have a strong family history of breast cancer and/or have certain other risk factors for the disease; some recommend preventive mastectomy, while others recommend very close observation (monthly breast self-examination, checkups every 3 months, and periodic mammograms) instead. In addition, doctors are concerned that women who have preventive surgery may have a false sense of security. Some patients mistakenly believe that

---

NCI Cancerfax 208/600075.

the operation is a complete guarantee against breast cancer. However, it is almost impossible to remove all breast tissue with any type of mastectomy, and breast cancer can develop in any remaining tissue.

Because every woman is different, the use of prophylactic mastectomy should be considered in the context of each woman's unique risk factors as well as her feelings about mastectomy and breast reconstruction. A woman considering preventive mastectomy should discuss her risk factors, the mastectomy procedure, the likely outcome of reconstructive surgery, potential complications, and follow-up care with her doctor and plastic surgeon. She should also consider getting a second medical opinion.

When a woman decides to have preventive mastectomy and reconstructive surgery, a plastic surgeon carefully examines her breasts, taking into consideration what tissue will be needed for reconstruction. She should discuss with the doctor the types of reconstructive procedures that are appropriate for her and decide with which procedure she feels most comfortable. Breast tissue removed during surgery is examined by a pathologist to make sure that no cancer cells are present. To restore the shape of the breast, the surgeon then inserts an implant under the skin and the chest muscles. Another option is to create the shape of a breast using skin, fat, and muscle from the patient's abdomen or back.

The surgeon will discuss with the patient any limitations on exercise or arm motion after surgery. The patient will be followed carefully in the post-operative period to detect and treat complications, such as infection, movement of the implant, or contracture (the formation of a firm, fibrous shell around the implant caused by the body's reaction to it). Routine screening for breast cancer should also be part of the post-operative follow-up because the risk of cancer cannot be completely eliminated.

Women who are considering reconstructive surgery may find it helpful to contact the American Society of Plastic and Reconstructive Surgeons and ask for the names of qualified plastic surgeons in their area. The address of the Society is 444 East Algonquin Road, Arlington Heights, IL 60005; the toll-free referral service number is 1-800-635-0635. Calls are answered between 9 a.m. and 3 p.m. eastern time. At other times, callers may leave a message.

Chapter 33

Mammography Facilities Must Meet Quality Standards

No news is good news, the maxim goes, and when a woman is told that her mammogram shows no evidence of cancer, that's good news indeed. But the "good news" can turn into bad if tumors are missed because of poor mammography. Undetected, and thus untreated, the cancer advances.

In December, 1993, the Food and Drug Administration published in the *Federal Register* interim final regulations intended to ensure that all mammography done in the United States is safe and reliable. They are a crucial step in implementing the Mammography Quality Standards Act (MQSA), enacted by Congress in 1992 in response to concerns that mammography was not being practiced to uniformly high standards at all facilities. Senator Barbara Mikulski (D-Md.), who co-sponsored the bill, was instrumental in ensuring its passage and funding. In June 1993, the assistant secretary for health delegated to FDA responsibility for implementing and enforcing the new law.

Breast cancer is the second leading cause of cancer deaths in American women. According to U.S. Public Health Service (PHS) figures, nearly half a million women will die of breast cancer in the 1990s, and more than one-and-a-half million new cases will be diagnosed in that time.

Mammography—a special x-ray examination of the breast—is the most effective method for detecting breast tumors early, when the

---

FDA Consumer Magazine Reprint FDA Pub No. 94-8284.

disease is most successfully treated. It can find 85 to 90 percent of breast cancers in women over 50 and can discover a tumor up to two years before a lump can be felt.

Widespread screening of women over 50, followed by prompt treatment when needed, can reduce breast cancer deaths by as much as 30 percent, according to PHS. This striking statistic underscores the need for accurate mammography. The x-ray images must be of high quality, they must be read by physicians proficient in interpreting them, and the results must be reported promptly.

Under the MQSA, no mammography facility—whether in a hospital, doctor's office, mobile van, military base, or any other public or private enterprise—will be able to operate legally after Oct. 1, 1994, unless it is accredited and federally certified as meeting quality standards. All will be subject to federal inspection and certification. After initial certification, facilities must pass annual inspections by approved federal or state inspectors (Veterans Administration hospitals are exempt from the law. However, the House Committee on Veterans Affairs has stated it will take steps to ensure that mammography in veterans facilities is subject to the same quality standards required by the MQSA.)

The regulations published in December, 1993, became effective in February, 1994. Facilities must comply with standards covering:

- quality assurance and quality control

- radiological equipment

- personnel qualifications for the technicians who perform mammography, physicians who interpret the mammograms, and medical physicists who are required to survey the facilities annually

- medical record-keeping and disposition of written reports of mammography examinations.

The regulations also include standards for approval of accrediting bodies that will evaluate the facilities and review films for image quality.

Also as required by the MQSA, FDA established a National Mammography Quality Assurance Advisory Committee, which advises the agency on developing quality and personnel standards, and on monitoring the entire program.

Time Crunch

FDA found a challenge in implementing the MQSA by the mandated deadlines. The law contains two significant dates: July 22, 1993, for completion of all federal mammography standards, and Oct. 1, 1994, for certification of facilities. "These dates were virtually impossible to meet if we followed standard procedures," says Richard Gross, an assistant director in FDA's Office of Training and Assistance in the Center for Devices and Radiological Health. "The administrative procedures for writing and publishing complex standards typically take two years. They require notice of a draft rule, opportunity for public comment, analysis of the comments and revision of the rule, and publication in the Federal Register with an effective date. Establishing an advisory committee also requires time to follow procedures set by the Federal Advisory Committee Act."

Nevertheless, standards had to be published so that facilities could be certified by the Oct. 1 deadline. Facilities not certified could not lawfully operate.

Working together, Congress—particularly Senator Mikulski and Representative John Dingell (D-Mich.) and the Department of Health and Human Services solved the problem by giving FDA authority to issue an interim final rule, enforceable 60 days after publication. The interim final regulations include standards essentially the same as those developed by the American College of Radiology (ACR) for its voluntary program of mammography accreditation. (With minor modifications to its standards, ACR can apply for and be approved as an accrediting body.) Since more than half the facilities have already been accredited by ACR and another 20 to 30 percent had applied by the time the interim final regulations were published, federal certification is expected to proceed smoothly and quickly.

"The interim final regulation is like a draft rule," Gross says, "except it got us to the point of being able to issue the certificates. We don't expect a final rule to be in place until maybe a year down the road—so it might be October 1995 before final standards are published."

During that time, the advisory committee will assess what the agency has done and what changes it thinks need to be made. FDA will also receive comments from the public and will consider mammography guidelines recently developed by the Public Health Service's Agency for Health Care Policy and Research. After incorporating relevant information and opinions from comments, FDA will issue a final rule.

Inspections will start after Oct. 1, 1994, Gross says, adding that both federal and state inspectors must complete an FDA training program and be certified.

Most of the inspections will be done in cooperation with the states, and it is likely that once the standards are final and the training programs established, much of the program can be administered by the states.

Lireka Joseph, Dr.P.H., an assistant director in the Center for Devices and Radiological Health's Office of Training and Assistance, says that if a facility is not in compliance with the standards it will be given an opportunity to develop a corrective action plan, which FDA will review. "Then, we'll work with the facility to bring it up to speed," she says. "Our intention is not to close facilities, but to improve mammography."

Facilities that can't or won't comply, however, will face sanctions, says Joseph, who was the center's interim director for mammography quality radiation programs. (Florence Houn, M.D., began as permanent director last Dec. 14.) Noncompliant facilities may be fined, have their certification suspended or revoked, or be enjoined by a court to stop operating.

Quality Control Before the MQSA

Mammography has not been totally without oversight until now. In fact, Gross says, the MQSA actually is a "marriage of sorts" between two existing mammography standards programs—ACR's accreditation program and the Health Care Financing Administration's Medicare certification program.

FDA's involvement with mammography is not new either. The agency turned its focus on the procedure following a report in 1974 by Henry Bicehouse, a Pennsylvania state inspector. Bicehouse had done some mammography surveys in eastern Pennsylvania, measuring radiation exposures to women from mammography techniques used in different facilities. The report showed a few extremely high doses.

Mammography Facilities Must Meet Quality Standards

"That was the first time there had ever been any real attention paid to mammography—how it was being conducted and what was happening," Gross says.

In 1975, the Center for Devices and Radiological Health started a national program in cooperation with the states—the Breast Exposure Nationwide Trends (BENT). The program's objective was to locate facilities giving excessively high radiation exposures and to assist them in reducing the exposures.

During this voluntary program, industry also worked to improve equipment and films, and mammography techniques began to change. As a result, radiation doses began to decrease.

"But we were concerned that much of the pressure to reduce the dose might have the effect of compromising image quality," Gross says. "So in 1983 we began to develop a more reliable phantom—the one used in the BENT program was fairly crude."

(A phantom is a plastic device embedded with objects of varying materials and size that is used to evaluate image quality. The device is x-rayed as though it were a breast, and the image score is determined by the number of objects picked up by the x-ray film.)

"Since 1974, FDA has had performance standards for special-purpose mammography equipment, so that mammography x-ray machines had to meet specific requirements. But quality and patient issues were left to the state programs," Gross says.

In 1985, using the new phantom, FDA and the state governments conducted a mammography survey under the Nationwide Evaluation of X-ray Trends (NEXT) program. A cooperative federal-state survey program of the Conference of Radiation Control Program Directors, NEXT measures average radiation exposures from various diagnostic x-ray procedures. For mammography, image quality is also evaluated.

"We found a wide range of image quality, from good to bad, but at that time we didn't have a generally accepted way of determining what was acceptable and what was not," Gross says. "But we found some images so bad that it would have been very difficult to detect anything. The problem was not with the equipment—the machines were performing accurately—so we presented our findings to the ACR, suggesting that the problem needed to be dealt with and leaving it in their hands."

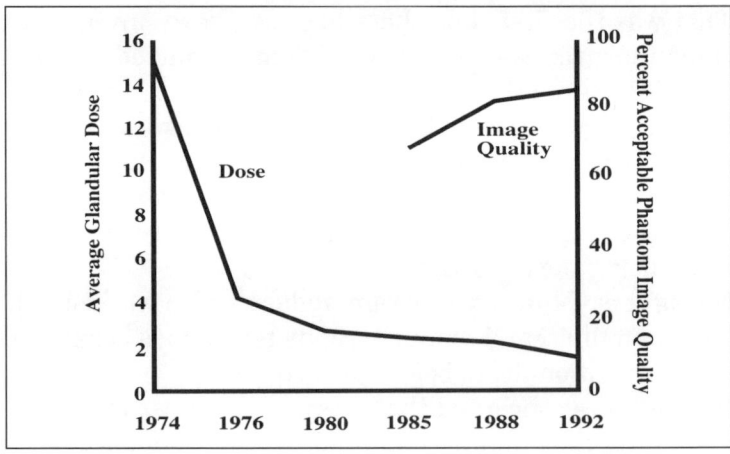

Figure 33.1. Dose Decreases, Image Improves. With advances in mammography equipment and techniques, the average radiation dose has declined dramatically, while image quality has improved. In 1985, 64 percent of mammography images evaluated using phantom devices were of acceptable quality; by 1992, the percent of acceptable images had risen to 86 percent. (Measurement of image quality was not adequately reliable until the 1985 survey, in which improved phantom devices were used.) Radiation exposure to women declined from an average 15.1 glandular dose (mGy) in 1974 to an average 1.8 mGy in 1992. (I mGy = 0.1 rad)

Poor Techniques

The problems were due to poor techniques, such as improper film processing and improper use of image receptors. These were issues over which FDA, at that time, had no regulatory authority, Gross says, and which had to be corrected within the facility.

ACR agreed to try to help correct the problem and, in 1987, established its mammography accrediting program. FDA regulated the equipment, and ACR policed the facilities. But the accrediting program was voluntary, and not all facilities participated.

At about the same time, the Health Care Financing Administration was establishing standards facilities would have to meet in order to receive Medicare reimbursement for screening mammography. (Medicare already covered diagnostic mammography, but there were no specific standards requirements.) The agency's new certification

Mammography Facilities Must Meet Quality Standards

program was mandatory, but only for facilities that wanted to provide screening mammography services to Medicare patients.

"There were pieces from both the ACR and the Medicare programs people liked that were in one but not the other," Gross says. In "marrying" the two, the MQSA contains the better features of both, including annual inspections and an accreditation requirement that includes image review. Furthermore, accreditation and certification are mandatory for all mammography facilities in the country.

Room for Improvement

Even in the best circumstances, some tumors are missed by mammography. If, for instance, a woman's tumor at the particular time she has a mammogram is the same density as the surrounding breast tissue, it may not show up on the x-ray.

"Mammography is not perfect," says Joseph, "but it's the best method we now have. With the MQSA we can hope to see possibly a 30 percent reduction in mortality for older women who receive mammograms. We're trying to make sure that women 50 and older go to accredited, certified facilities where they receive quality mammograms and quality interpretations of the mammograms, so that in the long run we can see that mortality drop from breast cancer. But even the best facility can't help a woman if she doesn't use it."

Who Should Get a Mammogram

There has been some debate recently about who should have mammograms and how often. In late 1991, the National Cancer Institute (NCI) began a review of clinical data to assess the value of screening mammography in reducing breast cancer deaths.

In a statement issued last December, NCI noted that experts generally agree that in women over 50, screening every one to two years can reduce breast cancer deaths by about one-third. Experts do not agree on the usefulness of screening mammography in women 40 to 49, as clinical trials have not shown a clear benefit in reduced mortality for women under 50, according to the institute.

Some organizations, including the American College of Physicians, recommend that women begin to have mammograms at age 50 and have them every year. Others, including the American Cancer Society, recommend mammograms every one to two years beginning at age 40, and every year after age 50. There is no dispute among organizations that women over 50 should be encouraged to get routine mammograms.

These screening recommendations apply to women who have no symptoms of breast cancer, and who are not at higher risk for the disease. Any woman, regardless of age, should see her doctor immediately if she has symptoms, such as a lump or other change in the breast. And for women who have no symptoms but may be at higher risk because of family history, obesity, or late childbearing, for example. a physician may recommend earlier and more frequent mammograms.

—by Marian Segal

Marian Segal is a member of FDA's public affairs staff.

Chapter 34

Chances Are You Need a Mammogram: A Guide for Midlife and Older Women

If you are a woman 50 years of age or over, the chances are very good that you need a mammogram, but haven't had one. The National Cancer Institute, along with twelve other medical organizations, recommends that women have this simple test once a year starting at age 50 in order to detect breast cancer. Studies show, however, that only one-third of women 50 and over actually do.

Perhaps you think you don't need a mammogram. You do. One out of nine American women will develop breast cancer. As you age, your chances of getting it actually increase every year. In fact, two-thirds of all breast cancers occur in women over the age of 50.

Regular mammograms are one of the best weapons you can have against breast cancer. It is important to do monthly breast self-examinations and get breast exams at your clinic or doctor's office at regular check-ups, but be sure to also get regular screening mammograms. A screening mammogram can detect cancer at its earliest stages, up to two years before a lump can be felt. Up to 90 percent of breast cancers can be treated successfully if they are found early and have not spread beyond the breast. So you do need a mammogram!

If you are 65 years of age or older, there is some good news about the cost of mammograms. Medicare now helps cover the cost of screening mammograms every other year for women 65 and over. It is important that women learn about mammography, but they aren't the only ones who need to learn about it. It is important for men who care

---

National Cancer Institute Pub No. PF4730(1094)•D14502.

about the health of their partners, sisters, mothers, or daughters to learn about early detection as well. Men can encourage the women in their lives to take advantage of this life-saving opportunity.

What Is A Mammogram?

A mammogram is an x-ray picture that can show a lump in a breast two years before a woman or health professional can feel it. Finding a lump early increases a woman's chance of surviving breast cancer and allows more treatment choices. Because the mammogram is a low-dose x-ray, the risk from radiation is very low and clearly better than not finding breast cancer early. During a mammogram, a technologist will ask you to undress above the waist and wear a jacket or gown that opens in the front. You will stand in front of an x-ray machine and the technologist will place each breast, one at a time, on a small platform. The breast is flattened for the x-ray picture with a device called a paddle. After having your mammogram, be sure to ask how you can get a copy if you need it in the future.

Chances are, you need a mammogram. Many women do not get mammograms. Why not? Do any of the following statements sound familiar to you?

"I don't need a mammogram, no one in my family has ever had breast cancer."

It is true that family history is a risk factor for breast cancer. If a woman's mother or sister has had breast cancer, her chances of getting breast cancer double. But 80 percent of women who get breast cancer have no family history. All women need to take advantage of screening.

"If I haven't gotten breast cancer so far, I won't get it now. I'm too old!"

Age itself is a risk factor. The incidence of breast cancer actually increases with age. Two-thirds of all breast cancers occur in women over the age of 50. In fact, being a woman and getting older are the main risk factors for breast cancer; women 65 and older are 6 times as likely as those under 65 to have breast cancer.

"I spend so much money on doctors already. I hear it can cost over one hundred dollars! I just can't afford to have one."

Cost plays an important role in a woman's ability to get a mammogram. The average cost of a mammogram is between $100.00 and $125.00; however, the cost can range from less than $50.00 to $250.00. While free mammograms are rare, there are some low-cost programs with fees determined on a sliding scale based on ability to pay. Some private doctors or facilities may also lower fees if a woman cannot afford the usual fee. Many communities have facilities that just do mammography and are beginning to offer lower cost mammograms. Also watch for special low-cost programs during Breast Cancer Awareness Month in October each year.

Mammograms may be covered by private insurance. Many states have passed legislation that requires private insurers to include screening mammograms in insurance benefits. Check with the American Cancer Society about legislation in your state.

As of January 1, 1991, Medicare covers part of the cost of screening mammography every other year for women 65 years and over. Certain payment limitations apply. For more information, call your local Medicare Carrier. (Refer to your Medicare Handbook for the name of your Medicare Carrier or call your local Social Security Office.)

In order to have Medicare help pay for your screening, the clinic or center you use must be certified by Medicare to do mammography screening. You will need to ask the facility: *"Have you been certified by Medicare to perform screening mammograms for Medicare beneficiaries?"* If the answer is no, ask your doctor for the name of a certified facility.

While most women covered under Medicare are 65 or over, there are some cases when younger women receive Medicare benefits. For more information on mammography screening for younger women, contact your Medicare Carrier.

"If I have cancer; I don't think I can face it. I don't want to know."

Breast cancer is often called the disease women fear most. However, if breast cancer is detected early enough and has not spread beyond the breast, up to 90 percent of women can be treated successfully.

There have been many positive advances made in breast cancer treatment in the past 20 years. There are more treatment choices and a much better outlook for those who have breast cancer today. Many women are now able to choose treatment that does not require removal of the breast because their cancers have been detected in early stages. A variety of surgical techniques, which are combined with radiation or chemotherapy, make breast reconstruction easier. Keep in mind, however, that more treatment choices and improved survival rates depend greatly on early detection.

(For more information on treatment options, please refer to the "treatment" sections of this sourcebook or consult your physician.)

"I haven't the slightest idea where to get a mammogram."

The number of facilities offering mammograms is growing rapidly. The American College of Radiology (ACR), the professional organization that sets quality standards for and accredits mammography facilities, estimates that as of July 1991, there are 11,000 units nationwide. If a woman has her own physician, she should ask him or her to recommend a mammography facility In addition, many public health departments, hospitals, and women's clinics can perform mammography screening. To find mammography facilities in your area, check with:

- the National Cancer Institute's Cancer Information Service at 1–800-4-CANCER (1-800-422-6237);
- the American Cancer Society Cancer Response System at 1–800-227-2345;
- local hospitals—try clinics for Obstetrics and Gynecology, Family Planning or Family Medicine, or the Oncology Department;
- local/county public health departments;
- local women's groups;
- mobile vans that are operated by city or county health departments;
- visiting nurse or home health agencies

Chances Are You Need a Mammogram

How will I know if I'm getting a good mammogram?"

It's very important to get a mammogram from a quality facility. Call the facility of your choice and ask five simple questions. A quality facility will answer yes to all five questions.

1. Does the facility use machines specifically designed for mammography? *These are called "dedicated mammography machines." Women should not get mammograms from machines that also take pictures of the bones and chest.*

2. Is the person who provides the mammogram a registered technologist? *These people must be trained to position the breasts correctly to get a good picture. They should be certified by the American College of Radiological Technologists or be licensed by the state.*

3. Is the radiologist who reads the mammogram specially trained to do so? *The radiologist should be board-certified and should have taken special courses in mammography.*

4. Does the facility provide mammograms as part of its regular practice? *The American College of Radiology suggests choosing a facility that performs at least 10 mammograms per week.*

5. Is the mammography machine calibrated at least once a year? *When a machine is calibrated, it is checked against a standard to be sure that its measurements and doses are correct. Adjustments are made if necessary.*

"My doctor has never suggested it and when I asked, he didn't seem to think it was that important."

Physicians often do not refer older women for mammograms. Physicians may not refer because they are not aware of the guidelines recommended by the National Cancer Institute, are concerned about expense to their patients, or don't realize the low risk from the radiation involved. Women, especially older women, need to be assertive.

You need to ask your doctor to refer you for a mammogram. Most physicians are very receptive to patient requests for a referral.

You can also get a mammogram without a physician referral by contacting a local facility directly.

"I don't know how I'd get there."

Transportation can be a problem. Consider public transportation, if you are in an urban area, or ask a friend or relative to take you. Some communities may have programs in which volunteers will transport women to facilities. Call the Cancer Information Service at 1-800-422-6237 or the American Cancer Society at 1-800-227-2345 for more information on transportation services.

"I hear the test really hurts. They squeeze your breasts. I don't want to feel that kind of pain."

Some women experience discomfort during a mammogram. But the majority of women report no discomfort. The actual time of compression, when the breast is flattened and pain may occur, is less than 30 seconds. The compression is needed to get a good picture of the breast. The entire mammography procedure lasts about 15 minutes.

"It's an x-ray. I don't want to expose my body to any radiation unless I absolutely have to."

Over the past 20 years, x-ray technology has advanced substantially. As a result, a mammography x-ray uses a very low dose of radiation. Today's mammogram uses 1/40 the amount of radiation required 20 years ago. Clearly, the benefits far outweigh the risk. Remember, a quality facility with dedicated equipment and trained staff is the best way to assure a safe, accurate mammogram.

Don't take unnecessary chances with your health. Make an appointment for a mammogram today.

For more information on breast cancer and mammography, including facilities near you, contact the National Cancer Information Service at 1-800-4-CANCER (1-800-422-6237).

You can also write for these free brochures from the Office of Cancer Communications, National Cancer Institute, Publications, Bldg. 31, Rm. 10A24, Bethesda, MD 20892:

Chances Are You Need a Mammogram

"Breast Exams: What You Should Know"
"Breast Lumps: What You Should Know"
"Breast Cancer: Understanding Treatment Options"

For Medicare information, write to:

Office of Public Affairs
Health Care Financing Administration
Room 435-H, Humphrey Building
200 Independence Avenue, S.W.
Washington, DC 20201

Chapter 35

Screening as Cancer Prevention

Breast Cancer Screening

The National Cancer Institute (NCI) recently released the following statement concerning breast cancer screening:

- There is a general consensus among experts that routine screening every 1 to 2 years with mammography and clinical breast examination can reduce breast cancer mortality by about one-third for women ages 50 and over.

- Experts do not agree on the role of routine screening mammography for women ages 40 to 49. To date, randomized clinical trials have not shown a statistically significant reduction in mortality for women under the age of 50.

The statement represents a summary of scientific fact about effectiveness, that is, the ability of mammography, coupled with appropriate treatment, to reduce the mortality from breast cancer. It summarizes scientific knowledge derived from two decades of clinical trials research. The statement is a successor to a "working guideline" formulation drafted in 1987 and will be revised as new information is developed.

NCI Cancerfax 208/600513 and 208/05145 and 208/04728.

Background Information. The NCI is the lead Federal agency for research on the causes, prevention, diagnosis, and treatment of cancer. The NCI conducts ongoing evaluations of the results of cancer research and in late 1991, began the process of examining clinical trial evidence for the value of screening mammography.

The NCI convened an International Workshop on Breast Cancer Screening in February 1993. The results from eight randomized clinical trials were reviewed. The workshop conclusions reinforced the advisability of screening for women ages 50 to 69, and stated that the effects of screening in women ages 40 to 49 do not demonstrate a statistically significant reduction in mortality to date.

Between May and December 1993, scientific data from clinical trials, including the workshop results were reviewed by a number of scientific organizations, health groups, and advisory boards.

Screening for Ovarian Cancer

Summary of Evidence

There is insufficient evidence to establish that screening for ovarian cancer with serum markers such as CA-125 levels, transvaginal ultrasound, or pelvic examinations would result in a decrease in mortality from ovarian cancer.

Significance

Ovarian cancer is the fourth leading cause of cancer death among U.S. women and has the highest mortality rate of all gynecologic cancers. It is projected that 26,600 new cases of ovarian cancer will be diagnosed and 14,500 women will die of the disease in 1995. The prognosis for survival from ovarian cancer is largely dependent upon the extent of disease at diagnosis. Women diagnosed with local disease are over 4 times more likely to survive 5 years than women with distant disease. However, less than one-fourth of women present with localized disease at diagnosis. The overall 5-year survival rate for ovarian cancer is less than 40 percent. Incidence has increased only slightly from 1973 to 1989; mortality has decreased by about 8 percent in that same time period.

The etiology of ovarian cancer is poorly understood. The median age at diagnosis is 63. A decreased risk of ovarian cancer is associated with increased parity, oral contraceptive use, and breast feeding. A history of tubal ligation or hysterectomy with ovarian conservation is also associated with a decreased risk. Risk is increased in women with a family history of ovarian cancer and possibly among women who have used fertility drugs; however, this information has limited application in programs of selective screening due to the small number of women with these risk factors. Age at menarche, menopause, or first live birth are unrelated to the risk of ovarian cancer. Other factors, such as exposure to talcum powder, have also been suggested to increase risk.

Evidence of Benefit

Potential screening tests for ovarian cancer include bimanual pelvic examination, vaginal ultrasound, and CA-125 antigen as a tumor marker. The Pap smear may occasionally detect malignant ovarian cells, but is not sufficiently sensitive (reported sensitivity of 10-30 percent) or reliable to be used for the early detection of ovarian cancer. Another method of detection is cytologic examination of peritoneal lavage obtained by culdocentesis. Because of the technical difficulty, the discomfort of the procedure, and the reported low sensitivity for detecting early stage disease, it is inappropriate to consider this test for routine screening.

The sensitivity and specificity of pelvic examination for the detection of ovarian cancer is unknown. Generally, detection by this method reveals advanced disease.

Ultrasonography, particularly transvaginal ultrasonography, has been proposed as a screening method for ovarian cancer because of its ability to reliably measure ovarian size and detect small masses. The benefit of ultrasonography for the early detection of ovarian cancer has not been evaluated in controlled studies. Estimates of the yield and false positive rate are available from several cohort studies of women offered periodic screening. In a cohort of 801 women aged 40 to 70 who had one or more risk factors for ovarian cancer, 163 (20 percent) had an abnormal abdominal ultrasound. Surgery was performed in 30 cases for a yield of one borderline ovarian tumor and two endometrial carcinomas. In another study, 5,479 self-referred, asymptomatic women underwent periodic screening with abdominal ultrasonography with positive results obtained in 326 participants. After surgery, 5 women were diagnosed with stage Ia or Ib ovarian cancer; 4 women were diagnosed with metastatic ovarian cancer.

Transvaginal ultrasonography was used in a study of 3,220 asymptomatic, postmenopausal women. Forty-four women (1.4 percent) had persistent abnormal scans and underwent exploratory laparotomy. Three were found to have a primary ovarian carcinoma, two with stage IA disease. In one other study, transabdominal and transvaginal ultrasonography were both used to screen 1,601 self-referred women with a first- or second-degree relative with ovarian cancer. Sixty-one had positive screening tests; 6 had ovarian cancer that was detected at surgery (5 of 6 had stage I disease). Five additional cases of cancer (3 ovarian and 2 peritoneal) were reported 2 to 44 months after the last ultrasound test.

CA-125 is a tumor-associated antigen that has been used clinically to monitor patients with epithelial ovarian carcinomas. The measurement of CA-125 levels usually in combination with other modalities such as bimanual pelvic examination and transvaginal ultrasonography, has been proposed as a method for the early detection of ovarian cancer. Elevated CA-125 levels are not specific to ovarian cancer and have been observed in patients with non-gynecological cancers and in the presence of certain other conditions, such as the first trimester of pregnancy or endometriosis. The most commonly reported CA-125 reference value that designates a positive screening test is 35 U/ml. The sensitivity of CA-125 for the detection of ovarian cancer was determined in 2 nested case-control studies using serum banks. The sensitivity for CA-125 levels greater than or equal to 35 U/ml ranged from 20-57 percent for cases occurring within the first 3 years of follow-up; the specificity was 95 percent. A CA-125 screening program of 22,000 postmenopausal women with subsequent transabdominal ultrasound for those with elevated CA-125 levels (reference value of 30 U/ml) detected 11 of 19 cases of ovarian cancer occurring in the cohort for an apparent sensitivity of 588. The specificity for this screening study was 99.9 percent. Three of the 11 cases detected on screening were stage I disease. In one prospective screening study, the specificity of CA-125 levels of 35 U/ml was 97.6 percent.

The available evidence suggests that using CA-125 alone, particularly at a reference value of 35 U/ml, does not have a sufficiently high sensitivity to be recommended for routine screening of ovarian cancer. The use of multiple modalities including bimanual examination, transvaginal ultrasonography, and CA-125 serum levels may be a means to improve sensitivity and maintain an adequate level of specificity. The cost of tests such as ultrasonography, in addition to the risks and cost associated with subsequent surgical evaluation of false positive test results, is a potential impediment to routine screening. Recent reports from several ovarian cancer screening centers stress the difficulties of multimodulent screening in high-risk populations. A decision analysis model used to evaluate the potential effect of ovarian cancer screening predicted little improvement in life expectancy as a result of mass screening.

Whether measurement of CA-125 levels as a component of a multimodality screening program may be useful requires further evaluation in controlled clinical trials as none of these methods are of proven benefit for the early detection of ovarian cancer. A National Cancer Institute multicenter trial is underway to test the utility of transvaginal ultrasound and CA-125 measurement in reducing the mortality from ovarian cancer.

Screening for Cervical Cancer

Summary of Evidence

Evidence strongly suggests a decrease in mortality from regular screening with Pap tests in women who are sexually active or who have reached 18 years of age. The upper age limit at which to cease screening is unknown.

In 1995, an estimated 15,800 cases of invasive cervical cancer are expected to occur, with about 4,800 women dying from this disease. From 1950-1970, the incidence and mortality rates of invasive cervical cancer fell impressively by more than 70 percent. Since the early 1980s, however, the rates for incidence and mortality appear to be decreasing more slowly. According to incidence and mortality rates, screening for cervical cancer should start in the late teens when these rates begin their upward trend. Rates for carcinoma in situ reach a peak for both black and white women between 20 and 30 years of age.

After the age of 25, however, the incidence of invasive cancer in black women increases rapidly with age, while in white women the incidence rises more slowly. Mortality also increases with advancing age, with dramatic differences between black and white women.

Extra effort is warranted to reach older women who have not been screened. Over 25 percent of the total number of invasive cervical cancers occur in women older than 65, and 40-50 percent of all women who die from cervical cancer are over 65 years of age. A large proportion of women, particularly elderly black women and middle-aged poor women, have not had regular Pap smears. In some areas, as many as 75 percent of women over 65 have not had a Pap smear within the previous 5 years. These patterns underscore the importance of special screening efforts targeted to reach women who do not receive regular screening.

Evidence of Benefit

The widespread acceptance of the Pap smear makes the possibility of testing the efficacy of cervical cytology by randomized trials remote. There is, nevertheless, substantial evidence from observational studies that mortality from cervical cancer can be reduced by screening.

Mortality from cervical cancer has decreased in several large populations following the introduction of well-run screening programs. Data from several large Scandinavian studies show sharp reductions in incidence and mortality following the initiation of organized screening programs. Iceland reduced mortality rates by 80 percent over 20 years, and Finland and Sweden reduced their mortality 50 percent and 34 percent, respectively. Similar reductions have been found in large populations in the US and Canada.

Reductions in incidence and mortality seem to be proportional to the intensity of screening efforts. The Scandinavian countries with the highest rates of screening activity reported greater reductions in mortality than those countries with lower rates of screening. Mortality in the Canadian provinces was reduced most remarkably in British Columbia, which had screening rates two to five times that of the other provinces.

Case-control studies have found that the risk of developing invasive cervical cancer is 3-10 times greater in women who have not been screened. Risk also increases with longer duration following the last normal Pap smear, or similarly, with decreasing frequency of screening. Screening every 2-3 years, however, has not been found to increase significantly the risk of finding invasive cervical cancer above the risk expected with annual screening.

The analysis of survival data shows that survival appears to be directly related to the stage of disease at diagnosis. The 5-year relative survival rate for cervical cancer is 88 percent for women with an initial diagnosis of localized disease. For those initially diagnosed with distant disease, the survival is only 13 percent. Early detection, using cervical cytology, is currently the only practical means of detecting cervical cancer in localized or premalignant stages.

Targeting High-Risk Patients

Progress in mortality reduction will be accelerated most significantly by increasing the percentage of cervical neoplasms discovered in the precancerous or localized stages. This can be accomplished most effectively by screening women at greatest risk for cervical cancer, i.e. those who have not had a Pap test or those who have not had one for several years. These women are often older, are often of lower socioeconomic status, may be members of minority groups, and are often seen by physicians for a variety of acute and chronic conditions unrelated to preventive medical care. Other well-known risk factors, such as early age of first intercourse and multiple sexual partners, have less practical clinical significance due to the difficulty in obtaining adequate histories of these risk factors. Recent advances in understanding the relationship between specific HPV types and the risk of cervical cancer may have future applications in targeting high-risk groups for screening and other preventive interventions. For example, serologic markers of HPV infection may eventually prove useful in identifying women at risk for developing cervical cancer.

Chapter 36

Cancer Programs Make Good Business Sense

This fact sheet contains the information you will need to develop a rationale for implementing a breast cancer screening program in your corporation. It provides facts on the growing number of women in the workforce, the economic impact of breast cancer, and the costs and benefits of having an early detection program, both monetary and less tangible.

We encourage you to use this information as a tool to build support for a worksite screening program within your corporation. Some of the facts included would also be useful for employee newsletters, flyers, or during media contacts. Once you do develop a program, you can use this information to garner attention for your role as a responsible employer.

Introduction

Breast cancer continues to be a leading cause of cancer death among women, second only to lung cancer. The best way to detect breast cancer early is with screening mammography. Screening mammograms are breast x-rays for women who have no symptoms of breast cancer. These x-rays can detect breast cancer up to 2 years before a lump can be felt. Still, not enough women are getting regular mammograms. Too often women do not return every 1 to 2 years for

---

National Cancer Institute Pub. K/67, February 1994.

continued screening. The workplace provides an ideal setting to reach women with this lifesaving test.

More Women in the Workplace

All women are at risk for breast cancer. The two main risk factors are being a woman and getting older. Risk increases sharply after age 50.

An estimated 182,000 new cases of breast cancer and 46,000 deaths will occur in U.S. females in 1994.

Eighty percent of all breast cancer cases diagnosed occur in women ages 50 and older.

Almost 11 million women ages 50 and older were part of the U.S. workforce in 1993.

The National Cancer Institute reports that screening mammography for women ages 50 and older, when it is done every 1 to 2 years, potentially can reduce breast cancer deaths by one-third or more for women in this age group.

Breast Cancer Has an Enormous Economic Impact on Private Industry

1990 estimated costs of breast cancer borne by U.S. private industry employers and employees included: treatment costs—$937 million; disability costs—$567 million; and lost earnings due to premature death—$2.71 billion.

Costs that do not invoke dollar figures include the personal effects of cancer, such as pain and suffering, distress and anxiety, disruption of family life, and possible loss of life.

Breast Cancer Is More Costly If Treated Late

Recent unpublished estimates indicate that initial-treatment costs for breast cancer patients are greater if the disease is diagnosed at a more advanced stage, when it has begun to spread. The cost of initial treatment for cancer confined to the breast is $8,008; initial treatment of disease that has spread to nearby lymph nodes costs $8,132; and initial treatment of disease that has spread to other organs costs $10,300. These cost differences are based on Medicare charges. Cost differences for women under age 65 are, most likely, substantially larger.

Continuing medical costs for breast cancer survivors also increase if the disease is diagnosed at a more advanced stage. Disease confined to the breast costs $207/month; disease that has spread to nearby lymph nodes costs $281/month; and disease that has spread to other organs costs $282/month.

Care for a cancer patient during the last six months of life is approximately $14,000. This so-called terminal care for diseases other than cancer costs $10,000.

The differences in cost between early and advanced-stage breast cancer illustrate the financial importance of detecting cancer early, when treatment is less extensive and less costly.

Other costs that an employer can potentially avoid or minimize with early detection, include sick leave, disability payments, and costs of hiring and training temporary employees.

Adolph Coors Brewing Company calculated the cost impact of its breast cancer screening program, called Coorscreen. Based on the costs of direct medical care, short and longterm disability, hiring and training temporary replacements, and payment of ongoing benefits, the company calculated a difference of $132,000 between the cost of treating a woman with early stage breast cancer and a woman with late stage breast cancer.

Mammograms Need Not Be Costly

The average cost of a screening mammogram is approximately $90, but can range from less than $35 to $225. A number of corporations have negotiated $50 fees with local mammography facilities or mobile mammography vans.

Insurance coverage for mammography screening is becoming widespread. As of 1993, more than 40 states and the District of Columbia now have laws requiring health insurance companies to reimburse all or part of the cost of screening mammograms; for women 65 and older, the Federal Medicare program pays some of the costs for mammography every 2 years. In 1992, this program spent $204 million toward 4.4 million mammograms.

A workplace breast cancer screening program will incur initial start-up costs, which will vary based on the financial involvement chosen by the corporation. As the program continues through a number of years, program costs will decrease and benefits will continue to accrue. These benefits include years of life saved, savings in initial care costs and terminal care costs. Other benefits include improved employee morale and a corporate image reflecting responsibility and interest in employee welfare.

One Mammogram Is Not Enough

Only half of all women ages 50 and older have had a mammogram in the past 2 years and as few as 30 percent are having mammograms routinely. Older women, who are at greatest risk for breast cancer, are less likely to have mammograms as they age, and fewer than 25 percent of women over 65 have regular mammograms.

The reasons most often mentioned by women for not getting mammograms are "no need" and lack of a physician's recommendation.

Cost appears to be a barrier among women who have had one mammogram but have not returned for additional exams at the recommended interval.

A greater percentage of black women than white women have never had a mammogram (42% versus 35%).

Income and education levels correlate with mammogram use. Nearly half (43%) of women with annual household incomes under $15,000 and who have less than a high school degree have never had a mammogram, compared with less than a quarter (23%) of women with annual household incomes over $50,000 and a high school degree.

Corporations Cite Rationale for Screening/Wellness Programs

A recent survey showed that two-thirds of all U.S. worksites with 50 or more employees have at least one screening or wellness program in place.

A main reason corporations cite for initiating workplace screening or wellness programs is their potential to help contain rising health care costs.

Other reasons include better employee performance, less absenteeism, and the long-range benefits of a healthier workforce. Less tangible reasons include improved employee morale and providing employees with a sense of empowerment

Cancer Programs Make Good Business Sense

Screening and wellness programs are viewed by some corporations as more than a "perk"; rather, they are seen as an effective mechanism for attracting and retaining good, dedicated employees. Companies that regard their employees as their greatest resource know that maintaining and improving employee health is an important goal.

Getting Started Is Easy

Corporations interested in developing a breast cancer screening program can find help from a variety of sources. One is the National Cancer Institute's booklet: *Establishing Workplace Breast Cancer Screening Programs*. This publication provides detailed information about structuring the screening program, choosing a mammography provider, negotiating a contract, working with a corporate insurance plan, designing an educational component, selecting marketing strategies, and evaluating program effectiveness. *(This booklet is reproduced in the next chapter).*

Additional information and materials about breast cancer or any other cancer is available through NCI's Cancer Information Service at 1-800-4-CANCER (1-800-422-6237) Local divisions of the American Cancer Society can also provide information.

Chapter 37

Establishing Workplace Breast Cancer Screening Programs

Introduction

Breast cancer is a leading cause of cancer death among American women, second only to lung cancer. These deaths could be reduced significantly if all women had regular mammograms and breast exams by a doctor or nurse starting at age 50. Women are not taking full advantage of these early detection methods.

Almost 11 million women ages 50 and older were in the U.S. workforce in 1993. This makes the workplace an ideal setting to reach women with messages regarding the importance of early detection and to provide breast cancer screening programs.

A number of corporations already provide these services. Their insights on how to develop a breast cancer screening program are incorporated within this document. This chapter explains the benefits of a worksite program—both to the employer and employees and lists the "Top 10 Workplace Breast Cancer Activities." For a complete kit, including promotional materials and publication order forms, contact NCI at 1-800-4-Cancer (1-800-422-6237) or a local office.

These materials, used in conjunction with this planning document, will provide you with all of the information you will need to develop a screening program within your company and encourage female employees to take advantage of the company program.

National Cancer Institute Pub. K/60, February 1994.

Getting Started

Establish a Planning Committee

Most probably your corporation has already identified a department or division to lead and direct the breast cancer screening program. Companies with similar screening programs in place report working through their corporate medical departments/wellness programs, or human resources/benefits departments.

You will probably find it helpful to have a small committee to assist you in your planning efforts. A representative from each of the following areas would be appropriate:

- Corporate medical department or employee health services
- Human resources department
- Communications, marketing, or public relations department
- Legal department
- Union representative (should be able to represent the women you are trying to reach) or employee representative if your company is nonunion.

Gather Data on Demographics of Female Employees

To estimate program needs over a 3- to 5-year period, count the number of women in your company within the 50 or older age range. You could also survey your female employees ages 50 and older to determine their interest in a worksite screening program and find out what educational information and resources they need. This information would help provide internal support for the program as well as assist you in planning the program.

Prepare a Program Timetable

An important planning step is to develop a timetable or schedule for program development and implementation. The timetable should include the name of the person responsible, due date, and resources required for each task in your plan. Everyone on your planning committee should have a copy of the timetable. It should be considered a flexible management tool and should be updated regularly (e.g. monthly) so it can function to both manage and track progress.

Establishing Workplace Breast Cancer Screening Programs

Following NCI's Evaluation of Screening Mammography

Your corporation's screening program should encourage women employees, starting at age 50, to get screening mammograms. In a recent evaluation of the effectiveness of screening mammography worldwide, NCI concluded that routine mammograms every 1 to 2 years and clinical breast exams every year for women ages 50 and older could reduce the breast cancer death rate by 30 percent or more for this group of women.

Structuring the Screening Program

There are at least four options open to you as you begin to structure your breast cancer screening program. These options vary in the level of corporate involvement and each carries its own set of advantages and disadvantages. You will have to decide which option will be the most effective for your corporation.

1. **Corporation contracts with a mobile mammography van.** *Mobile van and staff come to corporation on pre-arranged dates, times; mammograms performed and interpreted by mobile van provider.*

    PRO:

    Often requires the least corporate involvement as some mobile van providers will schedule appointments, obtain patient consent forms, maintain records, send reports, and handle followup.

    Employees will not need time off from work to travel to screening site.

    CON:

    Corporation must handle administrative details if provider does not.

    Space must be available for parking of large mobile van.

2. **Corporation contracts with a mammography provider to bring portable mammography equipment to corporate offices.** *Provider supplies technologist; radiologist interprets mammograms offsite.*

   PRO

   Employees will not need time off from work to travel to screening site.

   CON

   Requires the temporary allocation of suitable space within the corporate offices.

   Corporation may be responsible for scheduling appointments, obtaining patient consent forms, maintaining records, sending reports, and handling followup as appropriate.

3. **Corporation contracts with an offsite mammography facility.** *Mammographic examinations are performed and intrepreted offsite. Scheduling appointments can be handled either by corporation or by mammography facility.*

   PRO:

   Less expensive than options cited above; involves less work for corporation. Outside provider obtains patient consent forms, maintains records, sends reports, and handles followup as appropriate.

   CON:

   May need to provide employees with time off from work to travel to screening site, unless evening or weekend hours can be negotiated.

Establishing Workplace Breast Cancer Screening Programs

4. **Corporation purchases mammography equipment and provides mammograms on site.** *Corporation hires a technologist to perform mammograms on-site, without a radiologist in attendance; contracts with an outside radiologist to interpret mammograms. In some states, corporations must receive approval from the department of health prior to purchasing equipment. All states require that radiologic equipment be registered.*

PRO:

Offers the most convenience to employees if equipment is a permanent fixture in corporation.

CON:

Only cost effective if corporation has a large number of eligible employees; requires a high level of corporate involvement for scheduling appointments, obtaining patient consent forms, maintaining records, sending reports, and handling followup.

There already are more mammography machines in the United States than consumer demand requires.

Corporation must ensure quality of machine and its operation.

Choosing a Mammography Company

The two most important issues to consider in choosing a company to provide the mammograms are quality and cost. One sign of quality is the American College of Radiology's (ACR) voluntary accreditation program for mammography facilities.

As of August 1993, 8,075 facilities have applied for accreditation of 10,758 units. Of those units, 5,619 have been accredited. The NCI's Cancer Information Service (CIS), 1-800-4-CANCER, can provide you with the names of accredited facilities in your area.

If there is no ACR-accredited facility in your area, you should contact your city or state health department, local hospital or medical center, American Cancer Society (ACS) division, the Cancer Information Service, or the Komen Foundation (at 1-800-I'M-AWARE) for a list of local breast cancer screening centers.

The following list of questions should be asked of non-accredited providers to be sure that their mammography machines are high quality and the technologist who conducts the exams and the radiologist who reads the films are well qualified. Choose a provider that answers "YES" to all five of these questions:

1. Does the facility use machines specifically designed for mammography? These are called "dedicated" mammography machines. You should not choose a company that uses a machine that also takes x-rays of the bones and other parts of the body.

2. Is the person who takes the mammograms a registered technologist? These people must be trained to position the breasts correctly to get a good image. They should be certified by the American Registry of Radiological Technologists or be licensed by the state.

3. Is the radiologist who reads the mammograms specially trained to do so? The radiologist should be board certified and should have taken special courses in mammography.

4. Does the facility provide mammograms as part of its regular practice? The ACR suggests choosing a facility that performs at least 10 mammograms each week.

5. Is the mammography machine calibrated at least once a year? The machine should be checked against a standard to be sure that its measurements and doses are correct. Adjustments are made if necessary.

Negotiating a Contract

Your next step is to meet with the chosen mammography company and negotiate a contract. Mammography screening should include two-view imaging of each breast to ensure a thorough exam. You will also have to determine the charge per mammogram exam and the length of the screening program. Depending on the size of your corporation, the program could operate for a specified period of time or continue indefinitely.

A critical principle in providing screening mammography is to schedule a large number of women in a short period of time so that the cost per woman is low. Quality performance and low cost are key elements. Although the average cost of a screening mammogram is usually between $100 and $125, a number of model programs have been developed for year-round mammography centers or mobile vans that charge $50 or less. If you are offering your screening program on-site, you will need a sufficiently large number of eligible women participating in the program for the provider to be able to offer you a competitive price. Some corporations that do not have a large number of eligible women have offered the program to spouses of male employees for a fee. Other small corporations have approached neighboring companies to establish a joint program, thereby gathering enough women to negotiate a low cost.

As a rule of thumb, past experiences show that 20 mammography exams per day are needed to minimize costs. By meeting this minimum number, you should be able to negotiate a contract in which the provider will perform screening mammograms within the $40 to $65 range.

If you are providing mammograms off-site, that is, at a radiologist's office, you still may be able to negotiate a low fee-especially if the radiologist has a sufficient number of clients from other sources to help contain costs.

Working With Corporate Insurance Plans

More than 40 states require insurance companies to provide some level of coverage for screening mammography. Medicare is also now providing some reimbursement to women 65 and older, as well as to disabled Medicare beneficiaries for regular screening mammograms.

You will have to determine the position of your corporate insurance provider. In either case, you must negotiate an acceptable arrangement between the insurance plan and the mammography provider.

If your company is one of the many that are self-insured, you will need to negotiate with those responsible for administering the program. On the other hand, if your corporation participates in an outside insurance plan (with or without co-payments), you will have to meet with a representative of the plan to negotiate this arrangement. Your corporation's human resources department should be able to put you in touch with the appropriate individual(s).

The actual cost of the mammogram can be shared by the company, the insurance plan, and, if you decide to charge the participants, by the participating employees. Some corporations sponsoring breast cancer screening programs charge each participating employee a small fee ranging from $5 to $15, citing the benefits of having employees "own" part of the program. Other corporations provide the screening free to all eligible employees. This decision should be made at the local level.

Ensuring Adequate Followup

What to Do with Suspicious Findings?

When developing your program, be sure to have in place a mechanism for ensuring that employees whose mammograms reveal a problem will receive appropriate followup care. This includes actions such as physician notification, and providing the employee with referral numbers to obtain more information.

Encourage Continued Screening Practices

Because early detection for breast cancer is only truly successful if practiced regularly, your corporation should provide an in-house promotion encouraging women to get screened and practice early detection regularly. The best case is for the corporation to provide the screening program from year to year. If that is impossible, reminders to employees, through regular corporate communications channels (payroll stuffers, newsletters, bulletin boards), could encourage them to seek continued breast cancer screenings and illustrate to them your continued concern for their health.

Designing an Educational Program

Many corporations include an educational segment in their breast screening programs to explain to employees the corporation's involvement in such a program, along with the importance of mammography, clinical breast exams, and breast self-exams (BSE). Some also provide instructions for performing breast self-exams and list information resources for other questions.

Set Program Objectives

The first step is to decide on the scope of your educational program and to set objectives. Suggested objectives of an educational program focusing on breast cancer screening are.

1. Increase knowledge of breast cancer risk factors—focusing mainly on the fact that all women are at risk.

2. Increase awareness of mammography screening guidelines.

3. Overcome barriers that keep women from getting regular mammograms.

4. Increase number of women who get regular mammograms starting at age 50.

5. Increase number of women who have yearly clinical breast exams.

6. Increase the number of women who practice BSE monthly.

Identify Target Audiences

The second step in planning an educational program is to determine the target audience. Since the risk of developing breast cancer increases with age, female employees age 50 and over should be considered the primary target audience and encouraged to take part in both the screening and education portions of the program.

All female employees over age 18 can be considered as a secondary target audience and invited to participate in the educational program. You may want to consider extending the education and/or screening program to eligible employees' wives and female retirees.

Male employees would also benefit from the education portion of the program, and should be encouraged to share the information with their female family members and friends.

Choose an Education Approach

There are a number of ways to reach your employees with breast cancer education messages. These include distribution of written materials, one-on-one discussion during an employee's physical exam, or classroom-type presentations integrating the use of audiovisual films or programs, and a personal presentation by a health professional or another credible source to educate and inform participants. Personal interaction is a desirable technique to teach women about breast cancer because of the complexity and sensitive nature of the subject.

It is often desirable to involve a health professional who can answer technical questions. Good resources include:

1. A representative from your corporate medical department (e.g. company nurse)

2. A qualified staff member from a local mammography facility

3. A representative from a local hospital or medical center, city or state health department, CIS, or ACS division.

Many resources are available to assist you in your education efforts. Contact the CIS for help in locating slide or videotape presentations about mammography and additional materials.

Develop Education Messages

The information to be communicated in an educational program on breast cancer screening includes:

Establishing Workplace Breast Cancer Screening Programs

1. All women are at risk for breast cancer—including those with no family history of the disease. The two main risk factors are being a woman and getting older.

2. For women ages 50 and older, early detection plus prompt treatment can improve significantly the chances for survival.

3. Mammography can find breast cancer in its earliest stages—up to 2 years before a lump can be felt.

4. Not enough women are getting regular mammograms. Only half of all women ages 50 and older have had a mammogram in the past 2 years, and as few as 30 percent are having mammograms routinely. Starting at age 50, a woman should get a mammogram every 1 to 2 years.

5. Mammography and clinical breast exams are the most effective methods for detecting breast cancer. These two methods are the primary screening procedures available to women. Breast self-examinations are secondary in importance when screening for breast cancer.

6. Mammograms are simple and the radiation risk is negligible.

These messages will help you break a main barrier that keeps women from getting mammograms—they do not think that they need them. Women have listed other barriers to getting mammograms that can be addressed in your education programs. These are:

- Lack of a physician referral or support
- No access to a screening program or access is too inconvenient
- Cost, especially for women who do not return for repeat mammograms as recommended
- Concern about the safety of the test and/or fear of radiation.

Select Marketing Strategies

Now that you have developed a plan for a successful program, the next step is to market the program within your corporation. These barriers will be overcome if you set appropriate educational objectives, invite a health professional to participate in your program, hold the program on site (or make it easily accessible), provide employees with time off from work to participate, and offer the program free or at minimal cost. These facts should be included in all of your promotional materials.

Marketing techniques that have proven successful in company sponsored breast cancer screening programs include:

1. Direct-mail campaign with information on the program sent to all eligible employees/dependents/retirees

2. Paycheck stuffers with similar information

3. Posters for company bulletin boards

4. Information sheets and sign-up forms placed on tables in reception areas, cafeterias, employee lounges, restrooms, locker rooms, and other places where women gather

5. Articles in employee magazine, newsletter, or newspaper.

Consider enlisting help from your employees. One corporation with a successful program organized a group of female employees who communicated the importance of breast cancer screening to other workers under the slogan "Talk to a Friend."

Plan to tie-in with National Breast Cancer Awareness Month in October. For information on how your corporation can get involved, contact the National Alliance of Breast Cancer Organizations (NABCO) at 1180 Avenue of the Americas, New York, NY 10036. Local media are often interested in covering corporate screening efforts. Consider contacting the media once your program is developed to garner positive recognition of your program.

Establishing Workplace Breast Cancer Screening Programs

Evaluating Program Effectiveness

Outcome evaluation usually consists of a comparison between the target audience's awareness, attitudes, and/or behavior before and after the program. These are quantitative measures that are necessary to allow you to draw conclusions about the effect or impact of the program. The measures may be self-reported (e.g. gathered by conducting interviews or using questionnaires to obtain information from members of your target audience) or they may be observational (e.g. noting changes in behavior among members of your target audience).

Refer Back to Program Objectives

To evaluate your program, refer back to the program objectives you developed at the beginning of the planning process. This list will give you a clear definition of the program's desired achievements.

For example, based on the objectives listed previously, the following are some suggested ways to measure program effectiveness:

1. Percentage of female employees who participate in the educational program component

2. Percentage of eligible women who participate in the breast cancer screening portion of the program

3. Percentage of women who return at recommended intervals for regular mammograms

4. Percentage of women who report requesting and/or obtaining a clinical breast exam during their routine checkups

5. Number of women with breast cancer detected by the program. (Rate should be approximately 2 to 4 cancers per 1,000 women screened.)

You will want to summarize pertinent data from this impact evaluation and present a written evaluation report to corporate management with recommendations about the future of the program.

Evaluation Constraints

Every program planner faces constraints to undertaking evaluation. These constraints may include limited funds, limited staff time and capabilities, and length of time allotted to the program. However, undertaking some measurement of program effectiveness will enable you to recommend continuation or termination of the program, make adjustments in the program design, and/or begin planning other health promotion initiatives.

For more information on breast cancer or information on other cancer control programs, such as smoking cessation, nutrition, or other screening programs, contact the National Cancer Institute's Cancer Information Service at 1-800-4-CANCER (1-800-422-6237) or your local division of the American Cancer Society.

For information on breast screening centers, call the Komen Foundation at 1-800-I'M-AWARE.

Top 10 List of Workplace Breast Cancer Activities

1. **Provide all employees with the 1-800-4-CANCER information phone number**

   The Cancer Information Service of the National Cancer Institute is a national network including 19 offices across the country. It provides callers access to up-to-date information about cancer causes and prevention, detection, diagnosis, treatment, rehabilitation, and continuing care. Anyone may call this number. By dialing 1-800-4-CANCER (1-800-422-6237), the caller is automatically put in touch with the CIS office in his or her area. The number can be posted in public areas, circulated in a memo, or even stamped on pay envelopes.

2. **Include stories about breast cancer education, detection, and treatment in the employee newsletter or video news.**

   Newsletter articles are available from the Cancer Information Service Companies with newsletter staff can write their own stories. Add local information such as where to get additional information, locations of mammography services etc..

3. **Post breast cancer information and the 1-800-4-CANCER number on bulletin boards, in cafeterias, women's restrooms, and other places employees are likely to see it. In addition, have breast cancer treatment information available for employees in the medical or benefits office.**

   Ready-to-copy brochures, posters, and newsletter articles are available from the National Cancer Institute's Cancer Information Service at 1-800-4-CANCER (1-800-422-6237) or local American Cancer Society chapters.

4. **Sponsor on-site breast cancer exhibits or information sessions. Ask the company physician or nurse and/ or representatives of a local cancer center to staff the exhibit/session to answer questions and distribute literature.**

5. **Gather information about local mammography facilities' quality, costs, and hours. Share this information with your employees in a letter, a brochure with additional educational information, in the employee newsletter, etc.**

6. **Cosponsor seminars on breast cancer prevention, detection, and treatment with a local hospital, medical society, or health maintenance organization. Schedule seminars on company time or immediately before or after the workday. Plan one version for employees and one for your company's medical staff. Distribute literature from the CIS at each.**

7. **Arrange for low cost or free onsite breast cancer screenings for employees by contacting local hospitals, health maintenance organizations, radiology groups, or American Cancer Society chapters.**

8. **Work with your health insurer to include insurance coverage for mammography if the plan does not currently include this benefit.**

9. **Have your company's directors and/or senior management make a permanent commitment to educating its female employees about the importance of early detection and treatment of breast cancer.**

    This can be done through a corporate resolution—a mandate from senior management to make educational materials and mammography services available to employees, spouses, and retirees.

10. **Become a model for other local companies to follow in the effort to save women's lives.**

Acknowledgments

This Blueprint for Action was developed with help from a number of corporations with innovative worksite screening programs, as well as health organizations that work to encourage and facilitate worksite screening efforts. Their assistance and willingness to share insights and knowledge made this document possible.

Thanks go to Adolph Coors Brewing Company, AT&T, DuPont Company, General Mills, ICI Pharmaceuticals Group, Manufacturers Hanover Trust, Martin Marietta Energy Systems, Metropolitan Life, Levi Strauss & Co., North Carolina National Bank, and Sara Lee Corporation.

Thanks go to the following health organizations as well. The American Cancer Society, Komen Foundation, National Alliance of Breast Cancer Organizations, National Cancer Care Foundation, Memorial Sloan-Kettering Cancer Center, Washington Business Group on Health, and the Wisconsin Division of Health's Department of Health and Social Services.

Chapter 38

The Papanicolaou Test: Routine Cancer Detection with the Pap Smear

The Controversial Pap Test: It Could Save Your Life

Sixty-five years ago, George Papanicolaou, M.D., observed that cervical cancer could be detected by studying cells taken from a woman's genital tract. His finding was put to use 25 years later with the development of the Pap test, named after him.

In the decades since then, the Pap test has become a routine part of gynecologic examinations and one of the most widely used procedures for detecting cancer. The American Cancer Society credits the Pap smear—so called because cells are "smeared" on a glass slide—and regular gynecologic check-ups with cutting deaths from cervical cancer by 70 percent over the last 40 years. Although 6,000 women will die from it this year, four decades ago cervical cancer claimed the lives of 20,000 American women annually. For years, Pap test results have reassured millions of women that they are either free of cervical cancer or it has been detected at an early stage, with a high probability of cure.

Recently, though, the Pap test has been surrounded by controversy. Reports suggest that 10 to 40 percent of cervical cancers or the cell abnormalities that precede them may be missed because of sloppy laboratory work or poor tissue sampling. The reports have prompted medical organizations and the federal government to investigate qual-

---

DHHS (FDA) 90-1159 and NCI Cancerfax 208/600156.

ity control in Pap testing and propose stricter standards to ensure more reliable test results for cervical cancer and other diseases and conditions.

Meanwhile, researchers are trying to devise more accurate ways to detect the early signs of cervical cancer and to zero in on who is at risk for it. At the same time, health and medical groups once at odds over guidelines for cervical cancer screening have joined forces to develop unified recommendations for how often women should have a Pap test.

The Best Screening Tool for Cancer

"For all the problems that have come to the forefront, the Pap smear is still by far the best screening tool we have for any cancer," says William Creasman, M.D., professor and head of the Department of Obstetrics and Gynecology at the University of South Carolina and head of the cancer screening task force of the American College of Obstetricians and Gynecologists.

The American Cancer Society estimates that in 1989, 47,000 American women will be diagnosed with uterine cancer. Of these, 13,000 will be found to have cancer of the cervix—the neck of the uterus, which opens into the vagina. The remaining 34,000 women will be diagnosed with cancer of the body of the uterus or of the endometrium, its lining.

Cervical cancer develops slowly over years, and when caught early is very curable. In the very earliest stages of cervical cancer, cells on the surface of the cervix change in structure—a condition known as dysplasia. Dysplasia is most often treated by cryosurgery (freezing) or laser therapy. In some cases, however, effective treatment calls for surgical excision of the lesion or hysterectomy—surgical removal of the entire uterus.

In the next step, abnormal cells develop into a localized cancer ("carcinoma in situ"). Carcinoma in situ is virtually 100 percent curable by surgery—either conization, in which a cone of tissue surrounding the cancer is removed, or a total hysterectomy. The choice of procedure often depends on whether the woman wants to have children. For patients diagnosed early but with more invasive cancer, the survival rate is from 80 to 90 percent, and treatment involves radiation, hysterectomy or both. The five-year survival rate for all cervical cancer patients is 66 percent, according to the American Cancer Soci-

The Papanicolaou Test: Routine Cancer Detection

ety, which implies that some cases are not being found and treated early.

Properly done, the Pap test is highly effective in detecting abnormal cervical cells before they become cancerous. (It is only about 50 percent effective in detecting endometrial cancer. Because endometrial cancer afflicts mostly middle-aged or older women, the American Cancer Society recommends that women at risk of this disease have tissue samples taken (curretage) at menopause. Their risk factors include infertility, obesity, failure to ovulate, and prolonged estrogen therapy.)

A Labor-Intensive Test

The accuracy of the Pap test depends on meticulous care in each of its steps, from cell collection, preparation, and staining on the slide to the interpretation of each specimen.

The test is a "uniquely labor intensive complex process" compared with other medical and laboratory tests, and its outcome "depends entirely on human judgment," states Leonard G. Koss, M.D., pathologist at the Albert Einstein College of Medicine, the Bronx, N.Y., in a recent issue of the Journal of the American Medical Association. Improperly done, the value of the test is "seriously compromised," notes the American Medical Association in a recent report on quality control in Pap testing.

The Pap smear is a seemingly easy procedure. A hollow tube-like instrument called a speculum is inserted into the vagina to spread the walls and expose the cervix. Then a cotton-tipped swab, wooden spatula, or cervical brush is used to collect cells from the opening of the cervix and its inner and outer surfaces. The cells are quickly pressed on a glass slide and "fixed" to prevent them from drying and changing appearance.

The doctor or nurse must take important information about the patient, such as age and obstetric and gynecologic history, which is forwarded along with the slide to the testing laboratory. There the sample is examined under a microscope by specially trained technologists who search for abnormalities among the 50,000 to 300,000 cells on each slide. Any suspicious slides are sent on to a pathologist.

In the past, Pap smear diagnoses were often reported as a class number, one through five. In 1988, a workshop sponsored by the National Cancer Institute developed a new format called the "Bethesda System," which uses descriptive terms for reporting Pap smear results. Cytopathology laboratories are encouraged to use such descriptive diagnoses in order to improve communication with the physician and patient.

Koss estimates that from 10 to 20 percent of Pap smears are inadequate from the first step. "It is generally assumed that obtaining a cervical smear is an easily executed, clinically simple procedure," says Koss. "This is not true."

Some practitioners don't do it properly—either not collecting enough cells, collecting them from the wrong place, or fixing them improperly on the slide—and so a flawed sample is sent for screening. And some laboratories, perhaps fearful of losing the physician's business, do not reject poor samples, according to Creasman.

Screening of the samples may be inadequate, too. In November 1987, the Wall Street Journal reported that some so-called "Pap mills" around the country screen smears much too quickly and in haphazard ways that may fail to reveal abnormalities. The Journal's report set off congressional and professional reviews of the quality control of medical testing and prompted legislation to tighten regulations of laboratories that do Pap screening.

Koss estimates that each smear requires at least five minutes of study. The American Society of Cytotechnology suggests that no technologist screen more than 12,000 cases annually—or 50 to 100 slides a day. (A case may consist of one or two slides.) Yet, the Wall Street Journal reported laboratories in which individual workers screened as many as 35,000 slides in a single year.

New Quality Control Regulations

The American College of Obstetricians and Gynecologists believes that up to 40 percent of Pap smears may fail to disclose cancer or the cellular abnormalities that can lead to it. As many as half of those errors may result from inadequate sampling; the rest are apparently caused by shortcomings in the laboratories.

Currently, the federal Centers for Disease Control requires that cytology laboratories engaged in interstate commerce (and thus subject to federal regulation) must rescreen 10 percent of negative Pap smears as a means of quality control. New York State licenses laboratories only after a mandatory examination of the cytotechnologists. A California law forbids that state's cytotechnologists from screening more than 75 slides a day. And Congress last year amended the 20-

The Papanicolaou Test: Routine Cancer Detection

year-old Clinical Laboratory Improvement Act to require quality standards for the estimated 12,000 labs receiving Medicare and Medicaid funding or engaging in interstate commerce. Congress also ordered the Health Care Financing Administration (HCFA) to regulate doctors' office laboratories that examine Pap smears.

In effect, HCFA officials say, the new rules will cover nearly all commercial laboratories and should go a long way toward improving cervical cancer detection. Among the requirements: proficiency testing for examiners and laboratories and a ceiling on the number of slides to be screened by each technician. The new regulations, still being formulated, will take effect Jan. 1, 1990.

Out of the controversy comes hope for greater survival. Increased attention to quality control, a new consensus on Pap test guidelines, and research on who is at risk and how testing can be improved could eventually lower deaths from cervical cancer still further. "We certainly could knock the incidence of invasive disease down to a greater degree," says Creasman. "But we'll never get rid of it entirely because some women won't get Pap smears or won't get them done when they should."

Who Should Be Tested—How Often?

For years, women and their doctors have been confused about how often Pap testing should be done because health organizations made different recommendations. Last year, seven medical, professional and scientific organizations announced new uniform guidelines for Pap testing.

The organizations, including the American Cancer Society and the American College of Obstetricians and Gynecologists (ACOG), determined that all women who are or have been sexually active or are over 18 should have an annual Pap test and pelvic examination. After three consecutive normal results, they said, the test could be done less often—if the woman and her doctor agree. However, the groups advised that all women at high risk for cervical cancer should have annual Pap tests.

If possible, the best time to have a Pap smear taken is 10 to 14 days after the first day of the last menstrual period. Women should avoid using vaginal douches or lubricants for 48 hours before the examination.

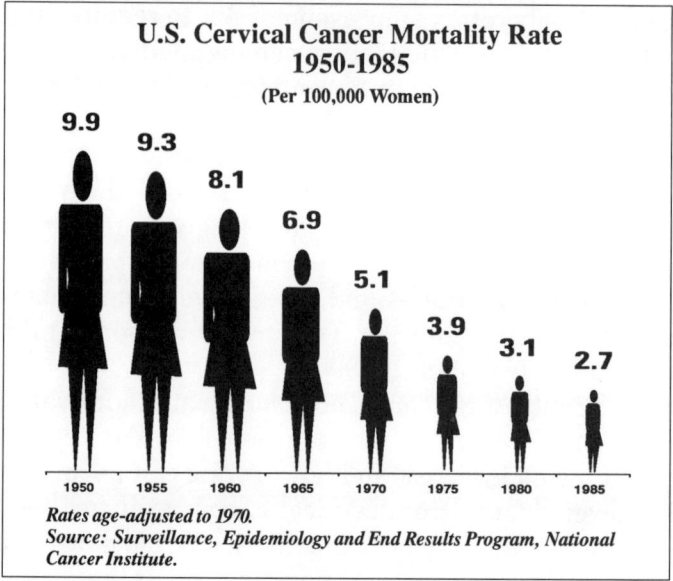

Figure 38.1. Cervical Cancer Mortality Rate.

Who Is at High Risk?

Studies show that women who become sexually active early in their teen years, who have multiple sex partners, who have their first child before the age of 20, and who have many pregnancies are at higher than average risk. Also at higher risk are women whose sex partners have other partners.

The risk of cervical cancer is much lower in women in monogamous relationships, and studies indicate that the disease occurs much less often in celibate women. But recent studies show that half of all married women and from 70 to 80 percent of married men have had multiple sex partners. About half of all teenagers have had more than one sexual partner by the time they reach 16, according to ACOG. In effect, then, the consortium of medical groups recommends that nearly all women who are sexually active have annual Pap tests regardless of age, according to Creasman.

"If a woman is in any of these high-risk groups, she should have annual Pap tests and cervical exams," says George Morley, M.D., the president of ACOG. "To do any less is to play Russian roulette with her life. The annual Pap test will be her early warning system to protect her health and perhaps her life."

The Papanicolaou Test: Routine Cancer Detection

Women whose mothers took the hormone diethylstilbestrol (DES) during pregnancy are at a higher risk of a rare form of vaginal cancer, which may be detected by a Pap test. Prescribed in the late 1940s and 1950s to prevent miscarriage, DES is no longer given for that purpose.

Some specialists estimate that most women who develop cervical cancer are infected with HPV. The incidence of HPV-caused genital warts has been increasing dramatically the last few years, suggesting an eventual increase in cervical cancer. Although a link between cervical cancer and herpes virus type 2 has also been suggested, it is far less certain than that between HPV and the disease.

In a study reported earlier this year in the Journal of the American Medical Association, University of Utah scientists noted another possible risk factor for cervical cancer: passive or active smoking. The researchers found that women who don't smoke but who are exposed to cigarette smoke for three hours or more a day were nearly three times more likely to get the disease. Women who smoke are more than three times as likely to get the disease. The Utah study has not yet been duplicated.

In the past, some doctors have suggested that women over 60 or 65 need not get Pap tests, but the new guidelines have no such cut-off. After three years of negative tests, older women, like younger ones, should discuss with their doctors how often they should have a Pap test.

Creasman also recommends that women who have had hysterectomies for treatment of a malignant cervical lesion should have an annual Pap test to make sure that the tumor has not recurred. If the hysterectomy was for a benign lesion, the risk is much lower and testing can be done every two to three years, he says.

Most important, say experts, is that every woman should discuss her risks with her physician and the two of them then should decide how often she should be tested.

Pap Test Saves Lives

Some instances of pre-cancerous cell changes are missed in Pap tests because changes in the cells are too slight for technologists to detect. Several companies are now working on tests that detect the human papilloma virus in cervical tissue before pre-cancerous lesions develop. The first such test, called Virapap, was approved by the Food and Drug Administration in January 1989 for use in high-risk women as an adjunct to the Pap smear.

Efforts are also under way to find better ways of reading the Pap smear. One technique involves using a computerized microscope to measure dye absorbed by cells—a potential clue to cancer or the cellular changes that precede it.

Still, Creasman believes there is nothing on the immediate horizon that will replace the Pap test. "We've been waiting for years to get a computer to do it . . . and we're still waiting." Says ACOG President Morley: "Our main defense against death from the disease is prevention. We can prevent death through early detection. We detect the disease through regular pelvic examinations and Pap tests. The earlier we detect it, the greater the chances for cure."

It may not be perfect, but the Pap test saves lives.

Where Goes That Smear?

Until better tests for cervical cancer come along and new federal guidelines controlling quality of laboratory testing are in place, William Creasman, M.D., head of the cancer screening task force for the American College of Obstetricians and Gynecologists, says women should question their physicians closely about Pap testing. He recommends the following:

- Ask where your specimen will be sent. Is the laboratory certified by a professional organization like the College of American Pathologists? If the lab does testing for Medicare—or Medicaid—funded patients, chances are it is accredited.

- Is the lab near your doctor? A doctor and laboratory that are close geographically are probably more likely to communicate. Also, if a lab is far away, it suggests that specimens are being sent that far to save money—not a good practice when your life is at stake.

The most important thing to remember, say experts, is that cervical cancer is one of the most curable of all cancers because the cellular changes that lead to it are slow to develop and can be detected by a Pap test.

—Ellen Hale

Ellen Hale is a free-lance writer in Washington, D.C.

The Papanicolaou Test: Routine Cancer Detection

Questions and Answers About the Pap Smear

What is a Pap smear?

The Pap smear, or Pap test, is a way to examine cells collected from the cervix and vagina. It can show the presence of infection, inflammation, abnormal cells, or cancer. A Pap smear and pelvic exam are important parts of a woman's routine health care.

What is a pelvic exam?

In a pelvic exam, the uterus, vagina, ovaries, fallopian tubes, bladder, and rectum are felt to find any abnormality in their shape or size. During a pelvic exam, an instrument called a speculum is used to widen the opening of the vagina so that the upper portion of the vagina and the cervix can be seen.

Why are a Pap smear and pelvic exam important?

As with many types of cancer, cancer of the cervix can be successfully treated and cured if it is detected early—before it becomes invasive. Regular Pap smears and pelvic exams could prevent most invasive cancers of the cervix.

Who performs a Pap smear?

Doctors and other specially trained health care professionals, such as physician assistants, nurse midwives, and nurse practitioners, may perform Pap smears and pelvic exams. These individuals are often called clinicians.

How is a Pap smear done?

A Pap smear is quick and painless; it can be done in a doctor's office, a clinic, or a hospital. While a woman lies on an exam table, the clinician inserts a speculum into her vagina to widen the opening. To do the test, a sample of cells is taken from in and around the cervix with a wooden scraper, a cotton swab, or a small cervical brush. The specimen is placed on a glass slide, which is sent to a laboratory for examination.

How often should a Pap smear be done?

Women who are or have been sexually active, or have reached age 18, should have a regular Pap smear and a physical exam. There is no upper age limit for Pap smears. Older women should continue to have regular physical exams, including a pelvic exam and a Pap smear. A woman who has had a hysterectomy (an operation to remove the uterus and cervix) should continue to have Pap smears. Her doctor may do a Pap smear less frequently, depending on the reason for the hysterectomy.

How are the results of a Pap smear reported?

The way of reporting Pap smear results has sometimes been confusing. For this reason, in 1988 a group of health care practitioners at a National Cancer Institute-sponsored workshop proposed a new reporting system. The "Bethesda system" is less ambiguous and provides clearer communication between the laboratory where the Pap smear is examined and the clinician who treats the patient.

What is the Bethesda system?

The Bethesda system uses specific, descriptive diagnoses rather than class numbers (1 to 5), which have been used to report Pap smear results in the past. The Bethesda system also includes an evaluation of the adequacy of the Pap smear, thereby reducing the likelihood of a false negative result due to an insufficient sample of cells. This system was described in the August 18, 1989, and the April 8, 1992, issues of the Journal of the American Medical Association. Many professional organizations have endorsed the Bethesda system, and it is becoming widely used.

How are the results of an abnormal Pap smear described?

Several different terms have been used to describe the abnormal cells that may be seen in Pap smears. In the Bethesda system, pre-cancerous conditions are called low-grade and high-grade squamous intraepithelial lesions. Other terms sometimes used to describe these abnormal cells are cervical intraepithelial neoplasia (CIN) and dysplasia.

The Papanicolaou Test: Routine Cancer Detection

What is dysplasia?

Dysplasia is one term that has been used to describe abnormal cells seen in a Pap smear. It is not cancer, although it may develop into very early cancer of the cervix. In dysplasia, normal cervical cells undergo a series of changes in their appearance. Although dysplastic cells look abnormal under the microscope, they do not invade nearby healthy tissue. Dysplasia is classified as mild, moderate, or severe, depending on how abnormal the cells appear under the microscope.

Part Four

Risk Factors and Current Research

Chapter 39

Breast Cancer and Low-Fat Diets

Women at high risk for breast cancer who adhered to a low-fat diet had less oxidative damage to DNA than did high-risk women who remained on their regular diets. Dr. Zora Djuric, assistant professor of medicine at Wayne State University in Detroit, Michigan, and her associates report that the DNA damage, suspected to be a factor in tumor promotion, may be used effectively as a marker of dietary fat intake.

The research was part of the Breast Cancer Prevention Program, a Detroit-based study begun in 1987 to examine if a change in diet might prevent cancer. Patients who are admitted to the program must meet at least one of these three criteria: Have one or more close relatives with breast cancer; have a biopsy of breast tissue that shows specific abnormalities; or have a mammogram that suggests a high risk for cancer.

Of the 194 women who participated in the diet program, 21 between the ages of 19 and 57 were selected for the DNA study as a consecutive group of 21 admissions. Dr. Silvana Martino, director of the program and associate professor of medicine at Wayne State University, explains that the primary aim of the study was to identify measurable parameters that would correlate diet and risk for breast cancer just as blood cholesterol levels have been correlated to risk for heart disease.

Research Resources Reporter January 1992.

Studies conducted in animals-particularly rats-during the past half century have shown a relationship between dietary fat and the risk of developing tumors at various sites. Subsequent studies have reported similar associations for human breast and colon cancer. Additional evidence, obtained in animals, suggests that oxidative damage to DNA may be an important factor in aging and diseases, such as cancer, that are associated with aging.

Dr. Djuric and her colleagues determined the extent of oxidative damage by measuring levels of 5-hydroxymethyluracil in the DNA of the patients' white blood cells. An oxidation product of DNA, 5-hydroxymethyluracil might be associated with carcinogenesis, according to the investigators. This oxidation of DNA may occur as a result of fat metabolism. The DNA analysis was performed by gas chromatography/mass spectrometry at the Michigan State University Mass Spectrometry Facility in East Lansing.

After grouping by age, the 21 patients in the DNA damage/diet study were randomly assigned, 12 to remain on their own diet and 9 to the Low-Fat Eating Plan, a diet developed by the American Health Foundation and the University of Minnesota Nutrition Coordinating Center. In this diet only 15 percent of the daily calories are provided by fat. As a point of reference, the current dietary guidelines from the National Academy of Sciences recommend reducing fat intake to 30 percent or less of daily calories.

Blood studies were performed at 3- to 6-month intervals during the course of the 2-year study. When blood was drawn, the women also completed a 24-hour diet recall and a 3-day food record with a registered dietician.

Dr. Djuric notes that "by 3 months fat intake goes down and stays down for those on the low-fat diet. Therefore, further changes in the levels of oxidative DNA damage are not expected after 3 months on the diet. That is to be expected because blood cells are turned over rapidly."

Both the average total fat intake and the average percent of body fat were significantly lower in the low-fat diet group than in the non-intervention group, although there were no significant differences in the two groups' daily intake of calories. The study sample was too small to allow statistical interpretation of the differences between the groups in their intake of specific fatty acids, but the low-fat diet group did report a 52 to 58 percent lower intake of saturated fat, monounsaturated fat, and polyunsaturated fat than did the nonintervention group.

The average level of 5-hydroxymethyluracil in the DNA of women who followed the low-fat diet was three times lower than the level in the non-intervention group. Dr. Martino stresses that this is the first study to link oxidative DNA damage and ingestion of dietary fat as a "potential marker for fat intake." In addition, oxidative DNA damage may be a marker of cancer risk. "It is hoped that the women who are at increased breast cancer risk due to genetic factors can decrease their risk by decreasing fat in the diet," she notes.

To see if similar results could be obtained from an animal model, Dr. Djuric and her coworkers recently completed a study in which mammary gland and liver tissue were examined in rats maintained on a normal diet or a low-fat diet. "DNA damage in both the mammary gland and liver was decreased by a low-fat diet," notes Dr. Djuric. "Now that we have this animal model we would like to look at whether certain fats are more protective than others." The investigators will examine various fatty acids with respect to their roles in eliciting DNA damage, and the mechanisms by which fatty acids influence tumor growth. Finally, the relative importance of caloric restriction versus fat intake will be examined in rats.

"We are now adding to our human study by looking at normal volunteers who do not have a family history of cancer and at women who already have breast cancer. We can then compare these three groups: The control, the high risk, and the women with cancer," says Dr. Djuric. "We will try to establish whether oxidative DNA damage is indeed a marker of risk."

"Additionally, the dietary program used in the study will be made available to people who wish to change the fat content of their diets or lose weight. It may be that body weight is as important in determining risk as is the fat content of one's diet," notes Dr. Martino. Future studies will also consider whether age and smoking influence the DNA damage levels in humans. Oxidative DNA damage also may be linked to estrogen levels.

"What is remarkable in this study," Dr. Martino points out, "is that in a very small study group there were clear differences. It only took 21 subjects to show that there was a correlation of fat consumption to DNA damage. This relationship may be used as a check or verification for the amount of fat reported to have been consumed in the diet."

—by Linda B. Berman

Additional reading:

1. Djuric, Z., Heilbrun, L. K., Reading, B. A., et al., Effects of low-fat diet on levels of oxidative damage to DNA in human peripheral nucleated blood cells. *Journal of the National Cancer Institute* 83:766-769, 1991.

2. Welsch, C. W., House, J. L., Herr, B. L., et al., Enhancement of mammary carcinogenesis by high levels of dietary fat: A phenomenon dependent on *ad libitum* feeding. *Journal of the National Cancer Institute* 82:1615-1620, 1990.

3. Hietanen, E., Bartsch, H., Bereziat, J.-C., et al., Quantity and saturation degree of dietary fats as modulators of oxidative stress and chemically induced liver tumors in rats. *International Journal of Cancer* 46:640-647,1990.

4. Ewertz, M., and Gill, C., Dietary factors and breast-cancer risk in Denmark. *International Journal of Cancer* 46:779-784, 1990.

5. Howe, G. R., Hirohata, T., Hislop, T. G., et al., Dietary factors and risk of breast cancer: Combined analysis of 12 case-control studies. *Journal of the National Cancer Institute* 82:561-569, 1990.

The research described in this article was supported by the Biomedical Research Technology Program of the National Center for Research Resources, the National Cancer Institute, and the Wayne State University Ken Kasle Trust for Cancer Research.

Chapter 40

Lifetime Probability of Breast Cancer in American Women

A report from the National Cancer Institute (NCI) estimates that about 1 in 8 women in the United States will develop breast cancer during her lifetime.

The present estimate is higher than the 1-in-9 figure reported previously by the American Cancer Society (ACS), primarily due to the inclusion of the oldest age groups in the new calculations. The 1-in-9 estimate used a cutoff age of 85 years, but the new 1-in-8 figure (approximately 12.6 percent) includes all age groups in 5-year intervals up to an open-ended interval of 95 years and over. Each age interval is assigned a weight in the calculations based on the proportion of the population living to that age. The probability of developing breast cancer before age 85 remains approximately 1 in 9

NCI's Eric Feuer, Ph.D., and Lap-Ming Wun, Ph.D., and Catherine C. Boring of ACS derived the new estimate using 1987-1988 cancer incidence rates from NCI's Surveillance, Epidemiology, and End Results Program. Their work, which appears in summary form in NCI's Cancer Statistics Review 1973-1989, was published in full in the June 2, 1993, issue of the Journal of the National Cancer Institute.

In evaluating cancer risk for a cancer-free individual at a specific point in time, age-specific (conditional) probabilities are more appropriate than lifetime probabilities. For example, at age 50, a cancer-free black woman has about a 2-percent chance of developing breast can-

NCI Cancerfax 208/600056.

cer by age 60, and a cancer-free white woman has about a 2.5-percent chance.

"I think there's been too much focus on this single number, the lifetime risk," Feuer said. "We don't know what incidence rates will be in the future, so it's something of a hypothetical number. Conditional probabilities over a decade or two are probably a better reflection of somebody's actual risk."

These probabilities are based on population averages. An individual woman's breast cancer risk may be higher or lower, depending upon a variety of factors, including family history, reproductive history, and other factors yet to be identified.

The NCI is directing special attention to women with disproportionately high rates of breast cancer and poor survival rates, including members of certain minority groups and the medically underserved. Efforts targeted at these groups are under way in all components of NCI's program: basic research, early detection, clinical trials, rehabilitation, education and information dissemination, and cancer centers.

Chances of Developing Breast Cancer

By age 25: 1 in 19,608
By age 30: 1 in 2,525
By age 35: 1 in 622
By age 40: 1 in 217
By age 45: 1 in 93
By age 50: 1 in 50
By age 55: 1 in 33
By age 60: 1 in 24
By age 65: 1 in 17
By age 70: 1 in 14
By age 75: 1 in 11
By age 80: 1 in 10
By age 85: 1 in 9
Ever: 1 in 8

Chapter 41

Research To Improve Methods of Breast Cancer Detection

The National Cancer Institute (NCI) funds numerous research projects to improve conventional mammography and develop alternative imaging technologies to detect and characterize breast tumors.

For breast cancer screening, high-quality mammography (an x-ray technique to visualize the internal structure of the breast) is the most effective technology presently available. Studies have shown that in women ages 50 and older, mammography coupled with clinical breast examination is effective in detecting breast cancer and, with treatment, can result in as much as a 30- to 35-percent reduction in deaths in this age group.

Efforts to improve conventional mammography center on refinements of the technology and quality assurance in the administration and interpretation of the x-ray films. To advance the technology, NCI is funding research to reduce the already low radiation dosage; enhance image quality; develop digital mammography as an improvement over the conventional, film-based technique; develop statistical techniques for computer-assisted interpretation of digitized images; and enable long-distance image transmission technology for clinical consultations.

Digital Mammography

Digital mammography, a computerized technique that displays images using an infinite scale of gray tones, is of keen research inter-

NCI Cancerfax 208/600514.

est. Mammography x-ray films can contain subtle information not easily discernible to the radiologist. Digital images potentially could enhance the quality of the image and even magnify the view of specific areas of the breast. This is expected to improve the sensitivity of mammography especially in radiographically dense breast tissue, which renders visualization of cancer problematic and to decrease the radiation dose per mammogram. Digital mammography also will allow computer-aided diagnosis and teleradiology.

The NCI funds many studies of this technology, including those of the National Digital Mammography Development Group. This multidisciplinary academic and industrial group is developing and evaluating methods to increase image quality and technologies such as image processing for improved lesion visualization, computer-aided diagnosis for enhanced image interpretation, and telemammography (electronic image transmission providing access to specialized clinical experts at remote sites).

Novel Non-Ionizing Radiation Imaging

While a very useful technology, mammography is not perfect. It cannot produce clear x-ray images of dense (more glandular) breast tissue, and its effectiveness is limited in women with breast implants. Younger women tend to have dense breast tissue, which does not provide as clear a mammographic image as needed for diagnosis of early breast cancer. Looking for an abnormality on an image of dense breast tissue is somewhat like trying to detect an individual brush stroke of paint in a modern art painting where many overlapping splashes of the same shade of color are splattered all over the canvas. One cannot see under a splash of color, and it is hard to make distinctions between individual brush strokes of paint.

Mammography also cannot distinguish with absolute certainty benign from cancerous lesions. For such reasons, scientists are exploring novel non-ionizing imaging technologies including magnetic resonance imaging (MRI), ultrasound, optical imaging, and other technologies. The NCI-funded studies encompass basic technology and instrumentation development through preclinical and clinical testing. These studies aim to define the precise role of the technologies in detecting and characterizing breast tumors.

MRI and Ultrasound

Of novel non-ionizing technologies, conventional MRI and ultrasound have been the most studied as ways to improve the sensitivity of breast cancer detection and staging in certain groups of women. Both have shown potential for distinguishing between benign and malignant lesions and in detecting tumors in dense breast tissue. Furthermore, contrast-enhanced MRI may offer promise as an adjunct test in cases where mammography and physical examination are inconclusive, such as in distinguishing benign cell growth (dysplasia) from cancer.

The MRI and ultrasound technologies have their limitations too. An MRI cannot detect micro-calcifications (minute calcium deposits), which may indicate a small cancer. About one-half of cancers detected by mammography appear as a cluster of micro-calcifications. Likewise, ultrasound does not consistently detect micro-calcifications, nor can it detect very small tumors.

Breast Biopsies

Imaging is also being tested as an aid in performing biopsies. Of the women in the United States who undergo surgical breast biopsies, the majority (80 percent) do not have cancer. As an alternative to surgery, mammography-guided, stereotactic needle breast biopsy is being studied for women with non-palpable lesions. (Women who have large, palpable lesions usually undergo needle aspirations to determine if their lesions are solid or fluid-filled cysts.) Stereotactic needle biopsy offers the potential advantages of minimized tissue damage, reduced waiting time until diagnosis, and cost savings. A multi-institutional research program is now testing the efficacy of the large-core and fine-needle biopsies.

Other Areas of Study

In addition to research on imaging technologies, other research is developing methods to detect products of breast cancer (antigens) in blood, urine, or nipple aspirates, and to detect genetic alterations in women who are at increased risk for breast cancer. Once cancer is diagnosed, studies of these types contribute to characterization of breast tumors and can be useful in treatment planning. Still other NCI-funded projects seek to increase the utilization of mammography among women in age groups for which mammography has proven benefit.

Another emphasis is to increase utilization among minority and medically underserved women.

Chapter 42

Reducing the Risk of Mammography

When a woman goes to her doctor for a mammogram, she's taking a bit of a gamble. Although the cards are stacked overwhelmingly in her favor, even the low doses of radiation used in mammography can shuffle cancer-causing mutations into a cell. Lowering the radiation dose even further can only be good news for patients.

Now, with the aid of a novel mathematical analysis program, scientists have developed an improved mammography system that may cut the patient's radiation dose by more than half. Known as the FDA/NIH Optimized Mammography System, it features an improved antiscatter device built by Dr. Alec Eidsath and his colleagues in NCRR's Biomedical Engineering and Instrumentation Program (BEIP). The antiscatter device helps produce a sharper picture by absorbing stray X-rays that can cloud the image on the film.

The optimized mammography system has not yet been tested on humans, but a clinical study is expected to begin this year under the technical supervision of James Vucich, a medical physicist in the Diagnostic Radiology Department at the NIH Clinical Center. If it proves clinically useful, the instrument could be especially beneficial for younger women, who tend to have dense breasts, and for women who have large or fibrous breasts, which are difficult to image because they inhibit passage of the low-energy X-rays used in mammography. Although the radiation dose for most patients is typically quite low, it climbs rapidly for such women. And for women at risk for breast can-

---

NCRR *Reporter* November/December 1994.

cer, who might start getting mammograms while younger and thus receive many more exposures during their lifetimes, lower doses offer additional advantages, since the damaging effects of radiation can be cumulative.

Design of the system began more than a decade ago, when Dr. E. Philip Muntz, professor of radiology and of aerospace engineering at USC, laid out a plan for mathematically analyzing the standard mammography examination. He and his colleagues developed a complex computer program that numerically analyzed, and optimized, nine aspects of a standard mammography unit. The program showed that by altering the distances between parts, using a tungsten rather than a molybdenum x-ray source, and making additional adjustments, the optimized machine could significantly reduce the radiation dose yet produce an image at least as clear as that of a standard instrument. A prototype machine built at FDA confirmed the program's predictions.

"Many aspects of this system are unconventional: There are a lot of special parts, but 90 percent of it is a standard mammography unit," says Dr. Robert Jennings, a supervisory research physicist at the FDA. One of the system's more unusual components is the arc-shaped antiscatter device constructed according to FDA specifications by NCRR's Dr. Eidsath.

X-ray machines are essentially high-tech shadow-making devices, Dr. Eidsath explains. They work by shining a beam of X-rays through a part of the body and then capturing the resulting image on photographic film. X-rays pass more easily through softer tissues, like fat, than through fibrous or glandular tissues or calcifications. Thus the beam transmitted by the breast creates a pattern of light and dark areas on the film that represent the distribution of different tissues. When radiologists examine a mammogram, they look for suspicious white objects that may indicate a tumor, a fluid-filled cyst, or tiny calcifications that could signify cancer.

Unfortunately, X-rays are not limited to passing straight through the body or stopping completely. A significant portion bounce off the body's tissues, thus exposing the wrong region of film and reducing the image contrast. To absorb wayward X-rays, most mammography systems feature antiscatter devices, called grids, which lie beneath the breast-support pad and above the film. Typical grids consist of arrays of thin lead strips, about 1 millimeter tall, that stand along the paths of unscattered X-rays. The soft lead strips, sandwiched with paper strips that help maintain their shape, absorb scattered rays that approach at sharp angles. Although the paper serves a critical structural function, it also has a negative side effect: It absorbs some of the unscattered X-rays. Thus a higher dose of radiation is needed to produce a clear mammogram.

Dr. Muntz's optimization program suggested that a change in grid architecture would intercept stray X-rays even more effectively while cutting absorption of unscattered rays. The new design called for a curved grid, comprising thin stainless steel vanes arranged to point toward the x-ray source. Because stainless steel is more rigid than lead, no paper is needed to support the vanes. Working with and mounting these thin metal strips, each 14 inches long and a ten-thousandth of an inch thick—or thin enough to readily slice fingers—proved to be a challenge for Dr. Eidsath and colleagues Ronald Seldon and James Sullivan of BEIP's Precision Instrument Unit. Ultimately the scientists fashioned the grid by using small dowels to hold the vanes to their arc-shaped supports.

Another critical improvement to the antiscatter device is the deeper and narrower slots between the vanes, explains Dr. Jennings. "Only those scattered rays that enter at a very small angle to the primary photon direction—the unscattered photon direction—can get through the grid," which improves the contrast of the image. To prevent the vanes from being imaged and creating a series of unwanted straight lines on the film, the grid swings in an arc while in use. "The grid makes a single pass during the exposure, which could last as long as 2 or 3 seconds, or be as short as half a second," says Dr. Eidsath. "When the vanes move at a constant velocity, and the x-ray exposure is synchronized with the grid motion, none of the lines show up."

Preliminary testing of the new mammography system, conducted at FDA's laboratories in Rockville, Maryland, showed that it can reduce the radiation dose delivered by a standard mammography unit by as much as two-thirds. The instrument is now at the Clinical Center awaiting final adjustments and its first clinical tests. "We hope to show that the system's diagnostic effectiveness is at least as good as current mammography systems, but with substantially reduced doses to the patient," says Dr. Jennings.

—by Victoria L. Contie

Additional Reading

Eidsath, A., Gopalan, R, Jennings, R., and Vucich, J. Mechanical design of the NIH mammography anti-scatter device. In Advances in *Bioengineering*, Volume 20 (Vanderby, R., ed.). New York: American Society of Mechanical Engineering, 1991, pp. 199-202.

Jennings, R. J., Fewell, T. R., Jafroudi, H., and Muntz, E. R, Laboratory evaluation of an optimized mammographic imaging system. In SPIE Vol. 914—*Medical Imaging 11: Image Formation, Detection, Processing, and Interpretation*. Bellingham, WA: Society of Photo-Optical instrumentation Engineers, 1988, pp. 176-181.

Chapter 43

Oral Contraceptives and Breast Cancer

In the April 6 issue of The Journal of the National Cancer Institute (JNCI), researchers at Fred Hutchinson Cancer Research Center, Seattle, report on an increased risk for breast cancer among women under age 35 who used oral contraceptives for more than 10 years. [Note: The study is "Breast Cancer Among Young U.S. Women in Relation to Oral Contraceptive Use," Emily White, Kathleen E. Malone. Noel S. Weiss, Janet R. Daling, JNCI, April 6, 1994.]

The findings add to evidence accumulating from other studies that long-term use of oral contraceptives may increase risk for early-onset breast cancer. Although scientists are concerned about these findings, inconsistencies among study results remain to be reconciled. The National Cancer Institute (NCI) is carefully watching research developments in this area and is conducting its own study on oral contraceptives and risk for breast cancer, which will be completed by late this year.

Most studies have found no overall increased risk for breast cancer associated with oral contraceptive use. But during the 1980s, findings began to emerge that suggested a link between early-onset breast cancer and both long-term use of oral contraceptives and use at young ages. Some studies also suggested that women of all ages who have a family history of breast cancer or a personal history of benign breast disease and who have used oral contraceptives may be at a particularly increased risk for breast cancer.

NCI Cancerfax 208/600313.

Oral contraceptives were first marketed in the United States in 1960. Sufficient time has now elapsed to permit studies with large numbers of women who took the pill for many years beginning at a young age, and to follow them as they become middle-aged. Fred Hutchinson's Emily White, Ph.D., and colleagues focused on women born since the mid-1940s because they had the pill available during their entire reproductive lives.

White and colleagues found that women under age 35 who used oral contraceptives for more than 10 years had a 70 percent increased risk for breast cancer compared to women who had never taken them or had taken them for less than one year. They also found a 30 percent increased risk for breast cancer among those who took the pill within five years after menarche (start of menstruation). Some earlier studies suggested that risk may be increased by taking the pill either before age 25 or before the first full-term pregnancy, but White, like investigators of other recent studies, did not find these relationships.

Ninety-eight of the study participants had used combination pills, which contain two synthetic versions of the female hormones estrogen and progesterone that are similar to the hormones the ovaries normally produce. The combination pill, which has differed in estrogen/progesterone composition over the years, is the most frequently prescribed oral contraceptive in the United States. White found a 50 percent increased risk associated with taking pills containing high amounts of progestin (synthetic progesterone) for at least one year under age 35. Pills containing high levels of synthetic estrogen did not appear to pose an additional risk. Furthermore, no difference in risk was observed between pills containing the two types of synthetic estrogen used in oral contraceptives, ethinyl estradiol and mestranol.

Earlier Studies. White noted that six published reviews of studies have raised concern about the use of oral contraceptives and the risk of breast cancer for women under age 45. Two meta-analyses (studies in which data from many studies are pooled and analyzed) found similar 11 percent increased risks for breast cancer for women under age 45 who had ever used oral contraceptives, and 40 percent increased risks for women in this age group who were long-term users.

Research is focusing on whether long-term use or use at an early age increases risk for breast cancer, and if there is a risk, at what age an effect appears. Findings from some recent studies on oral contraceptives and breast cancer in young women illustrate the efforts being made to clarify the risk:

- An analysis of data from the U.S. Cancer and Steroid Hormone (CASH) Study found that women aged 20-34 years who had ever used the pill had a 40 percent increased risk of breast cancer. But the investigators cautioned against over interpretation of the data, noting the absence of a dose-response relationship and the complexities involved in evaluating changing pill composition over time. No increased risk was found for women aged 35-44 years, and a slightly decreased risk for breast cancer was seen for women aged 45-54 years, a finding that has not been reported in many studies.

- A Boston study found an overall two-fold increased risk for breast cancer among women under age 45 who used oral contraceptives. Risk was increased for short-term as well as long-term users, and risk increased as duration of use increased (a dose-response relationship). There was a two-fold increased risk of breast cancer for women who took the pill for fewer than 10 years, and a four-fold increased risk for women who took the pill for more than 10 years.

- A New Zealand study found a 20 percent increased risk for breast cancer associated with taking the pill in women under age 35. Risk was slightly, although not statistically significantly, increased during the first few years after starting use of the pill.

- A study in England found that women under age 36 who had taken the pill for 4 to 8 years had a 40 percent increased risk for breast cancer, while those taking it for more than 8 years had a 70 percent increased risk.

- In a Swedish study, researchers found that starting oral contraceptive use before age 25 increased risk for breast cancer, but total duration of pill use did not appear to increase risk. Women who started using oral contraceptives before age 20 had nearly a six-fold increased risk for breast cancer, and the risk was increased five-fold for using the pill more than 5 years before age 25.

- A study conducted in Sweden and Norway found that the risk for breast cancer was doubled for women under age 45 who had taken the pill for 12 years or more.

While the relationship between oral contraceptives and breast cancer risk is still under study, women who may be at increased risk of developing cancer—those who have used the pill long-term, began use at an early age, or have a family or personal history of breast cancer or a personal history of benign breast disease—should discuss the risks and benefits of oral contraceptive use with their doctors.

NCI Study. NCI is conducting a case-control study of oral contraceptives, as well as of alcohol and diet, as possible risk factors for breast cancer. The study involves about 2,000 U.S. women newly diagnosed with breast cancer (cases) and 3,000 women who do not have the disease (controls). The study focuses primarily on determining the influence of hormones and other factors on breast cancer risk in women under age 45. Of the study population, 1,500 of the women who have breast cancer are 45 years of age or younger. Results of the oral contraceptive analysis will be available in late 1994.

Background. A woman's risk of developing breast cancer depends in part on hormone-related factors, such as age at first menstruation, age at first live birth, and age at menopause. For this reason, a number of studies have examined the relationship between use of oral contraceptives and risk of breast and other cancers.

Estrogen stimulates the growth and development of the uterus at puberty, thickens the endometrium (the inner lining of the uterus) during the first half of the menstrual cycle, and stimulates changes in breast tissue at puberty and childbirth.

Progesterone, which is produced during the last half of the menstrual cycle, prepares the endometrium to receive the egg. If the egg is fertilized, progesterone secretion continues, preventing release of additional eggs from the ovaries. For this reason, progesterone is called the "pregnancy supporting hormone," and scientists believe it may have valuable contraceptive effects. The synthetic progesterone used in oral contraceptives is called progestogen or progestin.

References

Chilvers C, McPherson K, Pike MC, et al: Oral contraceptive use and breast cancer risk in young women. Lancet, 1:973-982, 1989. (United Kingdom)

Meirik O, Lund E, Adami HO, et al: Oral contraceptive use and breast cancer in young women. Lancet 2:650-654, 1986. (Sweden and Norway)

Miller DR, Rosenberg L, Kaufman DW, et al: Breast cancer before age 45 and oral contraceptive use: New findings. American Journal of Epidemiology 129(2):269-280, 1989. (Boston)

Olsson H, Moller TR, Ranstam J: Early oral contraceptive use and breast cancer among premenopausal women: Final report from a study in southern Sweden. JNCI 81(13):1000-1004, 1989.

Paul C, Skegg DCG, Spears GFS: Oral contraceptives and risk of breast cancer. International Journal of Cancer 46, 366-373, 1990. (New Zealand)

Romiu I, Berlin JA, Colditz G: Oral contraceptives and breast cancer: Review and meta-analysis. Cancer 66:2253-2263, 1990.

Thomas DR: Oral contraceptives and breast cancer: Review of the epidemiologic literature. Contraception 43(6):597-642, 1991.

Wingo PA, Lee NC, Ory HW, et al: Age-specific differences in the relationship between oral contraceptive use and breast cancer. Cancer Supplement, 71(4):1506-1517, 1993. (CASH Study)

Chapter 44

Abortion and Possible Risk for Breast Cancer: Analysis and Inconsistencies

A study reported in the Nov. 2 issue of the *Journal of the National Cancer Institute* ("JNCI") on induced abortion and risk for breast cancer discusses whether an association exists, but the findings are not conclusive. Further research is needed to interpret the results. The research was independently conducted by Janet Daling, Ph.D , Fred Hutchinson Cancer Research Center, University of Washington, Seattle, and colleagues. [Note: The paper is titled "Risk of breast cancer among young women: Relationship to induced abortion." The authors are Janet R. Daling, Kathleen E. Malone, Lynda F. Voigt, Emily White, and Noel S. Weiss, of the Fred Hutchinson Cancer Research Center, University of Washington, Seattle.]

The study suggests that women age 45 or younger who have had induced abortions have a relative risk of 1.5 (50 percent increased risk) for breast cancer compared to women who had been pregnant but never had an induced abortion.

In epidemiologic research, relative risks of less than 2 are considered small and are usually difficult to interpret. Such increases may be due to chance, statistical bias, or effects of confounding factors that are sometimes not evident. In an editorial accompanying the study, Lynn Rosenberg, Sc.D., Boston University School of Medicine, points out that a "difference in risk of 50 percent (relative risk of 1.5) is small in epidemiologic terms [human population studies], and severely chal-

---

NCI Cancerfax 208/600342.

lenges our ability to distinguish whether it reflects cause and effect or whether it simply reflects bias."

Rosenberg notes that "the overall results as well as the particulars are far from conclusive, and it is difficult to see how they will be informative to the public."

Daling and colleagues did not find a consistent pattern of increasing or decreasing risk associated with age at abortion, as would be expected by many scientists. [Risk was greater for women who had their first induced abortion before age 18 (relative risk of 2.5) and for women who were 30 years of age or older (relative risk of 2.1).] Furthermore, the risk did not vary by number of abortions, whether abortion preceded or followed a full-term pregnancy, or by length of time to diagnosis of breast cancer. One key point is that women aged 45 or younger who had miscarriages were not found to be at increased risk for breast cancer.

Taken together, the inconsistencies and scarcity of existing research do not permit scientific conclusions.

In the Daling study, the researchers analyzed data on 845 white women who were diagnosed with invasive or *in situ* breast cancer from 1983 to 1990 and 961 control subjects. All the women were born after 1944. Data were collected on reproductive history, family history of breast and other cancers, and lifestyle and other factors. The study population was from three counties in Washington State. Only white women were included in the study because of the small minority population in this area.

The researchers also found that risk for breast cancer was more enhanced for women having an induced abortion prior to age 18 if their pregnancy was interrupted during the 9-to-24-week period of gestation. However, this finding was based on small numbers.

Studies published in the "JNCI" are peer-reviewed by scientists and represent the views of the authors. Papers published in the journal do not necessarily reflect the views held by NCI or any other component of the federal government.

Chapter 45

Fertility Drugs As a Risk Factor for Ovarian Cancer

The possibility that the use of fertility drugs may increase the risk of ovarian cancer has prompted researchers to conduct studies to determine the long-term effects of such drugs. The most recent report on this topic was published in the September 22, 1994 issue of the "New England Journal of Medicine" by Mary Anne Rossing and her coworkers at the Fred Hutchinson Cancer Research Center in Seattle. These researchers found that prolonged use of the fertility drug clomiphene citrate may increase the risk of developing ovarian tumors, particularly tumors of low malignant potential that respond better to treatment than the more common type of ovarian cancer.

This study followed 3,837 women who had been evaluated for infertility in clinics in the Seattle area for an average of 11 years. Eleven women developed invasive or borderline malignant ovarian tumors, as compared with an expected number of 4.4 tumors. Nine of these women had taken clomiphene, with 5 taking the drug for 12 or more menstrual cycles. No excess risk was associated with the use of clomiphene for less than a year or with the use of human chorionic gonadotropin (HCG), another drug used to promote fertility. Because the number of women who developed ovarian tumors was small, larger studies are needed to confirm these results.

In 1992, an evaluation of previous studies of women who had ovarian cancer found that the risk for invasive epithelial ovarian cancer among women who had been diagnosed as being infertile and who had

---

NCI Cancerfax 208/600036.

received fertility drugs was nearly three times that of women who had no history of infertility. Infertile women who had not used fertility drugs had no increased risk. Those infertile women who used fertility drugs and became pregnant did not have a significantly increased risk for ovarian cancer. However, for infertile women who had never become pregnant, the use of fertility drugs was associated with a significantly increased risk of cancer compared with women who had no history of infertility. In the 1992 report, the authors were unable to distinguish which fertility drugs, combination of fertility drugs, or duration of treatment may have been associated with the increased risk of ovarian cancer.

The National Cancer Institute has begun further study into the epidemiology of ovarian cancer, including the use of fertility drugs. In addition, the National Institute of Child Health and Human Development (NICHD), another component of the National Institutes of Health, is supporting an expansion of the study by Rossing and her co-workers to include women evaluated for infertility in King County, Washington during the period 1974-93.

Women who have taken fertility drugs and who are concerned about their risk of developing ovarian cancer should discuss their previous treatment with these drugs with a gynecologist. At this time, however, there are no screening tests that are consistently accurate enough to detect ovarian cancer at an early stage when there are no symptoms. Research to identify better methods of diagnosing ovarian cancer and to evaluate currently available tests is under way.

For information about fertility drugs, write to the Office of Research Reporting, National Institute of Child Health and Human Development, Building 31, Room 2A32, Bethesda, MD 20892, or call 301-496-5133.

Chapter 46

Personal Use of Hair Coloring Products and Risk of Cancer

In the past few years, several studies have indicated that women and men who dye their hair frequently may be at increased risk for certain cancers. These studies showed an association between hair dye use and increased risks for multiple myeloma (cancer of cells in the bone marrow), non-Hodgkin's lymphoma (cancer of the lymph system), and leukemia (cancer of blood-forming cells) in both sexes, and ovarian cancer in women. Three recent studies support findings from earlier studies showing that increased risk might be restricted to long-term or frequent hair dye users, particularly users of dark hair dyes.

Hair coloring products are widely used in the United States by both men and women; estimates of current usage range from 20 percent to 60 percent of the population. These products may contain chemicals that are mutagenic (altering the structure of DNA) and carcinogenic (cancer-causing) in animals. The quantity and structure of these chemicals vary by product type and color; darker dyes tend to have greater amounts than lighter dyes.

Research has shown that some of the substances in hair dyes are readily absorbed through the skin and scalp during application.

Several studies of cosmetologists and other persons who apply hair dyes to others as part of their work have shown them to be at increased risk of non-Hodgkin's lymphoma, multiple myeloma, and leukemia. The International Agency for Research on Cancer, the research organization that classifies exposures as carcinogenic to humans, has

---

NCI Cancerfax 208/600332.

classified cosmetology as an occupation entailing exposures that are possibly carcinogenic.

Because the evidence from the studies of personal use of hair dyes is not conclusive, no recommendation to change hair dye use can be made at this time. However, because hair dye use is common in the United States, and because people who apply hair dyes as part of their work have been shown to be at increased risk of certain cancers, further research is needed to clarify whether there is a causal association.

Recent Reports

The most recent report, published in the February 2, 1994, issue of the *Journal of the National Cancer Institute*, shows that women who use permanent hair dyes do not have an overall increased risk of dying from cancer. However, women who used black hair dyes for more than 20 years had a slightly increased risk of dying from non-Hodgkin's lymphoma and multiple myeloma. Less than 1 percent of women in this study reported that they had used permanent black hair dyes for more than 20 years.

This study, carried out by Michael J. Thun, M.D., and colleagues at the American Cancer Society (ACS) and the U.S. Food and Drug Administration, included information from 573,369 women enrolled in a cancer prevention study. At the beginning of the study in 1982, the women answered a questionnaire that included questions on use of permanent hair dyes. The women were contacted periodically over the next 7 years, and those who had died were identified and their causes of death recorded.

The title of the study is "Hair Dye Use and Risk of Fatal Cancers in U.S. Women." The authors are M. J. Thun, S. F. Altekruse, M. M. Namboodiri, E. E. Calle, D. G. Myers, and C. W. Heath, Jr. The use of temporary, semi-permanent, or progressive hair dyes was not studied, and any women who began to use hair dyes after the initial questionnaire were not classified as hair dye users. This study of women may not apply to men because men tend to use hair dye products that differ chemically from women's hair dyes. The ACS study also looked at cancer deaths and not at cancer incidence (new diagnoses), which was the measurement used in previous studies of personal use of hair dyes.

Another recent report, published as an abstract in the October 15, 1993, issue of the *American Journal of Epidemiology*, showed that men and women who used permanent or semi-permanent hair dyes for 16 or more years had an increased risk for leukemia. The title of the study is "Hair Dye Use and Leukemia." The authors are D. P. Sandler, D. L. Shore, C. D. Bloomfield, and Cancer and Leukemia Group B Investigators.

Dale Sandler, Ph.D., and colleagues at the National Institute of Environmental Health Sciences (NIEHS) compared hair dye use among 615 leukemia patients and 630 people without the disease. The researchers found that those who had used any type of hair dye had a 50-percent increased risk of developing leukemia, compared with people who never dyed their hair.

Most of the risk shown in this NIEHS study was associated with permanent and semi-permanent dyes, which increased risk by 60 percent and 40 percent, respectively. Temporary rinses increased risk by 20 percent. Long-term users, who used hair dyes for 16 or more years, were 2 1/2 times more likely to develop leukemia than those who never used hair dyes.

A study by Anastasia Tzonou, D.M.Sc., and colleagues at the Harvard School of Public Health and the University of Athens Medical School, reported in the September 30, 1993, issue of the *International Journal of Cancer*, suggested that regular use of hair dyes might increase the risk of ovarian cancer. The name of the study is "Hair Dyes, Analgesics, Tranquilizers and Perineal Talc Application as Risk Factors for Ovarian Cancer." The authors are A. Tzonou, A. Polychronopoulou, C. Hsieh, A. Rebelakos, A. Karakatsani, and D. Trichopoulos.

The researchers asked 189 cancer patients and 200 hospital visitors how often they dyed their hair each year. Compared with women who had never dyed their hair, women who dyed their hair one to four times a year had a 70-percent increased risk for ovarian cancer. Women who used hair dyes five times or more per year had twice the risk of developing ovarian cancer than women who never used hair dyes.

Previous National Cancer Institute Studies

Linda Morris Brown, M.P.H., and her colleagues at the National Cancer Institute (NCI) and the University of Iowa published a report in the December 1992 issue of the *American Journal of Public Health* that showed a 90-percent increased risk for multiple myeloma in a study of 173 men with the disease and 650 men without it. The title of the study is "Hair Dye Use in White Men and Risk of Multiple Myeloma." The authors are L. M. Brown, G. D. Everett, L. F. Burmeister, and A. Blair. More than 8 percent of the men diagnosed with multiple myeloma reported using hair dyes, compared with less than 5 percent of the men without the disease. In addition to the overall increased risk of multiple myeloma, risk increased among men who had used hair dyes at least monthly for a year, compared with men who used dyes less frequently or for a shorter time.

In an NCI study conducted by Shelia Hoar Zahm, Sc.D., published in the July 1992 issue of *American Journal of Public Health*, women who used hair dyes had a 50-percent higher risk for developing non-Hodgkin's lymphoma and an 80-percent higher risk of multiple myeloma than women who never dyed their hair. The title of the study is "Use of Hair Coloring Products and the Risk of Lymphoma, Multiple Myeloma, and Chronic Lymphocytic Leukemia." The authors are S. H. Zahm, D. D. Weisenburger, P. A. Babbitt, R. C. Saal, J. B. Vaught, and A. Blair. Among the 876 women in the study, the risk associated with permanent hair coloring products was higher than that for semi-permanent or non-permanent hair coloring products. Risk was increased 70 percent in women who used permanent hair dyes and 40 percent in women who used semi-permanent or non-permanent dyes. Risk did not increase with frequency of hair dye use, although risk increased with the number of years of use.

Women who used black, brown/brunette, and red hair coloring products had a twofold to fourfold increased risk of being diagnosed with these cancers compared with no increased risk of cancer in women who dyed their hair with lighter colors. Other cancer risk factors, such as family history of cancer, cigarette smoking, and herbicide or pesticide exposure, did not change the risks calculated for hair dye use.

An earlier NCI study published in the May 1988 issue of the *American Journal of Public Health* showed that men who had used hair dyes had a twofold risk for non-Hodgkin's lymphoma and almost double the risk for leukemia. The title of the study is "Hair Dye Use and Risk of Leukemia and Lymphoma." The authors are K.P. Cantor, A. Blair, G. Everett, S. VanLier, L. Burmeister, F. R. Dick, R. W. Gibson, and L. Schuman. Kenneth P. Cantor, Ph.D., and his colleagues at NCI, the University of Iowa, and the University of Minnesota found this increased risk by interviewing men with non-Hodgkin's lymphoma, men with leukemia, and men without cancer.

Statistics

In the United States, about 12,700 new cases of multiple myeloma (6,500 men and 6,200 women) will be diagnosed in 1994, and about 9,800 people (5,000 men and 4,800 women) will die of the disease.

About 45,000 new cases of non-Hodgkin's lymphoma will be diagnosed in 1994 (25,000 men and 20,000 women), and about 21,200 people will die of the disease (11,200 men and 10,000 women).

Leukemias of all kinds will account for about 28,600 new cases of cancer (16,200 men and 12,400 women) and about 19,100 cancer deaths (10,500 men and 8,600 women) in 1994.

About 24,000 women will be diagnosed with ovarian cancer in 1994, and about 13,600 women will die from the disease.

Chapter 47

Menopausal Hormone Replacement Therapy and Cancer Risk

Replacement hormones (estrogen or a combination of estrogen and progestin) have been shown to be effective in relieving conditions usually related to menopause. These conditions include hot flashes, vaginal tissue dryness, and osteoporosis (thinning of the bones). However, the use of estrogen during or after menopause has been linked to an increase in endometrial cancer (cancer of the lining of the uterus), and there is some suggestion that it is linked to breast cancer as well. Currently, however, most scientists think that for most women, the benefits of hormone replacement therapy (for example, a reduction in the risk of osteoporosis and possibly of cardiovascular disease) clearly outweigh the possible cancer risks.

Risk of Endometrial Cancer

Studies have shown that women taking replacement estrogen have a two to eight times higher risk of developing endometrial cancer than women who do not take estrogen. The risk increases after 2 to 4 years of estrogen use and seems to be greatest when large doses are taken or when the preparations are used for long periods of time. Using a combination of estrogen and progestin appears to decrease the risk linked to use of estrogen alone.

Because the use of estrogen has been associated with an increased incidence of endometrial cancer, the U.S. Food and Drug Ad-

---

NCI Cancerfax 208/600310.

ministration requires that a special brochure about the drug accompany each prescription for it. The brochure explains that the risk of cancer of the lining of the uterus increases with the duration of use and the strength of the dose. It also points out that estrogen has not been shown to be effective in the treatment of nervousness and depression, conditions sometimes associated with menopause.

Women who have undergone a total hysterectomy (complete removal of the uterus) are in no danger of developing endometrial cancer. Use of estrogen may not be appropriate, however, for women who have already had endometrial cancer. Until more information becomes available from current clinical studies of this question, decisions for these women must be made on a case-by-case basis.

Risk of Breast Cancer

The association between hormone replacement therapy and breast cancer is less clear. In a study carried out by the National Cancer Institute (NCI), postmenopausal women who had taken estrogen for 20 or more years had a 50-percent increase in risk of developing breast cancer compared with women who had not taken it. A number of other studies support this association.

In another study, More than 23,000 Swedish women who used replacement hormones (both estrogen and estrogen-progestin combinations) were followed. These women had about a 10-percent higher incidence of breast cancer than expected. A more detailed study of all the women in the group who developed breast cancer and a random sample of women who did not develop the disease showed that the risk increased to 70 percent compared with the expected level among women who used the hormones for 9 years or more. This risk did not sees to be offset by the addition of progestin, as had been suggested by the study of estrogen-associated cancers of the lining of the uterus.

It is unclear whether estrogen has an adverse effect on women who are already at high risk for breast cancer. However, women who have had breast cancer are usually advised not to take replacement estrogen.

Deciding on Replacement Therapy

The NCI advises a woman to thoroughly discuss the question of hormone replacement therapy with her doctor. If she and her doctor decide that this treatment is appropriate, the dosage as well as the duration of use should be carefully considered in relation to the benefits and risks.

Before hormone replacement therapy is begun, a pre-treatment mammogram (x-ray of the breast) usually is taken. It is especially important that a woman on hormone replacement therapy be checked each year by her doctor for any signs of cancer. Vaginal bleeding should be reported to the doctor at once. Also, a woman on hormone replacement therapy should examine her breasts monthly for lumps or changes in appearance that may be warning signs of cancer.

Chapter 48

Inheritance of Proliferative Breast Disease in Families with Breast Cancer

More cases of breast cancer than previously thought may be due to genetic predisposition, according to Dr. Mark Skolnick and his colleagues at the University of Utah Medical Center in Salt Lake City. But unlike the rare form of breast cancer that strikes young women and is clearly a dominant genetic trait, these cancers may be one possible outcome of a subtler susceptibility to malignant disease.

This susceptibility, the researchers suggest, first expresses itself as a benign condition called proliferative breast disease (PBD), which is characterized by a benign but excessive multiplication of cells in mammary tissue. Although the condition encompasses a spectrum of changes, even in more severe cases the proliferating cells do not entirely lose their distinctive features or invade other tissues as do cancerous cells.

Although many PBD cases do not develop into cancer, studies involving several thousand women have demonstrated an increased incidence of breast cancer in women with PBD present in earlier breast biopsies. Dr. Skolnick's group is the first one to show that PBD is an inherited trait in families that have a high prevalence of either premenopausal or postmenopausal breast cancer.

Dr. Skolnick, a geneticist, and his co-investigators studied 103 women from 20 extended families, or kindreds, in which at least two first-degree relatives (mother, sister, or daughter) had breast cancer

---

Research Resources Reporter June 1991.

and, for the control group, studied 31 genetically unrelated women. Of the 103 women, 77 were first-degree relatives of the women with cancer. The 31 controls consisted of wives of men in the families (sisters-in-law) and their female relatives. Thirty-five percent of the 77 clinically normal women who were first-degree relatives of women with breast cancer showed cytologic evidence of PBD that ranged from moderate to severe cell proliferation. In contrast, only 13 percent of the controls had any of these signs of PBD.

The Utah team used a new variation on a technique called fine-needle aspiration, in which a narrow-gauge needle is used to aspirate cells from mammary tissue. Usually surgeons take cells only from a tumor site, but for this study the entire area of both breasts was sampled. Once the cell samples had been categorized the researchers began a genetic analysis to determine any association between inheritance of PBD and an increased risk of breast cancer.

According to the investigators, the simplest genetic model of susceptibility to PBD consisted of a single gene that might be present in a normal form or in a variant form-or allele- that might confer susceptibility to PBD. From this general model Dr. Skolnick and his colleagues devised more specific models that compared five possible combinations of susceptibilities to PBD and breast cancer. The data were incompatible with all the combinations except one that proposed a genetic link between inherited PBD and inherited excess breast cancer ("excess" meaning a higher number of cases than seen in the general population of Utah). This suggests, the researchers state, that genetic susceptibility to PBD may predispose some women to develop breast cancer.

If a woman has the gene for susceptibility to PBD she has approximately a 60-percent chance of developing PBD because not everyone who carries the gene is affected by it, Dr. Skolnick explains. Carriers of the suspect gene also are about 10 times likelier to develop breast cancer at a given age than is the general population of Utah. Combining these two factors, women with a genetic susceptibility to PBD who have PBD appear to have a 52- to 63-percent lifetime probability of developing breast cancer, concludes Dr. Skolnick.

Since the mid-1800s scientists have recognized that breast cancer runs in certain families. Until recently, most of the evidence to support this observation was based on population statistics. Now, however, the principles of statistics and the techniques of molecular biology have joined forces. In addition, genetic findings are supporting and expanding earlier evidence as well as contributing to a general understanding of cancer.

The Utah study illustrates the first stage of genetic analysis. Later stages involve linking of a trait to a chromosomal site and, finally, pinpointing a gene. In the first stage, Dr. Skolnick explains, the investigators try to understand how a disease or trait segregates within a family; that is, the pattern of affected versus unaffected family members.

The Utah investigators' work differs in orientation from other recent genetic studies of breast cancer. Others have concentrated on subtypes of the disease itself; the Utah study focuses on a potential precursor to the disease in its more general form—both premenopausal and postmenopausal. Genetic predisposition to cancer ranges from being very apparent to being far less obvious, according to Dr. Skolnick. The first category includes breast cancer in women (and sometimes men) in their twenties and thirties, often affecting both breasts—the early-onset subtype of the disease. Says Dr. Skolnick, "Everybody knows that those are genetic cases of breast cancer. But the majority of genetic predisposition, in my opinion, is of a subtler form and is much more common. That was what we were trying to point out. We should not think of a disease as non-genetic because we don't see obvious Mendelian patterns."

Population genetics studies of breast cancer and other cancers sometimes cause apprehension in clinicians. Even when predisposing factors are well established, it is difficult to distinguish individual from statistical risk. Although the evidence heavily favors PBD as a possible precursor of breast cancer, co-investigator Dr. John H. Ward, associate professor of hematology and oncology, prefers to reserve judgment until an actual genetic mechanism linking the two conditions is uncovered.

"We have not proven by any means that PBD is a precursor lesion. I'm very optimistic. I just don't want to create false hope," he says.

The Utah group continues to work in several directions. The hypothetical gene for PBD must now be mapped, and correlations made between cytological and histological findings. Subjects' breast tissue will be resampled to test consistency of results. The definition of PBD may change, says Dr. Skolnick, when he replaces standard clinical analysis of samples with an analytical image processing system he is now developing.

—by Nancy Heneson

Additional reading:

1. Skolnick, M. H., Cannon-Albright, L. A., Goldgar, D. E., et al., Inheritance of proliferative breast disease in breast cancer kindreds. *Science* 250:1715-1720, 1990.

2. Hall, J. M., Lee, M. K., Newman, B., et al., Linkage of early onset familial breast cancer to chromosome 17q21. *Science* 250:1684-1689, 1990.

3. Malkin, D., Li, F. P., Strong, L. C., et al., Germ line p53 mutations in a familial syndrome of breast cancer, sarcomas, and other neoplasms. *Science* 250;1233-1238, 1990.

4. Dupont, W. D. and Page, D. L., Risk factors for breast cancer in women with proliferative breast disease. *New England Journal of Medicine* 312:146-151, 1985.

The research described in this article was supported by the General Clinical Research Centers Program of the National Center for Research Resources, the National Cancer Institute, and the Willard L. Eccles Charitable Foundation.

Chapter 49

Scientists Nab Breast Cancer Gene

In independent discoveries, scientists have identified one candidate gene for familial breast cancer and narrowed the search for a second. Inherited gene defects are thought to cause about 5-10 percent of the estimated 180,000 breast cancer cases diagnosed each year in American women.

The first finding ends a 4-year race to capture the gene known as BRCA1, which in 1990 was linked to the long arm of chromosome 17. Scientists have now connected flaws in this gene with multiple cases of breast and ovarian cancer in five extended families. Within these families, women who inherit BRCA1 face an estimated 85 percent risk of developing breast cancer by age 65 and a 63 percent risk of ovarian cancer by age 70. Identification of BRCA1 should aid early diagnosis and treatment of the inherited conditions, but the gene does not appear to play a role in non-inherited cancers.

Through studies of 15 breast cancer-prone families who tested negative for BRCA1, another scientific team has found a region on the long arm of chromosome 13 likely to house a second gene for familial breast cancer. Scientists report that this gene, called BRCA2, does not seem to raise ovarian cancer risk. Preliminary estimates suggest that BRCA1 and BRCA2 each affect about 1 in every 200 women.

Reference: *Science* 265:2088-2090,1994; *Science* 266:66-71, 1994.

NCRR *Reporter* November/December 1994.

Part Five

Glossary

Chapter 50

Glossary of Common Medical Terms

Abdomen (AB-do-men): The part of the body that contains the stomach, intestines, liver, reproductive organs, and other organs.

Adjuvant therapy (AD-joo-vent): Treatment that is given following the primary treatment, such as chemotherapy after surgery.

Anesthesia (an-es-THEE-zha): Loss of feeling, awareness, or sensation resulting from the administration of drugs or gases. A local anesthetic causes loss of feeling in a part of the body. A general anesthetic puts the person to sleep.

Anesthesiologist: a doctor who administers drugs or gases to put a patient to sleep before surgery.

Areola (a-REE-oe-la): The area of dark-colored skin that surrounds the nipple.

Ascites (a-SYE-teez): Abnormal buildup of fluid in the abdomen.

Aspiration (as-per-AY-shun): Removal of fluid from a lump, often a cyst, with a needle.

Atypical hyperplasia (hy-per-PLAY-zha): A benign (non-cancerous) condition in which breast tissue has certain abnormal features. This condition increases the risk of breast cancer.

Axilla (ak-SIL-a): The underarm.

Axillary sampling: Removal of some of the underarm lymph nodes.

Axillary dissection: Removal of all the underarm lymph nodes.

Barium enema: A series of x-rays of the lower intestine. The x-rays are taken after the patient is given an enema with a white, chalky solution that contains barium. The barium outlines the intestines on the x-rays.

Benign (bee-NINE): Not cancerous; does not invade nearby tissue or spread to other parts of the body.

Benign tumor (bee-NINE): A non-cancerous growth that does not invade nearby tissue or spread to other parts of the body.

Biological therapy (by-o-LOJ-i-kul): Treatment to stimulate or restore the ability of the immune system to fight infection and disease. Also called immunotherapy.

Biopsy (BY-op-see): The removal of a sample of tissue that is then examined under a microscope to check for cancer cells. Excisional biopsy is surgery to remove an entire lump and a margin of normal tissue around it. In incisional biopsy, which is done less often for breast tumors, the surgeon removes part of the tumor. Removal of tissue with a needle is called a needle biopsy.

Bladder: The hollow organ that stores urine.

Bone marrow transplantation (tranz-plan-TAY-shun): A procedure in which doctors replace marrow destroyed by high doses of anticancer drugs or radiation. The replacement marrow may be taken from the patient before treatment or may be donated by another person. When the patient's own marrow is used, the procedure is called autologous (aw-TAHL-o-gus) bone marrow transplantation.

Bone marrow: The soft, sponge-like material inside some bones. Blood cells are produced in the bone marrow.

Glossary of Common Medical Terms

Bowel: The intestine.

Breast implant: a round or teardrop-shaped sac inserted in the body to restore a breast form.

Breast enlargement: an operation in which an implant is inserted under normal breast tissues to make the breast larger.

Breast reduction: an operation in which breast skin and tissue are removed and the nipple is moved up onto the newly contoured breast to make the breast smaller.

Cancer: A general term for more than 100 diseases that are characterized by uncontrolled, abnormal growth of cells. Cancer cells can invade nearby tissue and can spread through the bloodstream and lymphatic system to other parts of the body.

CancerFax: A government sponsored telephone network that provides information and direction on all aspects of cancer through its regional network. Provides variety of free publications.

Carcinoma in situ (kar-si-NO-ma in SY-too): Cancer that involves only the cells in which it began and that has not spread to other tissues. Lobular carcinoma in situ develops in the lobules of the breast. Ductal carcinoma in situ (also called intraductal carcinoma) arises in the ducts.

Carcinoma (kar-si-NO-ma): Cancer that begins in the lining or covering of an organ.

Catheter (KATH-e-ter): A flexible tube that is placed in a body cavity to insert or withdraw fluids.

Cauterization (kaw-ter-i-ZAY-shun): The use of heat to destroy abnormal cells. Also called diathermy or electrodiathermy.

Cervical intraepithelial neoplasia (SER-vi-kul in-trae-pi-THEEL-ee-ul NEE-o-play-zha): A general term for the growth of abnormal cells on the surface of the cervix. Numbers from 1 to 3 may be used to describe how much of the cervix contains abnormal cells. Also called CIN.

Cervix (SER-viks): The lower, narrow end of the uterus that forms a canal between the uterus and the vagina.

Chemotherapy: Treatment with drugs to destroy cancer cells. Most often used to supplement surgery or radiation therapy. Chemotherapy may be taken by pill, or it may be put into the body by a needle in a vein. Chemotherapy is called a systemic treatment because the drugs enter the bloodstream, travel through the body, and can kill cancer cells outside the original infection site.

Clinical trials: Medical research studies conducted with volunteers. Each study is designed to find better ways to prevent, detect, or treat cancer and to answer scientific questions.

Colon (KO-lon): The section of the large intestine above the rectum.

Colony-stimulating factors: Laboratory-made substances similar to substances in the body that stimulate the production of blood cells. Treatment with colony-stimulating factors can help cells in the bone marrow recover from the effects of chemotherapy and radiation therapy.

Colposcopy (kul-POSS-ko-pee): A procedure in which a lighted magnifying instrument (called a colposcope) is used to examine the vagina and cervix.

Computed tomography (tom-OG-rahfee): An x-ray procedure that uses a computer to produce a detailed picture of a cross section of the body; also called CAT or CT scan.

Condylomata acuminata (kon-di-LOW-ma-ta a-kyoomi-NA-ta): Genital warts caused by certain human papillomaviruses.

Conization (ko-ni-ZAY-shun): Conization means taking out a cone-shaped piece of tissue where the cancer is found. Conization may be used to take out a piece of tissue for biopsy, but it can also be used to treat early cancers of the cervix. Also called cone biopsy.

Glossary of Common Medical Terms

Corpus: The body of the uterus.

Cryosurgery (KRY-o-SERjer-ee): Treatment performed with an instrument that freezes and destroys abnormal tissue. Cryosurgery kills the cancer by freezing it.

CT (or CAT) scan: A series of detailed pictures of areas inside the body created by a computer linked to an x-ray machine. Also called computed tomography or computed axial tomography.

Cyst (sist): A closed sac or capsule filled with fluid.

Cystoscopy (sist-OSS-ko-pee): A procedure in which the doctor inserts a lighted instrument into the urethra (the tube leading from the bladder to the outside of the body) to look at the bladder.

Diaphanography (dy-a-fan-OG-ra-fee): An exam that involves shining a bright light through the breast to reveal features of the tissues inside. This technique is under study; its value in detecting breast cancer has not been proven. Also called transillumination.

Diaphragm (DYE-a-fram): The muscle that separates the chest from the abdomen.

Diathermy (DIE-a-ther-mee): The use of heat to destroy abnormal cells. Also called cauterization or electrodiathermy. Diathermy kills the cancer by heat from electrical or magnetic currents.

Diethylstilbestrol (die-ETH-ul-stil-BES-trol): A drug that was once widely prescribed to prevent miscarriage. Also called DES.

Dilatation and curettage (dil-a-TAYshun and KYOO-re-tahzh): A minor operation in which the cervix is expanded enough (dilatation) to permit the cervical canal and uterine lining to be scraped with a spoon-shaped instrument called a curette (curettage). This procedure also is called D and C.

Dilator (DIE-lay-tor): A device used to stretch or enlarge an opening.

Douching (DOO-shing): Using water or a medicated solution to clean the vagina and cervix.

Duct: A tube in the breast through which milk passes from the lobules to the nipple. Cancer that begins in a duct is called ductal carcinoma.

Dysplasia (dis-PLAY-zha): Abnormal cells that are not cancer.

Endocervical curettage (en-do-SER-vi-kul kyoo-reTAZH): The removal of tissue from the inside of the cervix using a spoon-shaped instrument called a curette.

Endometriosis (en-do-mee-tree-O-sis): A benign condition in which tissue that looks like endometrial tissue grows in abnormal places in the abdomen.

Endometrium (en-do-MEE-tree-um): The layer of tissue that lines the uterus.

Epithelial carcinoma (ep-i-THEE-lee-ul kar-si-NO-ma): Cancer that begins in the cells that line an organ.

Estrogen (ES-troejin): A female hormone.

Fallopian tubes (fa-LO-pee-in): Tubes (one on each side of the uterus) that transport the egg cells from the ovaries to the uterus.

Fetus (FEET-us): The young in the uterus or womb, of viviparous animals, in the later stages of development; specifically, in women, from the end of the second month, prior to which it is called an embryo. Also spelled *foetus*.

Fibroid (FY-broid): A benign uterine tumor.

Gynecologic oncologists (guy-ne-ko-LAjik on-KOLojists): Doctors who specialize in treating cancers of the female reproductive organs.

Gynecologist (guy-ne-KOL-ojist): A doctor who specializes in treating diseases of the female reproductive organs.

Glossary of Common Medical Terms

Hair follicle (FOL-i-kul): A sac from which a hair grows.

Herpesvirus (HER-peez-VY-rus): A member of the herpes family of viruses. One type of herpesvirus is sexually transmitted and causes sores on the genitals.

Hormone therapy: Treatment of cancer by changing hormone levels in the body.

Hormone receptor test: A test to measure the amount of certain proteins, called hormone receptors, in breast cancer tissue. Hormones can attach to these proteins. A high level of hormone receptors means hormones probably help the cancer grow.

Hormones: Chemicals produced by glands in the body. Hormones control the way certain cells or organs function.

Human papillomaviruses (pap-i-LOW-ma-VY-rusez): Viruses that generally cause warts. Some papillomaviruses are sexually transmitted. Some of these sexually transmitted viruses cause wart-like growths on the genitals, and some are thought to cause abnormal changes in cells of the cervix.

Hyperplasia (hy-per-PLAY-zha): A precancerous condition in which there is an increase in the number of normal cells lining the uterus.

Hysterectomy: An operation in which the uterus and cervix are taken out along with the cancer. If the uterus is taken out through the vagina, the operation is called a vaginal hysterectomy. If the uterus is taken out through a cut (incision) in your abdomen, the operation is called a total abdominal hysterectomy. Sometimes the ovaries and fallopian tubes are also removed, which is called a bilateral salpingo-oophorectomy.

Infertility: The inability to have children.

Interferon (in-ter-FEER-on): A type of biological therapy, treatment that can improve the body's natural response to disease. It slows the rate of growth and division of cancer cells, causing them to become sluggish and die.

Intraepithelial (in-tra-e-pi-THEEL-ee-ul): Within the layer of cells that forms the surface or lining of an organ.

Intraperitoneal (in-tra-per-i-to-NEE-al): Within the abdominal cavity.

Intravenous pyelogram (in-tra-VEE-nus PIE-el-ogram): A series of x-rays of the kidneys and bladder. The x-rays are taken after a dye that shows up on x-ray film is injected into a vein. Also called IVP.

Intravenous (IV): being within or entering by way of the veins.

Invasive cervical cancer: Cancer that has spread from the surface of the cervix to tissue deeper in the cervix or to other parts of the body.

Laparoscopy (lap-a-RAH-sko-pee): A surgical procedure in which the doctor uses a lighted instrument to look at organs inside the abdomen through a small opening (incision).

Laparotomy (lap-a-ROT-o-mee): An operation to open the abdomen.

Laser (LAY-zer): A powerful beam of light used in some types of surgery to cut or destroy tissue.

Laser surgery: Surgery which uses a narrow beam of intense light to kill cancer cells.

Lesion (LEE-zhun): An area of abnormal tissue change. Local therapy: Treatment that affects cells in a tumor and the area close to it.

Lobe: A part of the breast; each breast contains 15 to 20 lobes.

Lobule (LOB-yool): A subdivision of the lobes of the breast. Cancer that begins in a lobule is called lobular carcinoma.

Local therapy: Treatment that affects cells in the tumor and the area close to it.

Glossary of Common Medical Terms

Lubricant (LOO-bri-kant): An oily or slippery substance. A vaginal lubricant may be helpful for women who feel pain during intercourse because of vaginal dryness.

Lumpectomy (lump-EK-toe-mee): Surgical removal of the lump or cancerous tissue in the breast and some or all of the underarm lymph nodes. Also sometimes called "local excision" or "tylectomy." Surgery to remove only the cancerous breast lump; usually followed by radiation therapy.

Lymph nodes: Small, bean-shaped organs located along the channels of the lymphatic system. Part of the lymphatic system that removes wastes from body tissue and carries fluids that help the body fight infection. Bacteria or cancer cells that enter the lymphatic system may be found in the nodes. Also called lymph glands. Lymph nodes in the underarm are those most likely to be invaded by cancer cells and are therefore often removed during breast cancer surgery.

Lymph (limf): The almost colorless fluid that travels through the lymphatic system and carries cells that help fight infection and disease.

Lymphatic system (lim-FAT-ik): The tissues and organs (including the bone marrow, spleen, thymus, and lymph nodes) that produce and store cells that fight infection and disease. The channels that carry lymph also are part of this system.

Lymphedema: swelling in the arm caused by excess fluid that collects when the lymph nodes and vessels are removed during surgery or damaged by radiation therapy. The patient's arm and hand become more prone to infection.

Malignant (ma-LIG-nant): Cancerous; can spread to other parts of the body.

Mammogram (MAM-o-gram): An x-ray of the breast.

Mammography (mam-OG-ra-fee): The use of x-rays to create a picture of the breast.

Mastectomy (mas-TEK-to-mee): Surgery to remove the breast.

Mastectomy, modified radical: the most common mastectomy performed today. Also called "total mastectomy with axillary dissection." The breast, breast skin, nipple, areola, and underarm lymph nodes are removed, while the chest muscles are saved.

Mastectomy, prophylactic: a procedure sometimes recommended for patients at very high risk of developing cancer in one or both breasts. One type, called a "subcutaneous" mastectomy, removes the breast tissue but leaves muscle, skin, and nipple.

Mastectomy, radical: the surgical removal of the breast, breast skin, nipple, areola, chest muscles, and underarm lymph nodes. This operation leaves a hollow area in the chest wall under the collarbone and in front of the armpit. Also called a "Halsted radical."

Menopause (MEN-o-pawz): The time in a woman's life when menstrual periods permanently stop. Also called "change of life."

Menstrual cycle (MEN-stroo-al): The hormone changes that lead up to a period (menstruation). For most women, one cycle takes about 28 days.

Metastasis (meh-TAS-ta-sis): The spread of cancer from one part of the body to another. Cells that have metastasized are like those in the original (primary) tumor.

Micro-calcifications (MY-krow-kal-si-fi-KA-shunz): Tiny deposits of calcium in the breast that cannot be felt but can be detected on a mammogram. A cluster of these very small specks of calcium may indicate that cancer is present.

MRI: A procedure that uses a magnet linked to a computer to create pictures of areas inside the body. Also called magnetic resonance imaging.

Myometrium (my-o-MEE-tree-um): The muscular outer layer of the uterus.

Glossary of Common Medical Terms

Neoplasia (nee-o-PLAY-zha): Abnormal new growth of cells.

Oncologist (on-KOL-ojist): A doctor who specializes in treating cancer. A gynecologic oncologist specializes in cancer of the female reproductive organs.

Oophorectomy (oo-for-EK-to-mee): The removal of one or both ovaries.

Ovaries (O-va-reez): The pair of female reproductive glands in which the ova, or eggs, are formed. The ovaries are located in the lower abdomen, one on each side of the uterus.

Palpation (pal-PAY-shun): A simple technique in which a doctor presses on the surface of the body to feel the organs or tissues underneath.

Pap smear (Pap test): Microscopic examination of a sample of cells collected from the cervix.

Pap test: Examination of a sample of cells collected from the cervix and the vagina. Also called Pap smear.

Pathologist (path-OL-o-jist): A doctor who specializes in the diagnosis of disease by studying cells and tissues removed from the body.

Pectoral muscles: muscles that overlay the chest wall

Pelvis: The lower part of the abdomen, located between the hip bones. Organs in the female pelvis include the uterus, vagina, ovaries, fallopian tubes, bladder, and rectum.

Peripheral stem cell support (per-IF-er-al): A method for replacing bone marrow destroyed by cancer treatment. Certain cells (stem cells) in the blood that are similar to those in bone marrow are removed from the patient's blood before treatment. The cells are given back to the patient after treatment to help the bone marrow recover and continue producing healthy blood cells.

Polyp: A mass of tissue that develops on the inside wall of a hollow organ.

Precancerous: Not cancerous, but may become cancerous with time.

Proctosigmoidoscopy (PROK-to-sig-moid-OSS-kopee): An examination of the rectum and the lower part of the colon using a thin, lighted instrument called a sigmoidoscope.

Progesterone (proe-JES-ter-own): A female hormone.

Prognosis (prog-NOE-sis): The probable outcome or course of a disease; the chance of recovery.

Prosthesis (pros-THEE-sis): An artificial replacement of a part of the body. A breast prosthesis is a breast form worn under clothing.

Rad: Stands for "radiation absorbed dose" A unit of measurement for radiation therapy.

Radiation oncologist (ray-dee-AY-shun on-KOL-ojist): A doctor who specializes in using radiation to treat cancer.

Radiation therapy (ray-dee-AY-shun THER-a-pee): Treatment with high-energy rays to kill cancer cells. External radiation is the use of a machine to aim high-energy rays at the cancer. Internal radiation therapy is the placing of materials that produce radiation (radioisotopes) through thin plastic tubes in the area where the cancer cells are found. Radiation may be used alone or in addition to surgery.

Radical hysterectomy: An operation in which the cervix, uterus, and part of the vagina are removed. Lymph nodes in the area may also be removed (this is called lymph node dissection). (Lymph nodes are small bean-shaped structures that are found throughout the body. They produce and store cells that fight infection).

Radiologist: A doctor who specializes in creating and interpreting pictures of areas inside the body. The pictures are produced with x-rays, sound waves, or other types of energy.

Glossary of Common Medical Terms

Rectum: The last 6 to 8 inches of the large intestine. The rectum stores solid waste until it leaves the body through the anus.

Remission: Disappearance of the signs and symptoms of cancer. When this happens, the disease is said to be "in remission." A remission can be temporary or permanent.

Reproductive system: In women, the organs that are directly involved in producing eggs and in conceiving and carrying babies.

Risk factor: Something that increases a person's chance of developing a disease.

Salpingo-oophorectomy (sal-PING-OOO-for-EK-to-mee): Surgical removal of the fallopian tubes and ovaries.

Schiller test (SHIL-er): A test in which iodine is applied to the cervix. The iodine colors healthy cells brown; abnormal cells remain unstained. usually appearing white or yellow.

Side effects: Problems that occur when treatment affects healthy cells. Common side effects of cancer treatment are fatigue, nausea, vomiting, decreased blood cell counts, hair loss, and mouth sores.

Silicone gel: medical-grade silicone rubber gel that has fluid qualities similar to the normal breast.

Speculum (SPEK-yoo-lum): An instrument used to widen the opening of the vagina so that the cervix is more easily visible.

Squamous intraepithelial lesion (SKWAY-mus intra-e-pi-THEEL-ee-ul LEE-zhun): A general term for the abnormal growth of squamous cells on the surface of the cervix. The changes in the cells are described as low grade or high grade, depending on how much of the cervix is affected and how abnormal the cells are. Also called SIL.

Squamous cell carcinoma (SKWAY-mus): Cancer that begins in squamous cells, which are thin, flat cells resembling fish scales. Squamous cells are found in the tissue that forms the surface of the skin, the lining of the hollow organs of the body, and the passages of the respiratory and digestive tracts.

Stage: The extent of the cancer. The stage of breast cancer depends on the size of the cancer and whether it has spread from its original site to other parts of the body.

Staging: The tests and exams needed to stage, or describe, the cancer by learning such things as its size, its exact location, and whether it has spread.

Stem cells: Cells that produce new cells that become specialized.

Surgery: An operation.

Systemic therapy (sis-TEM-ik): Treatment that reaches and affects cells all over the body.

Thermography (ther-MOG-ra-fee): A test to measure and display heat patterns of tissues near the surface of the breast. Abnormal tissue generally is warmer than healthy tissue. This technique is under study; its value in detecting breast cancer has not been proven.

Tissue (TISH-oo): A group or layer of cells that performs a specific function.

Transvaginal ultrasound: Sound waves sent out by a probe inserted in the vagina. The waves bounce off the ovaries, and a computer uses the echoes to create a picture called a sonogram. Also called TVS.

Tumor debulking: Surgically removing as much of the tumor as possible.

Tumor marker: A substance in blood or other body fluids that may suggest that a person has cancer.

Tumor: An abnormal mass of tissue.

Glossary of Common Medical Terms

Ultrasonography (ul-tra-son-OG-ra-fee): A test in which sound waves are bounced off tissues and the echoes are converted into a picture (sonogram). These pictures are shown on a monitor like a TV screen. Tissues of different densities look different in the picture because they reflect sound waves differently. A sonogram can show whether a breast lump is a fluid-filled cyst or a solid mass.

Ultrasound: A diagnostic procedure that projects high-frequency sound waves into the body and changes the echoes into pictures.

Ureter (yu-REE-ter): The tube that carries urine from each kidney to the bladder.

Uterus (YOO-ter-us): Often called the womb, this is the organ in which a fetus develops. During pregnancy, the uterus expands. But when a woman is not pregnant, the uterus is small, hollow, and shaped like a flattened pear.

Vagina: The muscular canal extending from the uterus to the exterior of the body.

Viruses (VY-rus-ez): Small living particles that can infect cells and change how the cells function. Infection with a virus can cause a person to develop symptoms. The disease and symptoms that are caused depend on the type of virus and the type of cells that are infected.

Wart: A raised growth on the surface of the skin or other organ.

X-ray: High-energy radiation. It is used in low doses to diagnose diseases and in high doses to treat cancer.

Xeroradiography (ZEE-roe-ray-dee-OG-ra-fee): A type of mammography in which a picture of the breast is recorded on paper rather than on film.

Index

Index

Index

A

Abdominal advancement reconstruction 224
Abortion 117-119, 477, 478
Acupuncture 308
Adenocarcinoma 123, 127, 128
Adnexal masses 349
African-American women 3
Age Groups 461, 466
  adolescents 212
  adults xiv, 256, 324, 393
  children xiv, xvi, xxii, xxv, 26, 51, 54, 57, 58, 61, 77, 84, 90-94, 107, 117, 121, 151, 188, 201, 211-213, 241, 250, 260, 269, 291, 292, 313, 320, 323-325, 328, 330, 444, 505
  elderly 387, 418
  infants 251, 256
  teenagers 291, 393, 448
AIDS 66, 314
Alcohol use and cancer xiii, xiv, 26, 152, 153, 241, 251, 474
Allergens 339
American Cancer Society xiii, xxii, 4, 24, 64, 82, 106, 149, 153, 179, 180, 211, 231, 232, 266, 270, 290, 291, 336, 339, 340, 366, 375, 403, 407, 408, 410, 425, 432, 440-445, 447, 461, 482

American College of Obstetricians and Gynecologists 444, 446, 447
American Society of Plastic and Reconstructive Surgeons 231
American Stop Smoking Intervention Study (ASSIST) 4
Anticancer drugs xvii, xix, 20, 28, 44, 56, 62, 74, 79, 104, 178, 289, 301, 304, 500
  5-fluorouracil xvii, xix, 20, 28, 44, 56, 62, 74, 79, 104, 178, 289, 301, 304, 500
  adriamycin 159, 298, 299
  cytoxan 159, 298
  doxorubicin 159, 298, 314, 355
  oncovin 298
  prednisone 298
  vincristine 298
Appetite 20, 21, 23, 62, 69, 80, 104, 159, 298, 308, 315
Asians/Pacific Islanders 388
Aspiration 11, 12, 33, 139, 140, 155, 185, 312, 492, 499
Axillary dissection 31, 33-35, 41, 199, 237, 281-283, 326, 500
Axillary sampling 281-283, 500

B

Barium enema 52, 70, 308, 312, 500

Benign tumors 7, 46, 68, 96
Bethesda System 49, 392, 393, 445, 452, 453
Biopsy 11, 12, 14, 33, 43, 50, 51, 70, 71, 77, 88, 98, 124, 129, 137, 139-141, 154, 155, 168-170, 176, 178, 186, 187, 189, 190, 192, 194-199, 201, 281, 296, 312, 352, 354, 391, 457, 465, 500, 502
   cone biopsy 50
   frozen section 11, 12, 14, 33, 43, 50, 51, 70, 71, 77, 88, 98, 124, 129, 137, 139-141, 154, 155, 168-170, 176, 178, 186, 187, 189, 190, 192, 194-199, 201, 281, 296, 312, 352, 354, 391, 457, 465, 500, 502
   one-step procedure 11, 12, 14, 33, 43, 50, 51, 70, 71, 77, 88, 98, 124, 129, 137, 139-141, 154, 155, 168-170, 176, 178, 186, 187, 189, 190, 192, 194-199, 201, 281, 296, 312, 352, 354, 391, 457, 465, 500, 502
   outpatient procedure 11, 12, 14, 33, 43, 50, 51, 70, 71, 77, 88, 98, 124, 129, 137, 139-141, 154, 155, 168-170, 176, 178, 186, 187, 189, 190, 192, 194-199, 201, 281, 296, 312, 352, 354, 391, 457, 465, 500, 502
   permanent section 168-170, 198
   two-step procedure 140, 155, 195-199
Birth control 26, 84, 108, 152, 153, 188, 309, 359
Black women 83, 188, 309, 367, 378, 380, 391, 417, 418, 424
Blood cells 20, 62, 79, 316, 458, 460, 500, 509
Bone marrow xvii, xix, 28, 161, 316, 357, 481, 500, 502, 507, 509
Bowel resection 353
BRCA1 495
BRCA2 495
Breast cancer xvi, xix-xxiii, 3-5, 7, 9, 10, 12-19, 21-32, 35, 37-39, 41, 43, 44, 84, 137, 140, 142-144, 149-162, 167-170, 172, 175-177, 179, 180, 183, 185, 187, 188, 190-194, 199-201, 203-205, 208, 211, 213, 219, 221, 231, 232, 237, 247, 251, 258, 259, 270, 271, 279, 281, 285, 287, 289-291, 295-300, 309, 310, 319-324, 327-329, 332, 333, 337, 345, 365,

Breast cancer, continued 367, 369, 373-378, 391, 392, 395-398, 403-408, 410, 411, 413, 414, 421-423, 425, 427-429, 432, 434-442, 457, 459-465, 471-475, 477, 478, 487, 488, 491-495, 499, 503, 505, 507, 512
   emotional support 24, 64, 82, 106, 217, 324
   follow-up care 63, 81, 105, 143, 243, 300, 396
   mastectomy xxiii, 15, 17-19, 22, 30-35, 41, 43, 147, 149, 155-159, 163-167, 169-173, 175-178, 180, 190, 196, 197, 199, 200, 202-205, 208-214, 219, 221, 222, 224, 227-232, 237, 238, 242, 245, 251, 255, 279, 324, 375, 395, 396, 508
   surgery xiv, xvi-xxi, xxiv-xxvi, 14-19, 21, 22, 30, 43, 49, 51, 54, 55, 57-61, 70, 73, 74, 76-79, 81, 88-94, 96, 97, 99-103, 106, 113-115, 120-122, 125-128, 131, 132, 134, 137, 140-142, 146, 147, 155-165, 169, 170, 172, 173, 175-178, 180, 189, 190, 196-198, 200, 203-207, 210, 212-216, 219-222, 224, 227, 229-234, 237, 238, 240-246, 250-253, 255, 258, 261, 262, 266, 267, 274, 278, 281-283, 289, 293, 295, 298, 313-316, 321, 324, 326-328, 330, 332, 349, 350, 352, 354-357, 360, 361, 385, 395, 396, 415, 416, 444, 465, 499, 500, 502, 506-508, 510, 512
   survival xv, xviii, xx, xxi, xxiii-xxvi, 30, 31, 33, 35, 41, 157, 161, 172, 200, 237, 238, 279, 296, 344, 346, 351, 352, 354, 356, 357, 361, 367, 374, 384, 408, 414, 418, 419, 437, 444, 447, 462
Breast Imaging Reporting and Data System 392
Breast Implants 164, 221, 228, 239-242, 244-254, 256-258, 260, 261, 263, 270, 273-275, 277, 464
   ruptures 250, 259
   saline 239, 240, 245-247, 250, 254, 256, 260, 265, 273, 277, 278, 312
   silicone gel 164, 165, 215, 221, 239, 240, 245-247, 249, 250, 252-254,

Index

Breast Implants, continued
  silicone gel, continued 256, 260, 273, 274, 277, 511
  trilucent 256
Breast reconstruction 22, 24, 33, 137, 141, 163-166, 171, 172, 175, 180, 196, 205, 206, 219-222, 227, 229-233, 244, 252, 253, 277, 332, 395, 396
Breast-feeding 188, 189, 191, 260, 348

C

CA 125 serum 125 164, 221, 228, 239-242, 244-254, 256-258, 260, 261, 263, 270, 273-275, 277, 344, 464
Capsular contracture 164, 227, 243, 245, 246, 250, 252, 259, 278
Carcinoma in situ xiv, xxiii, 17, 26, 48, 52, 100, 124, 130, 162, 384, 417, 444, 501
Cardiovascular disease 152, 349, 360, 487
CAT scan 52, 98, 308, 311
Cauterization 51, 501, 503
Cervical cancer
  cause and prevention 317
  treatment xiv-xxvi, 5, 6, 9, 11-24, 27, 28, 30-35, 37, 39, 41, 44, 47, 50-63, 66, 68, 70-82, 84, 87-94, 97, 99-108, 112-115, 118-122, 124-128, 130-134, 138, 140, 141, 143-146, 149, 155-161, 163, 167-172, 175-181, 187, 189-191, 195-201, 203-205, 209, 211, 221, 232, 233, 237, 238, 245, 279-281, 283-292, 294-300, 310, 312-316, 319-321, 323, 325, 326, 328-330, 332, 333, 335-339, 341, 343, 352, 355-358, 361, 365, 367, 374, 375, 379, 384, 387, 392, 398, 406, 408, 411, 413, 414, 422, 423, 437, 440-442, 444, 449, 463, 465, 479, 480, 488, 489, 495, 499, 500, 502, 503, 505, 506, 509-512
Cervical intraepithelial neoplasia 47, 393, 501
Chemotherapy xvii, xxi, xxiii, xxv, xxvi, 14, 16-18, 20, 21, 28, 32, 35-37, 40, 41, 43, 44, 54, 56, 59-62, 73, 74, 77-79, 81,

Chemotherapy, continued 89-94, 99-104, 108, 113-115, 119-122, 125-128, 131-134, 137, 141, 144, 145, 147, 156-161, 164, 177, 178, 180, 200, 213, 229, 241, 244, 245, 252, 289, 295-300, 313-316, 325, 326, 329-332, 335-341, 352, 354-357, 361, 408, 499, 502
  adjuvant 18, 30-32, 35-37, 39-41, 73, 157-159, 162, 177, 289, 295-299, 351, 352, 361, 499
  combination xiv, xxi, xxiii, xxiv, 14, 16, 19, 33, 35-37, 40, 41, 43, 54, 56, 74, 100, 108, 132, 156, 159, 248, 297, 298, 314, 315, 346, 349, 350, 352, 355, 356, 358, 416, 472, 480, 487
  hair loss 104, 159, 248, 262, 298, 316, 329, 330, 333, 336, 337, 511
  intra-arterial 303-305
  side effects 13, 17, 19-21, 27, 53, 56, 57, 60-63, 72, 74-76, 78-81, 90, 101, 103-106, 113, 121, 126, 132, 142, 144-147, 159, 160, 165, 179, 190, 204, 207, 227, 251, 280, 282, 284, 286, 287, 298, 299, 315, 316, 329, 330, 333, 335, 511
Childbearing 84, 95, 151, 348, 349, 352, 359, 404
Chinese 308, 367
Choriocarcinoma 117, 118
Clear cell adenocarcinoma 123
Clinical trials 5, 27, 28, 30, 32, 37, 39-41, 56, 57, 59, 75-78, 90, 91, 101-103, 108, 113-115, 134, 159, 180, 232, 247, 256, 277, 294, 297, 298, 303, 346, 351, 354, 355, 357, 358, 360, 361, 403, 413, 414, 417, 462, 502
Cobalt machine 284
Colonics 308
Colony-stimulating factors 28, 502
Color Doppler imaging 344
Colposcope 50, 502
Condylomata acuminata 65, 502
Conization 50, 51, 57, 58, 444, 502
Contraceptive 84, 108, 152, 153
Cosmetic side effect 337
Cranial prosthesis 337
Cryosurgery 51, 57, 444, 503
CT scans 353
Curretage 445

Cyclophosphamide 159, 298
Cytoxan 159, 298
Cyst 12, 68, 155, 168, 185, 186, 350, 468, 499, 503, 513
Cystoscopy 51, 503
Cytopathology 446

D

Danazol 190
Depression 157, 202, 299, 307, 308, 328, 488
DES (diethylstilbestrol) 65, 123, 449, 503
Diathermy 51, 57, 501, 503
Diet 26, 79, 80, 104, 150, 152, 153, 161, 190, 329, 457-460, 474, xx, xxii
Digital Mammography 463, 464
Distant disease xxvi, 19, 414, 419
Ductal carcinoma 501, 504
Dysplasia 47, 48, 384, 444, 453, 465, 504

E

ENCORE 211, 232
Endocervical curettage (ECC) 50
Endometrial cancer xxiv, xxv, 5, 47, 96, 102, 111, 345, 445, 487, 488
   detection xiv, xv, xix, xxi, xxii, xxiv-xxvi, 5, 9, 10, 27, 29, 35, 48, 66, 84, 154, 246, 266, 307, 310, 311, 313, 344, 356, 365, 367, 374-376, 384-387, 392, 406, 408, 415-417, 419, 421, 423, 427, 434, 437, 440-443, 447, 450, 462, 463, 465, 470
Endometriosis 96, 416, 504
Endometrium xxiv, 47, 50, 95, 96, 98, 100, 101, 111, 444, 474, 504
Epithelial carcinomas 68
Epithelial ovarian cancer 344, 355, 361
ERT 108, 152
Estrogen xix, xxii, xxiv, 4, 12, 20, 21, 26, 36, 38, 44, 67, 79, 101, 108, 140, 141, 152, 153, 160, 163, 169, 196, 200, 296, 298, 299, 315, 349, 360, 445, 459, 472, 474, 487, 488, 504
Ethnic Groups 366, 367, 369, 378, 379, 388, 391

Ethnic Groups, continued
   American Indians 388
   Blacks xxi, 151, 367, 369, 378-380, 388
   Black women 83, 188, 309, 367, 378, 380, 391, 417, 418, 424
   Chinese 308, 367
   Filipinos 367
   Hawaiians 367, 379
   Hispanics 388
   Japanese 152, 308, 367, 379
   Mexican Americans 366
   Native Americans 366, 367, 379
   North American 344
   non-Hispanic Whites 388
   Pacific Islanders 388
   Whites xxi, xxiii, 3, 50, 64, 70, 82, 83, 129, 153, 176, 198, 309, 316, 367, 369, 378, 380, 391, 417, 424, 458, 462, 468, 471, 472, 477, 478, 484, 500, 511
Excisional biopsy 186, 500
External radiation 16, 55, 58, 59, 61, 74, 75, 92, 99, 103, 113, 115, 126-128, 132, 176, 200, 281, 284, 285, 289, 510

F

Fallopian tubes xxvi, 48, 54, 71, 73, 76, 77, 88, 89, 91-93, 100-102, 113, 114, 126, 127, 312, 313, 451, 504, 505, 509, 511
Familial ovarian cancer 309
Food and Drug Administration (FDA) 149, 152, 160, 165, 221, 239, 240, 242, 247, 249-254, 256-258, 260-264, 271, 273-275, 277, 307, 309, 310, 314-316, 335, 338, 340, 397-402, 443, 449, 467, 468
Fertility drugs 84, 310, 345, 415, 479, 480
Fibroadenomas 188
Fibroids 96
Filipinos 367
5-fluorouracil (5-FU) 298
Frozen section 168, 169, 197, 198

Index

G

Genital herpes virus 65
Genital warts 46, 65, 502
Gestational Trophoblastic Tumor 440
Glass model research 301, 304, 305
Gynecologic examinations 443

H

Halsted radical 15, 155-157, 170, 204
Herpes virus type 2 449
Hispanics 388
Histologic Type 38, 163
HIV 66
Hormone receptor assays 296
Hormone replacement therapy 79, 487-489
Hot flashes xxiv, 20, 21, 103, 152, 159, 160, 299, 315, 330, 331, 487
Human immunodeficiency virus (HIV) 66
Human papilloma virus (HPV) 65, 117-119, 121, 384, 419, 449
Hyperplasia 27, 97, 499, 505
Hysterectomy xxvi, 49, 51, 54, 58-61, 73, 76, 77, 89, 91-94, 100-103, 113-115, 120-122, 126, 127, 351, 352, 415, 444, 449, 452, 488, 505, 510

I

Immune system xviii, 56, 65, 66, 248, 338, 500
Implants 22, 55, 164, 165, 200, 221, 228, 239-254, 256-265, 270, 272-275, 277, 278, 464
In situ xiv-xvi, xxiii, xxiv, 17, 26, 48, 52, 100, 124, 130, 154, 162, 177, 369, 380, 384, 417, 444, 478, 501
Incisional biopsy 33, 186, 500
Infertility xxiv, 20, 21, 84, 96, 310, 445, 479, 480, 505
Inflammatory breast cancer 43, 44, 162
Insurance xx, 53, 144-147, 191, 198, 216, 229, 255, 407, 423, 425, 433, 434, 442
Interferon xviii, 56, 505

Interleukin-2 xviii
Internal radiation 58, 61, 75, 99, 100, 103, 120, 126, 127, 132
Intimacy 201, 212, 291, 319, 323, 325, 326, 328, 331, 332
Intraductal cancer 40
Intraepithelial neoplasia 47, 388, 393, 453, 501, 506, 511
Intraperitoneal irradiation 74, 75, 77, 78, 355, 506
Intravenous pyelogram (IVP) 70
Invasive cancer xv, xxiii, 48, 417, 444
Invasive mole (choriocarcinoma destruens) 118
Iododeoxyuridine 303
Irritants 339
IUDR 303-305

J

Japanese 152, 308, 367, 379
Laparoscopy 312, 316, 350, 358, 506
Laparotomy 70, 71, 88-90, 312, 316, 346, 350, 352, 356, 361, 416, 506
Laser surgery 51, 57, 125, 127, 131, 132, 506
Latissimus Dorsi 164, 165, 222, 224, 225
Linear accelerator 284
Lipomas 189
Lobular carcinoma 9, 17, 501, 506
Local therapy 41, 54, 55, 74, 506
Look Good . . . Feel Better 336, 337, 340
Low-grade squamous intraepithelial lesion 388
Lower GI series 70
Lumpectomy xxii, 15, 31, 141, 156-158, 174-177, 205, 279, 324, 326, 330, 506
Lung Cancer xv, xx, 4, 29, 367, 421, 427
  incidence xiv, xv, xx-xxii, xxv, 3, 29, 32, 35, 36, 150, 152-154, 243, 308, 309, 344, 359, 365-367, 369, 378-380, 391, 392, 406, 414, 417, 418, 447, 449, 461, 462, 482, 487, 488, 491
Lymph nodes 18, 30, 58, 59, 102, 114, 115, 127, 144, 161, 162, 281, 283, 284, 293, 354, 510
Lymphedema 19, 22, 171, 209, 287, 330, 331, 507

Lynch syndrome II 345, 359

M

Magnetic resonance imaging (MRI) xviii, 52, 247, 259, 464, 465, 508
Malignant Tumor 7, 46, 68
Mammary duct ectasia 189
Mammography xx-xxii, 9-11, 22, 27, 29, 32, 35, 138, 139, 154, 164, 186, 230, 246, 247, 258, 259, 271, 278, 365, 369, 374-377, 387, 388, 391, 392, 395, 397-403, 405, 407-410, 413, 414, 421-423, 425, 429-433, 435-437, 441, 442, 463-470, 507, 513
Mastitis 189
Medicaid 447, 450
Medical Device Amendments of 1976 165
Medicare 400, 402, 403, 405, 407, 411, 422, 423, 433, 447, 450
MedWatch 260, 262-264
Melanoma xiv, xviii
Menarche xxii, xxiv, 373, 415, 472
Menopause xxii, xxiv, xxv, 10, 20, 21, 26, 49, 79, 87, 96, 97, 103, 107, 111, 150, 153, 160, 184, 188, 192, 315, 331, 360, 373, 415, 445, 474, 487, 488, 508
Metastases xxiii
Methotrexate 36, 159, 298
Methylxanthine 190
Mexican Americans 366
Micro-calcifications 10, 186, 191, 465, 508
Miscarriage 65, 123, 449, 503
Molar pregnancy 117
Mortality xv, xx-xxv, 5, 36, 153, 311, 321, 330, 345, 346, 348, 351, 357, 359, 360, 365-367, 369, 378-380, 386, 387, 392, 403, 413, 414, 417-419, 448
MRI xviii, 52, 247, 259, 464, 465, 508
Multicentric breast malignancies 32
Multifocal disease 32

N

Narcotic drugs 249, 481-485

National Breast and Cervical Cancer Early Detection Program 324, 386, 387, 392, 438
National Cancer Institute (NCI) xv, 6, 9, 30, 53, 55, 57, 61-63, 73, 75, 76, 78, 81, 137, 138, 150, 153, 170, 177, 179, 180, 185, 196, 213, 232, 249, 253, 271, 285, 289, 290, 293, 294, 298-303, 305, 311, 315, 343, 366, 376, 393, 403, 405, 408-410, 413, 417, 421, 422, 425, 427, 440-442, 445, 452, 460, 461, 463, 471, 477, 480, 482, 483, 494
Native Americans 366, 367, 379
Nausea xvii, xx, 20, 21, 62, 69, 79, 80, 102, 104, 115, 128, 134, 159, 160, 242-244, 298, 308, 315, 316, 329, 330, 511
Needle biopsy 11, 12, 186, 465
Nervousness 488
Nipple and areola 166, 221, 224, 227, 228, 243
North American 344
Nuclear Grade 38
Nutrition 21, 62, 80, 104, 440, 458

O

Obesity xxiv, 150, 404, 445
One-step procedure 155, 196, 197, 199
Oophorectomy xxvi, 58, 70, 73, 76, 77, 89-94, 100-102, 113, 114, 348, 349, 351, 359, 505, 509, 511
Optical imaging 464
Optimized Mammography System 467
Oral contraceptive 348, 415, 471-475
Organ transplant 66
Osteoporosis 152, 349, 360, 487
Outpatient 16, 56, 74, 103, 104, 140, 155, 164, 170, 176, 186, 187, 195, 197, 198, 221, 222, 242, 244
Ovarian Cancer xxv, xxvi, 5, 68-75, 79-81, 83-85, 272, 307-317, 343-351, 353, 355-362, 414-417, 479-481, 483, 485, 495

P

p53 gene 151

Index

Paget's disease 154
Pain xvii, xx, xxii-xxiv, 10, 15, 21, 23, 43, 49-51, 55, 59, 60, 69, 74, 79, 80, 96, 102, 115, 124, 128, 129, 134, 147, 184, 188, 190, 201, 207, 208, 242-247, 249, 250, 258, 259, 262, 282, 284, 286, 288, 303, 308, 313, 319, 321, 326, 332, 344, 410, 422, 506
Palpation 11, 154, 185, 186, 509
Pap smear (pap test) 391, 418, 446, 447, 451-453
Papanicolaou 365, 385, 387, 443
PDQ 28, 57, 76, 108, 109, 180, 232, 233, 277, 294, 298
Pelvic exam xxv, 48, 49, 51, 63, 69, 81, 98, 105, 310, 313, 345, 356, 451, 452
Peripheral stem cell support 28, 509
PET xviii
Phantom pain 207
Post-menopausal 36, 150
Postoperative treatment 352
Postpartum mastitis 189
Pre-cancerous lesions 51, 54, 60, 66, 391, 449
Pre-menopausal 36, 37, 152, 161, 162
Pregnancy 10, 57, 65, 67, 84, 96, 117-119, 152, 188, 192, 249, 260, 264, 297, 313, 348, 416, 449, 472, 474, 478, 513
Proctosigmoidoscopy 51, 510
Progesterone 12, 38, 67, 100, 140, 141, 163, 169, 196, 200, 296, 315, 472, 474, 510
Progestin 108, 472, 474, 487, 488
Progestogen 474
Proliferative breast disease 491, 494
Proliferative rate 38
Prophylactic mastectomy 190, 228, 395
Prophylactic oophorectomy 348, 349
Prosthesis 22, 205, 214-217, 234, 240, 241, 274, 292, 337, 510
Psycho-oncology 336

Q

Quality of life 35, 37, 41, 159, 256, 263, 316, 357, 359, 361

R

Radiation Therapy xviii, xxi, xxiii, xxvi, 16-21, 28, 30, 31, 33-35, 40, 43, 54, 55, 57-61, 73-75, 77, 78, 80, 89-92, 94, 99-104, 106, 108, 111, 113, 115, 120, 122, 125-128, 131-134, 137, 141, 143, 151, 160, 173-176, 178, 200, 205, 229, 279-281, 283-287, 289-292, 295, 298, 303, 314, 315, 330, 331, 357, 502, 506, 507, 510
  cervical cancer xxiii, xxiv, xxvi, 47-49, 51-54, 56-60, 64-66, 302, 303, 305, 365, 375, 378-380, 384-387, 392, 417-419, 443, 444, 447-450, 506
  gestational trophoblastic tumor 117-119, 121
  uterine sarcoma 111, 114, 115
  vaginal cancer 123, 126-128
  vulvar cancer 129, 132-134
Radiotherapy 16, 33, 55, 74, 99, 355
Reach to Recovery 24, 208, 211, 216, 232, 290
Rectus Abdominus 164, 165, 224, 226
Recurrent cancer 18, 354
Refractory disease 71
Rehabilitation xxiii, 6, 21, 24, 64, 82, 106, 178, 229, 440, 462
Reserpine 152
Risk factors xx, xxii-xxv, 25, 26, 64, 66, 83, 108, 150, 153, 154, 193, 251, 317, 344, 373, 379, 384, 395, 396, 406, 419, 435, 437, 445, 483, 484, 494
Rupture 164, 243, 246, 247, 250, 252, 253, 259, 261, 277, 278
  silent ruptures xx, xxii-xxv, 25, 26, 64, 66, 83, 108, 150, 153, 154, 193, 251, 317, 344, 373, 379, 384, 395, 396, 406, 419, 435, 437, 445, 483, 484, 494

S

Schiller test 50, 511
Screening xiv, xx, xxii, 5, 29, 259, 310, 311, 343-346, 348, 357-360, 365, 367, 369, 374-377, 379, 380, 384-388, 391,

Screening, continued 392, 396, 398, 402-408, 413-419, 421-425, 427-430, 432-440, 442, 444, 446, 450, 463, 480
Second-look laparotomy 90, 356, 361
Segmental mastectomy 31, 156, 173, 205
sexual activity 80, 323, 326, 327, 331, 333
Smoking xiii, xiv, xx, xxi, xxiii, 4, 65, 209, 241, 245, 251, 287, 384, 440, 449, 459, 484
Sonogram 11, 69, 308, 313, 512, 513
Sonographic 353
Squamous cell carcinomas 47
Squamous cells 511
Squamous intraepithelial lesion 47, 388, 511
Staging 34, 39, 51, 69, 70, 88, 89, 100, 112, 118, 124, 130, 281, 347, 350-354, 465, 512
Stereotactic needle biopsy 465
Streaming phenomenon 303
Subcutaneous mastectomy 395
Sun protection factor (SPF) 338
sunscreens 338
Systemic treatment 17, 18, 37, 56, 90, 120, 126, 132

T

Tamoxifen xix, xxiv, 4, 20, 27, 35-37, 40, 41, 160, 297-299, 357
Taxol xvii, 5, 314, 315
Telemammography 464
Thermography 186, 512
Tissue expander 222, 242
Traumatic fat necrosis 189
Tubal ligation 348, 415

Tumor debulking 73, 89, 91-93, 512
Tylectomy 156, 506

U

Ultrasonography xix, 11, 52, 68, 69, 345, 346, 350, 415, 416, 513
Ultrasound 84, 85, 87, 88, 118, 186, 247, 259, 308, 311, 317, 344, 346, 350, 353, 414-417, 464, 465, 512, 513

V

Vaginal Cancer xv-xvii, xxi-xxiii, 5, 11-14, 23, 33, 43, 49, 53, 69, 72, 97-99, 137, 140, 149, 167, 169, 178, 183, 186, 188, 191, 195, 198, 200, 201, 203, 204, 233, 241, 294, 310, 311, 313, 317, 319, 320, 325, 328, 330, 332, 333, 346, 354, 379, 414, 418, 440, 464, 465, 478, 495, 509
Vaginal discharge xxiii, 49, 96
Vaginal tissue dryness 487
Vaginectomy 126, 127
Virapap 449
Vitamin A xvii, 66
Vitamin E 190, 210, 283
Vitamins 308

W

White xxi, xxiii, 3, 50, 64, 70, 82, 83, 129, 153, 176, 198, 309, 316, 367, 369, 378, 380, 391, 417, 424, 458, 462, 468, 471, 472, 477, 478, 484, 500, 511
Wig 146, 330, 331, 335, 337, 338